Cosmetic Surgery for the Oral and Maxillofacial Surgeon

COSMETIC SURGERY

FOR THE ORAL AND MAXILLOFACIAL SURGEON

Edited by

John E. Griffin, DMD
Director of Fellowship Program
Facial Cosmetic and Reconstructive Surgery
Baptist Memorial Hospital, Golden Triangle

Private Practice
Oral and Maxillofacial Surgery
Columbus, Mississippi

King Kim, DMD
Adjunct Clinical Professor
Department of Oral and Maxillofacial Surgery
College of Dental Medicine
Nova Southeastern University and Broward General Medical Center
Fort Lauderdale, Florida

Private Practice
Oral and Maxillofacial Surgery
Melbourne, Florida

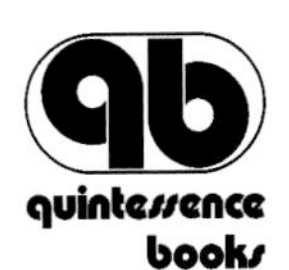

Quintessence Publishing Co, Inc
Chicago, Berlin, Tokyo, London, Paris, Milan, Barcelona, Istanbul, São Paulo, New Delhi, Moscow, Prague, and Warsaw

Library of Congress Cataloging-in-Publication Data

Griffin, John E., Jr.
Cosmetic surgery for the oral and maxillofacial surgeon / edited by John Griffin, King Kim.
p. ; cm.
ISBN 978-0-86715-490-0 (hardcover)
1. Face--Surgery. 2. Mouth--Surgery. 3. Surgery, Plastic. I. Kim, King. II. Title.
[DNLM: 1. Cosmetic Techniques. 2. Maxillofacial Abnormalities--surgery. 3. Maxillofacial Injuries--surgery. 4. Oral Surgical Procedures--methods. 5. Reconstructive Surgical Procedures--methods. WO 600 G851c 2010]
RD523.G766 2010
617.5'20592--dc22

2010023369

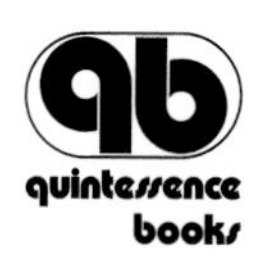

Quintessence Publishing Co Inc
4350 Chandler Drive
Hanover Park, IL 60133
www.quintpub.com

Editor: Bryn Grisham
Design: Gina Ruffolo
Production: Angelina Sanchez

Printed in China

Table of Contents

DEDICATION

I have had the greatest pleasure in working with the contributors to this book—most of whom have completed my fellowship program. It has been an honor and privilege to teach and learn from each of them. This book is dedicated to all of the past, present, and future fellows.

JOHN E. GRIFFIN

To all the folks who put up with me through the years, especially during this endeavor: Amber, Shayaan, Kichun, Chungok, and Alex. Without you, all of this would have been very difficult. Special thanks also to Joe, Steve, and John for teaching me surgery. My sincerest appreciation goes out to all of you.

KING KIM

Foreword

More than any other type of surgery, cosmetic surgery embodies the classical attribution of being both an art and a science. The art of facial cosmetic surgery has evolved through a long-term process of trial and error and gradual improvement based mostly on the technical acumen of the "masters." Conversely, the science of facial cosmetic surgery has recently undergone more of a revolution with rapid innovation in precision imaging and instrumentation as well as a more detailed understanding of the intricate anatomical planes, such as the superficial musculoaponeurotic system in rhytidectomy or the interdomal ligaments in rhinoplasty.

Now that facial cosmetic surgery has taken its rightful place within the scope of oral and maxillofacial surgery, it is important that the form of its art and the specifics of its science are understood within our profession, and this beautifully illustrated text provides an elegant yet practical way to accomplish this goal. The authors have written comprehensively on both the art and science of facial cosmetic surgery and detailed all of the known facial cosmetic procedures, including rhinoplasty, forehead and brow lift, blepharoplasty, facelift, and facial rejuvenation treatment. But what makes this book stand out most is the inclusion of discussions regarding possible complications associated with each procedure. The reader is provided with astute caveats on how to avoid complications as well as the essentials of how to manage them when they do occur.

As an educator with more than 30 years of experience in the field, I appreciate the importance of this book to oral and maxillofacial surgery residents as well as to established practitioners and educators who have an interest in this expanding sector of our profession.

Robert E. Marx, DDS
Professor and Chief
Division of Oral and Maxillofacial Surgery
Miller School of Medicine
University of Miami
Miami, Florida

Preface

Oral and maxillofacial surgeons are uniquely trained to manage the correction of traumatic injuries and deformities of the facial region. Because of our specialized training as well as the historical commitment within our discipline to research and product development, oral and maxillofacial surgeons also have the proficiency to manage cosmetic procedures that address age-related facial changes. Many oral and maxillofacial surgeons have opened up their practice to include treatment of the aging face. Those who have expanded their practice have already made significant contributions to the development of corrective procedures in this arena.

This clinical textbook is designed to outline proven techniques in a concise format. It does not explain the historical perspective for procedures but rather focuses on the actual surgical and adjunctive steps involved in common corrective procedures. Most of the chapter authors are previous fellows of Dr Griffin who have been trained in the proven techniques that are illustrated in this text. In keeping extraneous information to a minimum, the authors have attempted to describe these techniques in a very straightforward manner and to create a practical and easy-to-follow "how to" guide.

CONTRIBUTORS

CORTLAND S. CALDEMEYER, DDS
Private Practice
Oral and Facial Surgery
La Mesa, California

RON CALOSS, DDS, MD
Associate Professor and Program Director
Department of Oral-Maxillofacial Surgery and Pathology
School of Dentistry
University of Mississippi Medical Center
Jackson, Mississippi

ALEXANDRA DOWNEY
Aesthetician
Columbus, Mississippi

ELIE M. FERNEINI, DMD, MD, MHS
Clinical Instructor
Department of Oral and Maxillofacial Surgery
School of Dental Medicine
University of Connecticut
Storrs, Connecticut

Private Practice
Oral and Maxillofacial Surgery
Waterbury, Connecticut

JOHN E. GRIFFIN, DMD
Director of Fellowship Program
Facial Cosmetic and Reconstructive Surgery
Baptist Memorial Hospital, Golden Triangle
Columbus, Mississippi

Private Practice
Oral and Maxillofacial Surgery
Columbus, Mississippi

RAYMOND J. HAIGNEY II, DDS
Private Practice
Oral and Facial Surgery
Cornelius, North Carolina

DOUGLAS L. JOHNSON, DMD
Private Practice
Oral and Facial Surgery
Saint Augustine, Florida

KING KIM, DMD
Adjunct Clinical Professor
Department of Oral and Maxillofacial Surgery
College of Dental Medicine
Nova Southeastern University and Broward General Medical Center
Fort Lauderdale, Florida

Private Practice
Oral and Maxillofacial Surgery
Melbourne, Florida

MANOLIS G. MANOLAKAKIS, DMD
Co-Director of Facial Cosmetic Surgery
Department of Surgery
Cooper University Hospital
Camden, New Jersey

Clinical Assistant Professor
Temple University School of Medicine
Philadelphia, Pennsylvania

Private Practice
Oral and Facial Surgery
Shrewsbury, New Jersey

TAYLOR P. MCGUIRE, BSc, DDS, MSc, FRCD(C)
Associate Clinical Professor
Graduate Training Program in Oral and Maxillofacial Surgery
College of Dentistry
University of Tennessee Health Science Center
Memphis, Tennessee

Private Practice
Oral and Maxillofacial Surgery
Ottawa, Ontario, Canada

YVONNE STONE, RN
Patient Coordinator
Oral and Facial Surgery
Columbus, Mississippi

1

RHINOPLASTY

RON CALOSS, DDS, MD
KING KIM, DMD

The deviated nose is an asymmetric deformity in which the nose is positioned off the facial midline. It is a challenge to correct because of the complexity of both the esthetic and functional problems that typically coexist. The anatomical deformity usually involves the bony pyramid and/or septum and typically arises secondary to trauma, although it can occur congenitally or secondary to previous rhinoplasty surgery.[1] A major septal deviation commonly contributes to the deviation seen in the external nose and must be effectively managed.

There are several prerequisites to obtaining a good esthetic and functional outcome when managing a deviated nose. They include an understanding of anatomy and physiology, an accurate diagnosis of the deformity, a knowledge of cartilage healing, and the surgical skills needed to obtain a straight nose.

Applied Anatomy

It is imperative to have a thorough understanding of the various anatomical components of the nose and their interrelationship to one another when performing rhinoplasty. A discussion of basic anatomy is beyond the scope of this chapter; however, it is important to review the functional components of the airway because nasal deviation usually causes some level of airway compromise. Nasal patency depends on a number of interrelated factors, including the strength and integrity of the cartilaginous framework, the size of the inferior turbinates, and the status of the mucosal lining. Important anatomical components should be evaluated such as the septum, the internal and external nasal valves, and the inferior turbinates.

The septum is made up of the quadrangular cartilage, the vomer, the perpendicular plate of the ethmoid bone, the anterior nasal spine, and the maxillary crest (Fig 1-1). It is the structural foundation of the external nose and exerts a constant effect on airflow.[2,3] The extension of the perpendicular plate of the ethmoid bone under the nasal bones (the central complex) is another important component of the nasal skeleton that must be considered. If not addressed, it can contribute to residual deviation postoperatively.[4]

Fig 1-1 Septal anatomy. Cartilaginous and bony deviation frequently contributes to the deviation seen in the external nose.

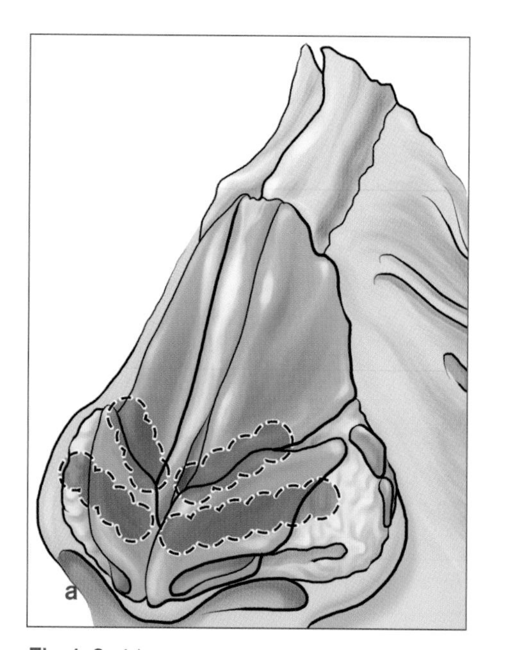

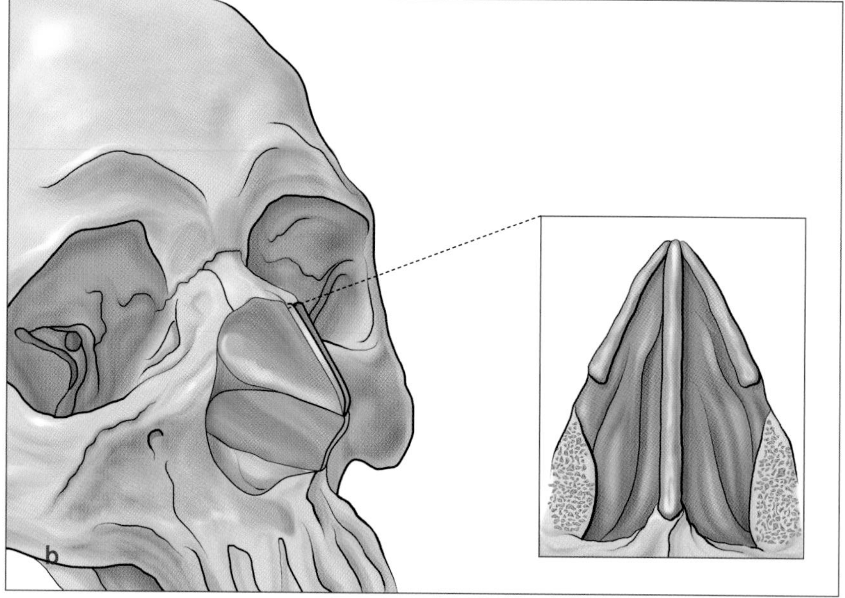

Fig 1-2 *(a)* Internal and external nasal valves. *(b)* The internal nasal valve angle is usually 10 to 15 degrees (see inset).

The internal nasal valve—the narrowest segment of the airway—is formed by the angle created between the caudal edge of the upper lateral cartilages and the dorsal septum (Fig 1-2). It accounts for the majority of total airway resistance and thus is a critical regulator of nasal airflow.[3] The rigidity and strength of the upper lateral cartilages support the nasal sidewalls, and their relationship to the dorsal septum is important for internal nasal valve integrity.[5] If trauma leads to disarticulation and collapse of the upper lateral cartilages or to caudal septum deviation and impingement on the valve region, there is increased potential for nasal valve dysfunction.

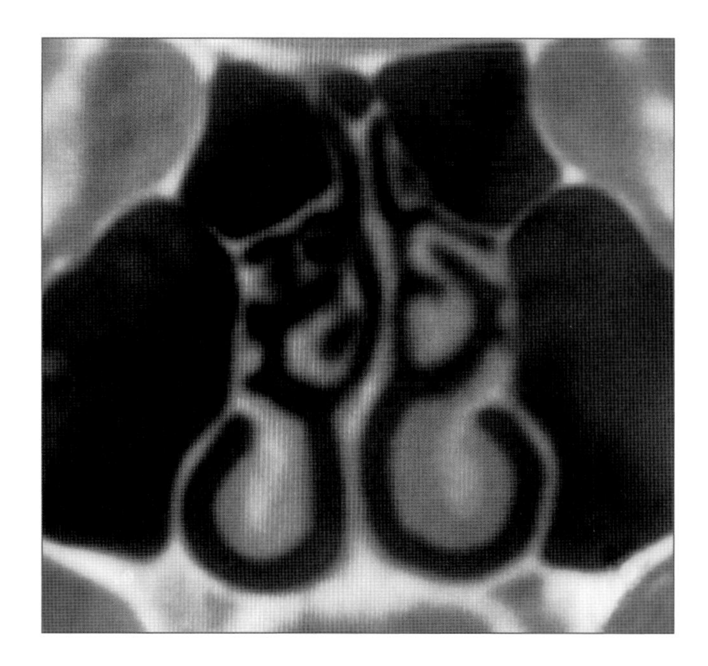

Fig 1-3 Computed tomography coronal image shows septal deviation to the right and compensatory left inferior turbinate hypertrophy.

The external nasal valve is a dynamic structure that lies caudal to the internal nasal valve (see Fig 1-2). As defined by Constantian,[6] it is composed of the cutaneous and skeletal support of the mobile alar wall, which includes the lower lateral cartilages and their investing external and vestibular skin cover. The size, strength, and anatomical position of the lower lateral cartilages and their associated fibrous attachments are important in maintaining the tip, ala, and external nasal valve stability necessary to resist collapse from negative transmural pressure generated on inspiration.[3] Enhancing the structural integrity of the internal and external nasal valve framework is a key principle in the surgical management of valve dysfunction that can accompany nasal deviation.

The anterior end of the inferior turbinate affects resistance at the internal nasal valve and thus is important in regulating airflow.[7] In patients with a severely deviated nasal septum, the inferior turbinate opposite the deviation frequently undergoes a compensatory enlargement in the body's attempt to equalize resistance in both airways (Fig 1-3).

Causes of deviation

Extrinsic and intrinsic forces lead to the septal deviation responsible for esthetic and functional deformity.[1,8] Extrinsic forces result from scar contracture and may occur subsequent to trauma or rhinoplasty. Extrinsic forces may also occur secondary to congenitally asymmetric attachments of the osteocartilaginous skeleton. These include attachments between the bony pyramid, the upper lateral cartilages, the lower lateral cartilages, and the septum. Intrinsic forces are those inherent or acquired abnormalities of the septal cartilage itself. With nasal trauma, these forces occur due to septal fracture.[9,10] Surgical maneuvers must release or overcome these deforming forces of the septum to successfully straighten the nose.

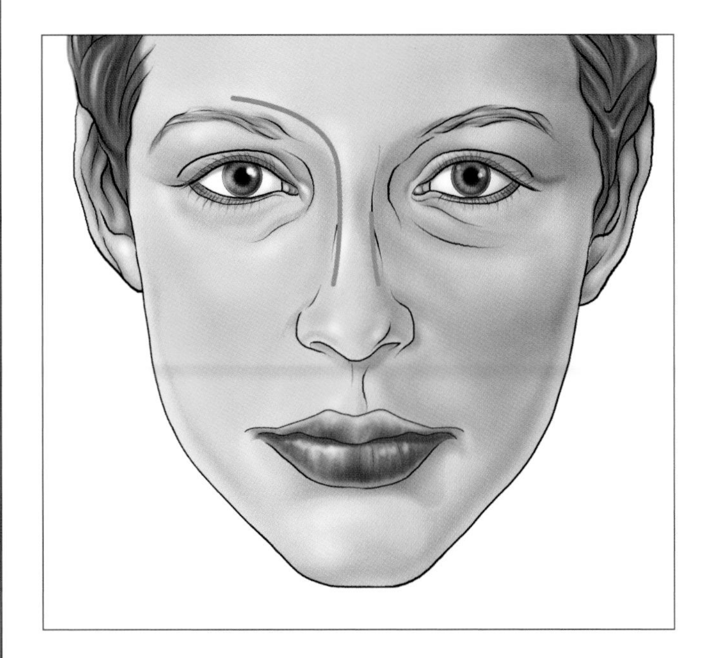

Fig 1-4 Dorsal esthetic lines. There should be a smooth, unbroken line extending from the medial brow down each line angle of the dorsum, which slightly flares out at the nasal tip.

Preoperative Evaluation

Clinical analysis is important in planning corrective surgery. History taking, physical examination, and photographs are needed. Standard photographs include frontal, three-quarter, profile, worm's-eye, and bird's-eye views. Reviewing photographs after an examination can enhance the overall assessment and appreciation of the patient's deformity.

In taking the history, it is important to determine if the patient has experienced previous nasal trauma or rhinoplasty surgery, medical therapy, or nasal illness, such as allergic rhinosinusitis. It is also important to assess if there is noticeable nasal obstruction and, if there is, to determine its temporal relationship to any noted trauma. In addition, relevant social history should include recreational intranasal drug use.[1]

The external physical examination starts with visual inspection of nasal shape, symmetry, and balance with the rest of the face. In particular, deviation of the nose from the facial midline should be noted as well as the quality and shape of the dorsal esthetic lines[1] (Fig 1-4). If the upper lateral cartilages disarticulate and collapse into the valve region, there will be disruption of the natural dorsal esthetic lines, collapse of the middle nasal vault, and probable nasal obstruction. Collapse can occur secondary to trauma, or postoperatively from dorsal hump reduction or other resective maneuvers, if the upper lateral cartilages are not preserved and resuspended to the dorsal septum (Fig 1-5). From a worm's-eye view, caudal septal deviation off the anterior nasal spine and associated nostril asymmetry should be noted (Fig 1-6).

Palpation of the nose is also an important part of the examination. The caudal septum is palpated to assess for deviation and/or dislocation off the anterior nasal spine. The external nose should be palpated to assess for bony pyramid step-offs suggesting previous fracture or upper lateral cartilage disarticulation at the keystone area. The skeletal support of the lower two-thirds (including the tip) and soft tissue

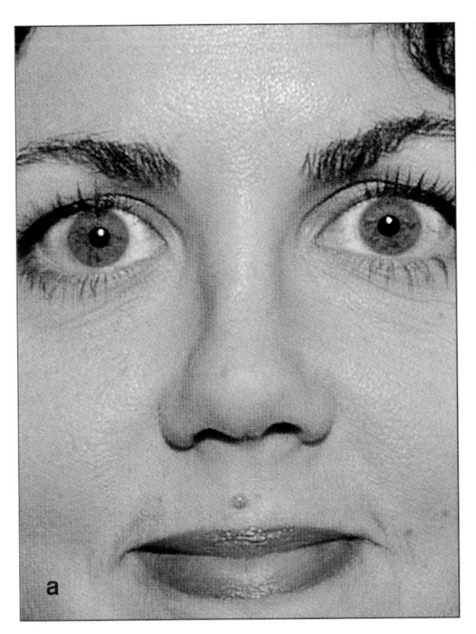

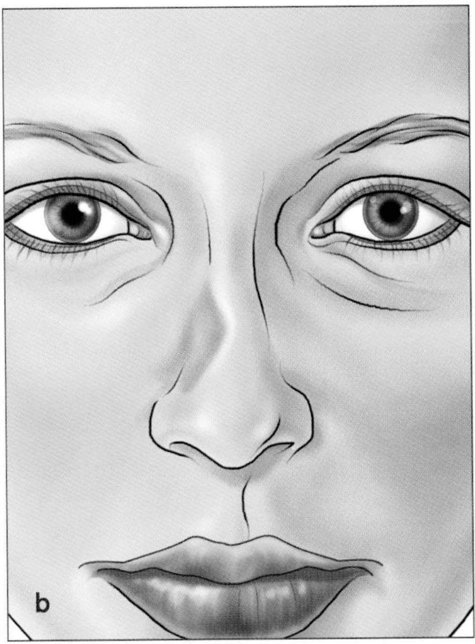

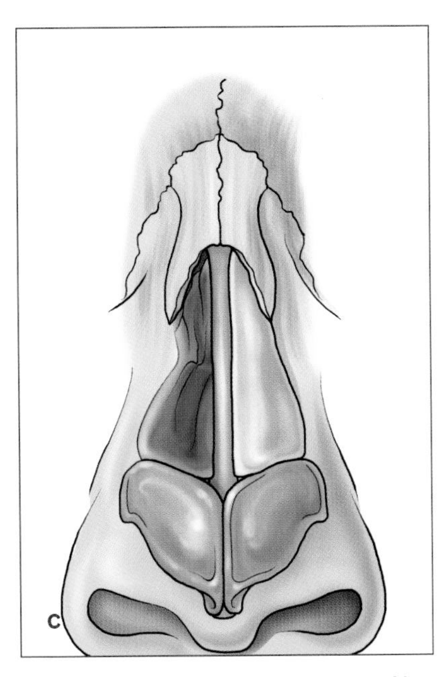

Fig 1-5 *(a)* This patient underwent a previous rhinoplasty for a deviated nasal deformity. *(b and c)* Postoperatively, she had a collapse of her right middle nasal vault due to disarticulation of the right upper lateral cartilage from the nasal bone and/or collapse of the upper lateral cartilage away from the dorsal septum.

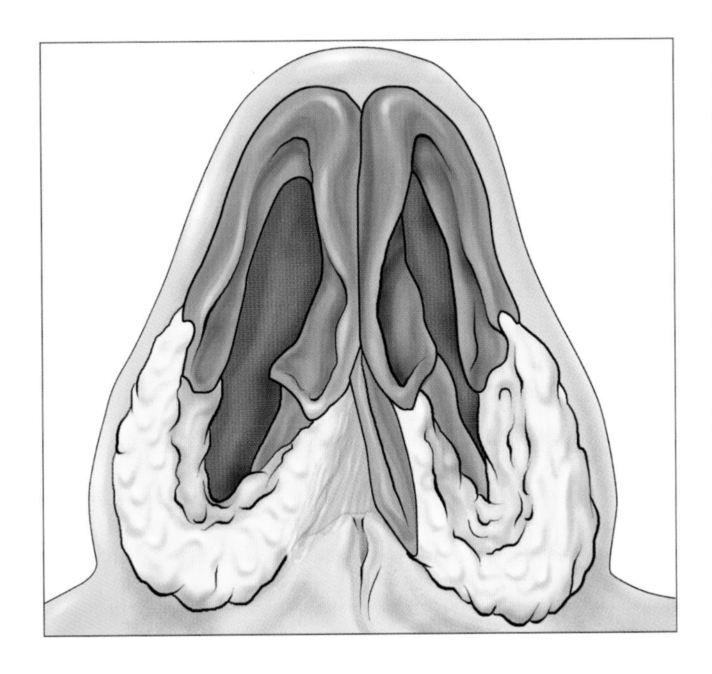

Fig 1-6 A dislocated caudal septum off the anterior nasal spine is obstructing the left nasal passage.

envelope thickness should be evaluated. The type, texture, and sebaceous content of the skin influences the effects of surgery. Thin skin more readily contracts and redrapes over the osteocartilaginous framework and shows slight contour imperfections than does thick sebaceous skin. Thick sebaceous skin and abundant intercartilaginous fibrofatty tissue tends to be associated with decreased strength of the underlying cartilaginous framework. Those with the latter skin type require more aggressive alteration of the underlying framework to effect change to the external definition of the nose.[11]

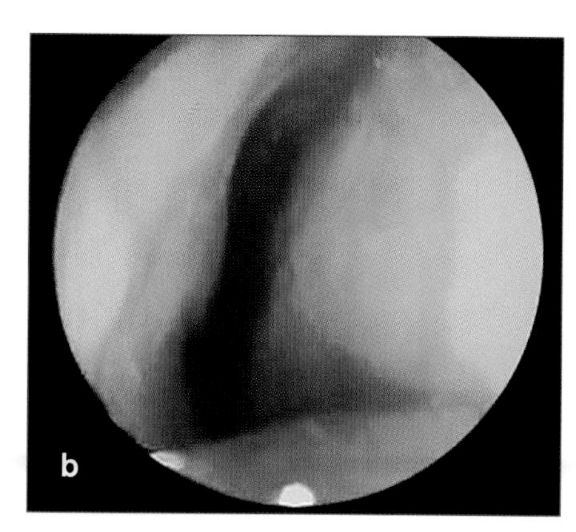

Fig 1-7 Rigid endoscopic images of the internal nasal valve region. *(a)* There is septal deviation with impingement on the left internal nasal valve. *(b)* The same patient has a more normal right internal nasal valve opposite the side of deviation.

Anterior rhinoscopy with a nasal speculum should be performed to visually inspect for septal deviation, inferior turbinate hypertrophy, bone spurs that may contribute to airway compromise, and overall mucosal health. Septal deviations may impinge on the internal nasal valve region and adversely affect nasal patency.[2] When assessing if there is impingement on the internal nasal valve, it is better to visually inspect the internal nasal valve area with the speculum withdrawn (Fig 1-7).

The integrity of the internal and external nasal valves should be evaluated during normal and deep inspiration (Figs 1-8 and 1-9). If the patient complains of obstruction and valve collapse is noted on deep inspiration, a cotton-tip applicator is used to manually distract the upper lateral cartilages and the lower lateral cartilages, sequentially, to assess where the patient experiences the greatest relief of obstruction (Fig 1-10). The exact site of external and/or internal nasal valve obstruction should be noted, the anatomical cause(s) of the obstruction should be identified, and the surgical plan must then be formulated to address the problem(s).[3,12,13]

Guyuron et al[14,15] has classified septonasal deviation. The type of septal deviation influences the external nasal deformity and, likewise, the treatment required to straighten the nose. The most common type of septal deviation is the *septal tilt* (40%). The cartilage and perpendicular plate of the ethmoid bone are free of internal curvature or fracture but are shifted to one side of the nose internally and to the opposite side externally. Often, there is compensatory hypertrophy of the inferior turbinate ipsilateral to the external deviation (Fig 1-11).

The second most common septal deviation is the *C-shaped anteroposterior deviation* (32%). The cartilage has a C-shaped curve, unlike the septal tilt where there is no curvature. The cartilage is often dislodged to one side of the maxillary crest, and externally, the nose deviates to the opposite side, similar to the septal tilt. Less commonly, there can be a *C-shaped cephalocaudal deviation* (4%), which externally presents as a C in the direction of the nose.

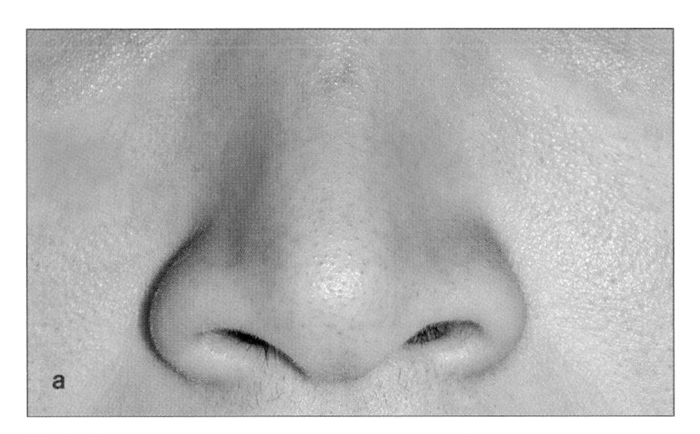

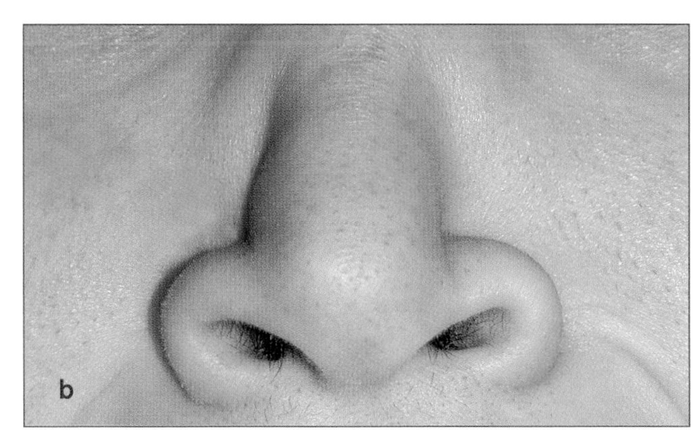

Fig 1-8 *(a)* Patient with flaccid nasal sidewalls. *(b)* On deep inspiration, the sidewalls and internal nasal valves collapse with deepening of the supra-alar groove. Note flaring of the alae to prevent further collapse at the external nasal valves.

Fig 1-9 *(a)* Patient with cephalic malposition of the lower lateral cartilages and a boxy nasal tip. *(b)* On deep inspiration, the alar rims and external nasal valves collapse inward. Cephalic malposition of the lateral crura leaves the alae devoid of cartilage and more susceptible to valve incompetence.

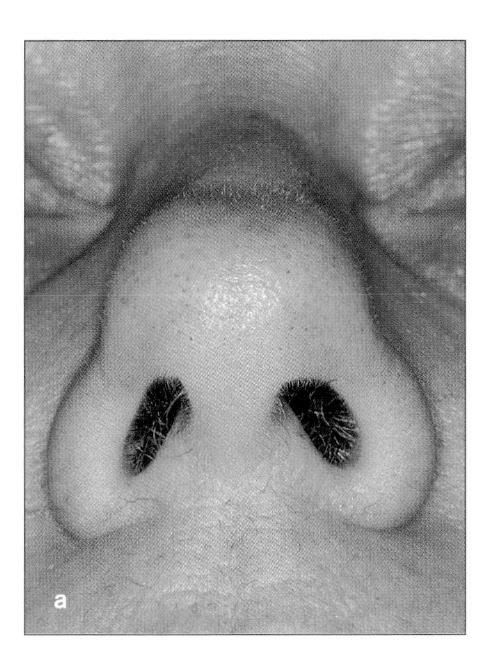

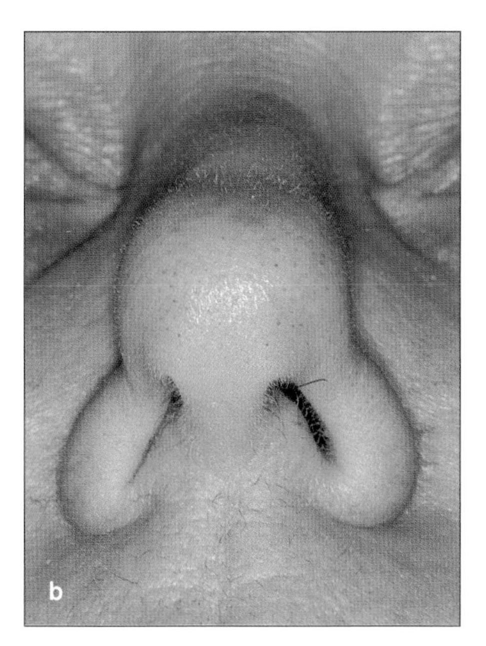

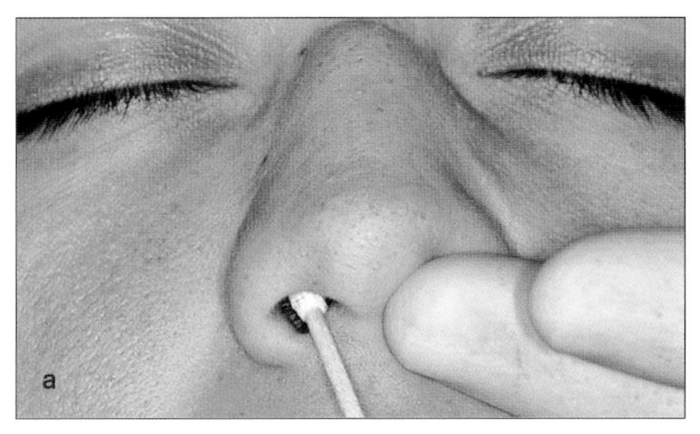

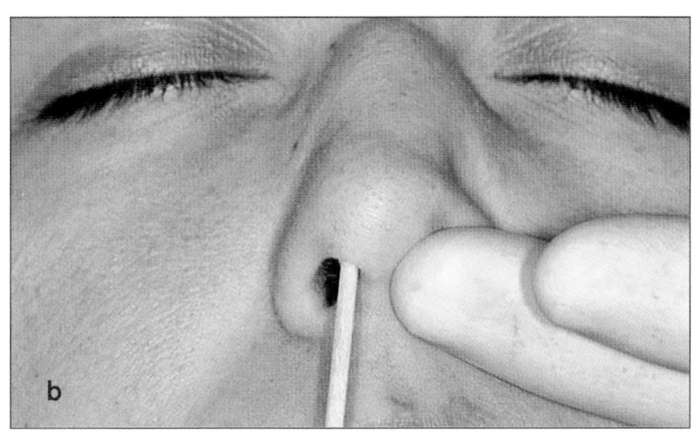

Fig 1-10 A cotton-tip applicator is used to manually support the *(a)* lower lateral cartilages/external nasal valves and *(b)* the upper lateral cartilages/internal nasal valves sequentially to assess where the patient experiences the greatest relief of obstruction.

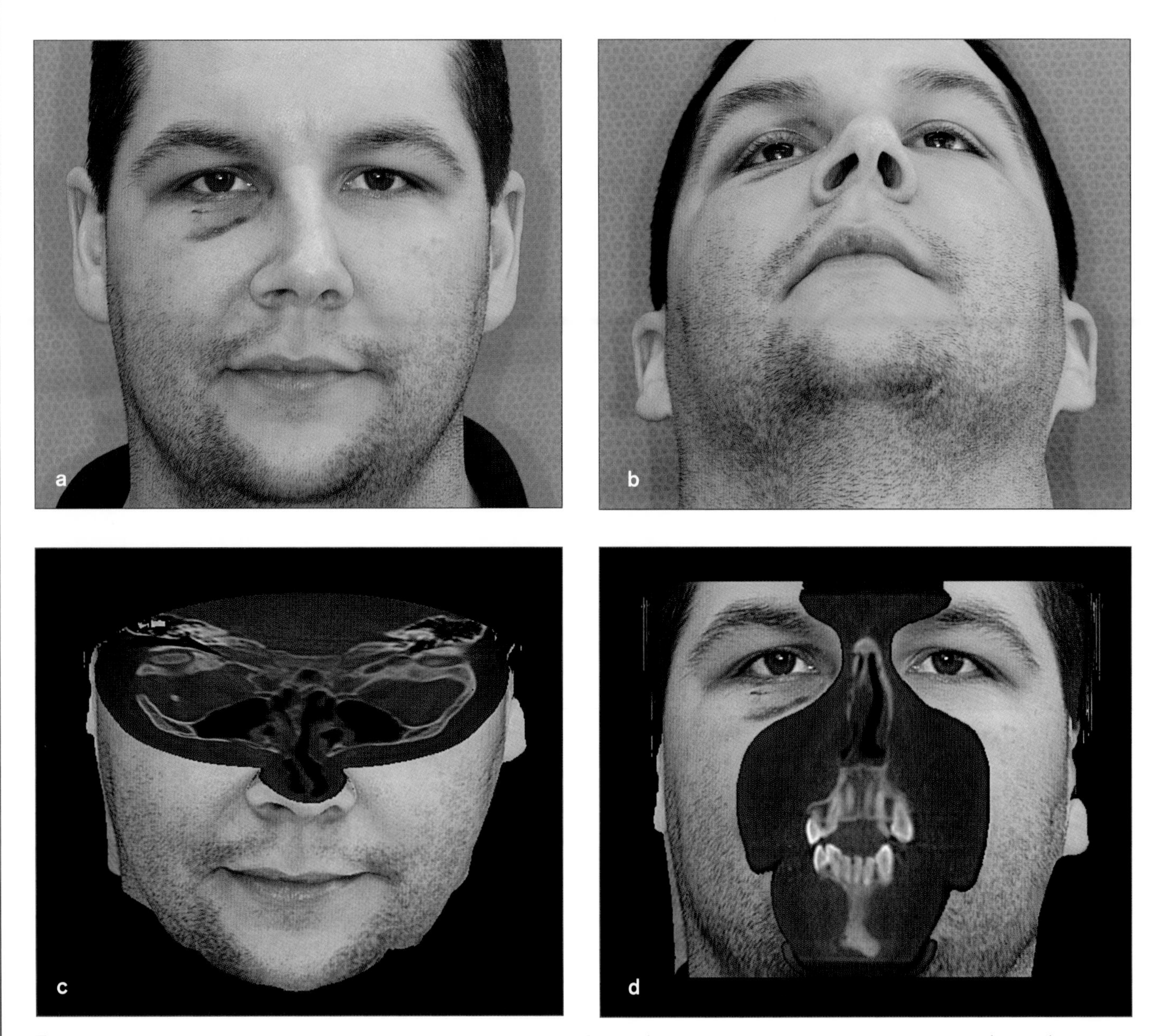

Fig 1-11 **Patient with an acute nasal trauma and septal tilt deformity.** *(a and b)* **Externally, the nose is deviated to the left.** *(c and d)* **Internally, the septum is deviated to the right.**

The *S-shaped anteroposterior* and *cephalocaudal deviations* (9%) are less common than C-shaped deformities. The anteroposterior S shape causes the external nose to shift to one side. The cephalocaudal S shape causes an S-shaped deviation to the external nose (Fig 1-12). The final category comprises localized septal deviations or spurs (15%). This is a purely functional problem and has no effect on the shape of the external nose.

The C-shaped and S-shaped septal deviations are more difficult to manage than the septal tilt. The intrinsic septal deforming forces must be eliminated to straighten the septum and external nose. Both the cartilaginous and bony septum may be deviated, and more extensive mobilization is necessary.

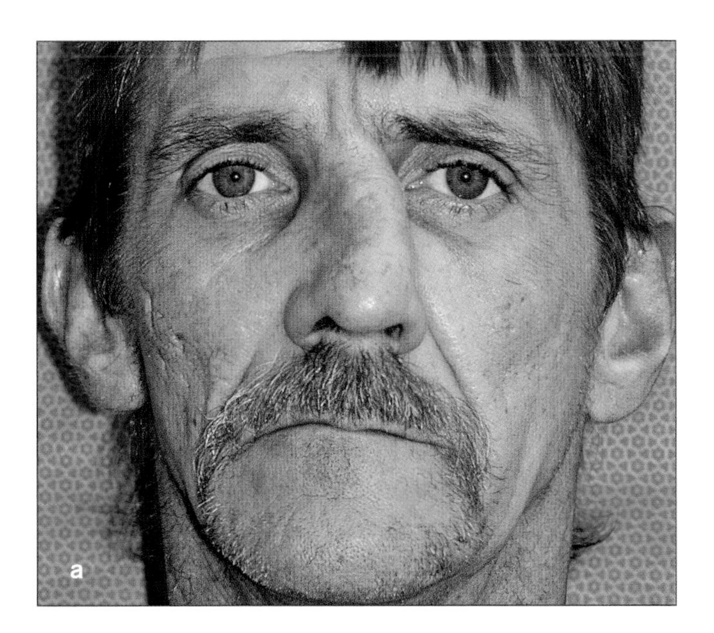
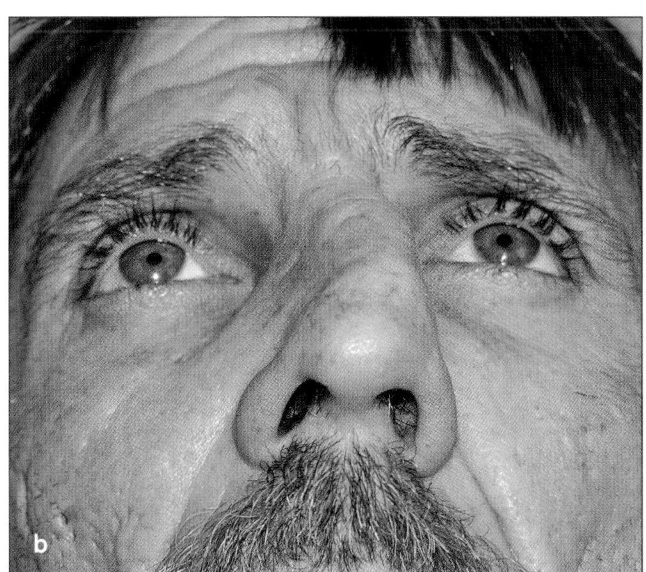

Fig 1-12 Patient with previous nasal trauma *(a)* and an S-shaped deviation of the external nose *(b)* and internal septum *(c)*.

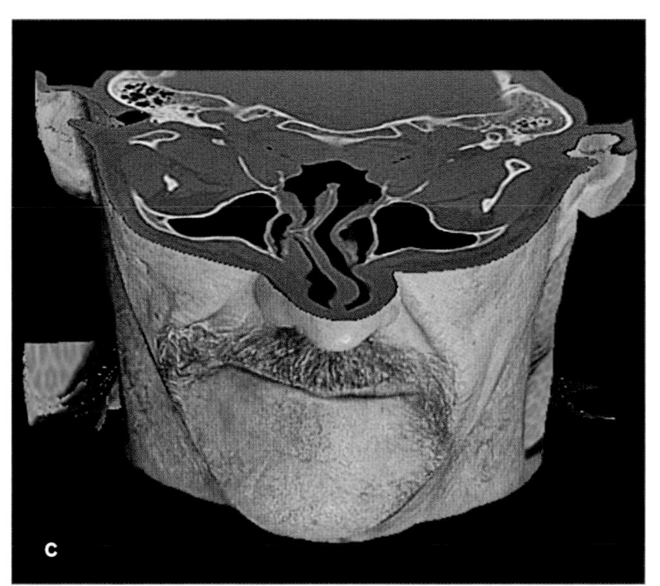

Treatment goals and principles

Both esthetic and functional treatment goals exist. Esthetic goals include straightening the bony pyramid and dorsum to improve dorsal esthetic lines and defining the tip to enhance tip esthetics. It is important to have a perfectly straight nose at the end of surgery. Functional goals aim to improve the nasal airway, including straightening the septum, restoring nasal valve integrity, and correcting inferior turbinate hypertrophy, if present.

Important treatment principles guide surgical correction of the deviated nose. Structures that are malpositioned must be freely mobilized of all attachments and placed into their correct anatomical positions. If the bony pyramid is deviated, osteotomies must be performed; if the upper lateral cartilages are displaced, they should be freed from the septum and the lower lateral cartilages. The deviated bony and cartilaginous septum must be widely exposed and mobilized to return it to the midline. Once extrinsic and intrinsic deforming forces are released, structural grafting is performed to reestablish skeletal support. Key treatment principles for managing the deviated nose have been previously outlined.[1,16,17] The following treatment algorithm is in part based on these principles:

- Open rhinoplasty for optimal exposure of deviated structures
- Wide release of deforming mucoperichondrial attachments
- Septoplasty for graft harvest and straightening the deviated septum
- Reduction of hypertrophied turbinate(s)
- Osteotomies of the bony pyramid
- Digital fracture of the central complex
- Restoration of dorsal septal support
- Stabilization of the nasal base
- Camouflaging crushed cartilage grafting of nasal sidewalls
- Structural alar grafting and tip refinement

Surgical Procedures

Open rhinoplasty for optimal exposure of deviated structures

The open rhinoplasty approach via transcolumellar and marginal incisions is preferred over the closed approach in most instances. Exposure afforded by the open approach allows maximal accuracy in diagnosis and control in performing the maneuvers necessary for repair of the deviated nose (Fig 1-13).

Wide release of deforming mucoperichondrial attachments

Wide exposure and release of mucoperichondrial attachments remove the deforming forces acting on the septum and nose. Extrinsic forces are sequentially released as needed. A cephalic trim is performed to free the lower lateral cartilages from the upper lateral cartilages at the scroll (Figs 1-14a and 1-14b). The caudal end of each upper lateral cartilage is identified at the anterior septal angle and then released from the dorsal septum in a subperichondrial plane (Figs 1-14c and 1-14d). If the upper lateral cartilages are contributing to septal deviation, this maneuver will straighten the septum.

The final step involves exposure of the septum itself to visualize and manage intrinsic forces causing septal deviation. Posterior or localized deviation can be approached through a hemitransfixion or Killian incision. For anterior or severe septal deviations, an open approach offers better access. The septum is exposed from the dorsal aspect after release of the upper lateral cartilages. The deviated portions of the cartilaginous and bony septum are fully exposed by releasing a full-thickness mucoperichondrial flap on both sides. If the caudal septum is deviated and must be accessed, the transdomal ligaments are released as well as the attachment of the medial crura to the septum down to the anterior nasal spine.

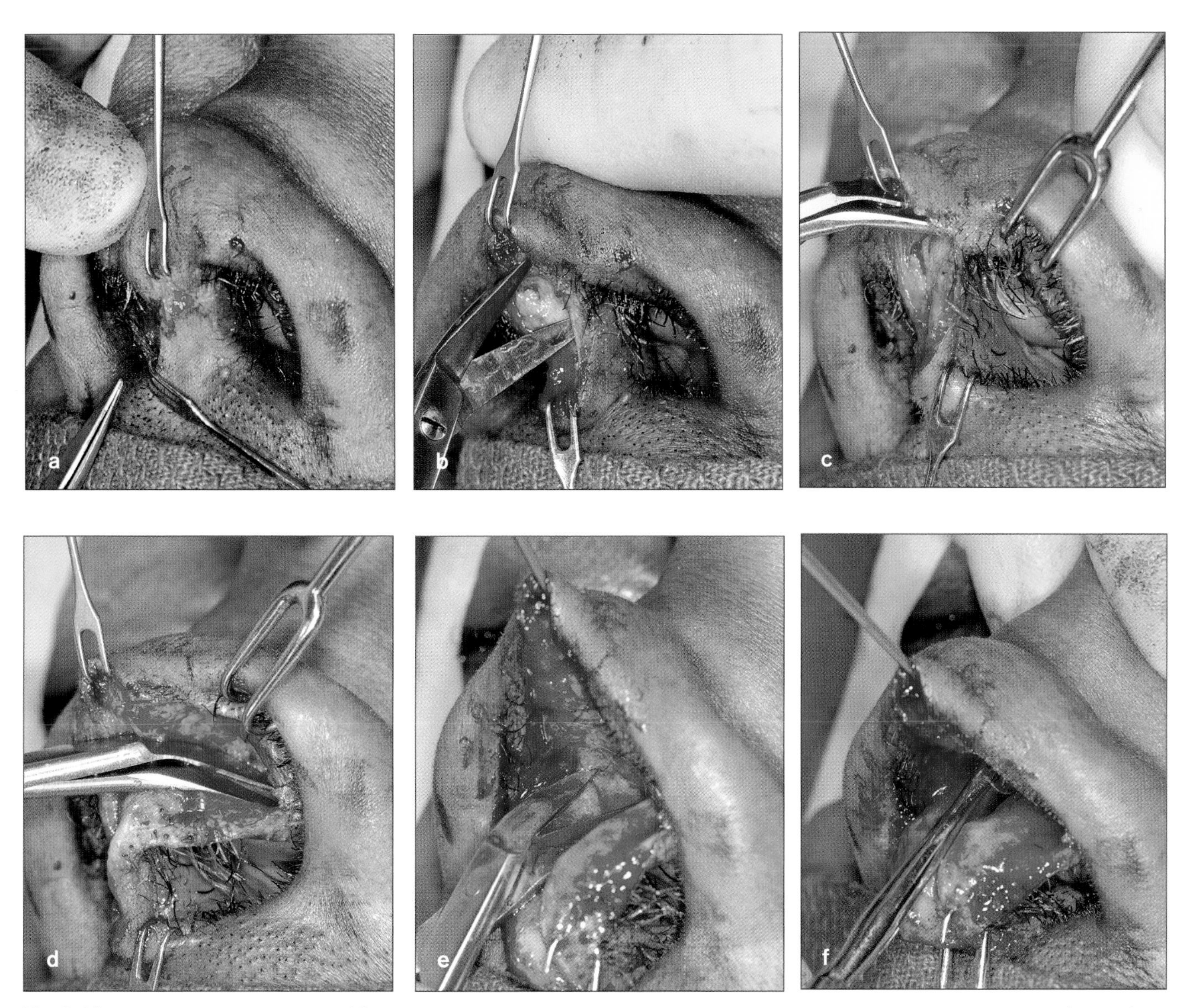

Fig 1-13 Open rhinoplasty approach. *(a)* An inverted V or stairstep transcolumellar incision is made across the midcolumella. *(b and c)* Bilateral marginal incisions are made just inferior/caudal to the medial crura and connect with the transcolumellar incision. A transcolumellar flap is reflected in a plane along the medial crura extending up into the domes. Blunt scissor dissection is carried out blindly in an avascular plane against the lateral crura. *(d)* The marginal incisions are then completed inferior/caudal to the lateral crura. *(e and f)* Once the lower lateral cartilages are exposed, blunt and sharp scissor dissection is carried out in the avascular plane overlying the cartilaginous dorsum and upper lateral cartilages. Once the bony dorsum is reached, dissection is carried out in a subperiosteal plane.

While often necessary, wide mucoperichondrial release reduces key nasal support to the lower two-thirds of the nose and blood supply to cartilage. Therefore, attachments should be preserved whenever possible to maintain support and minimize resorption that occurs with loss of blood supply.

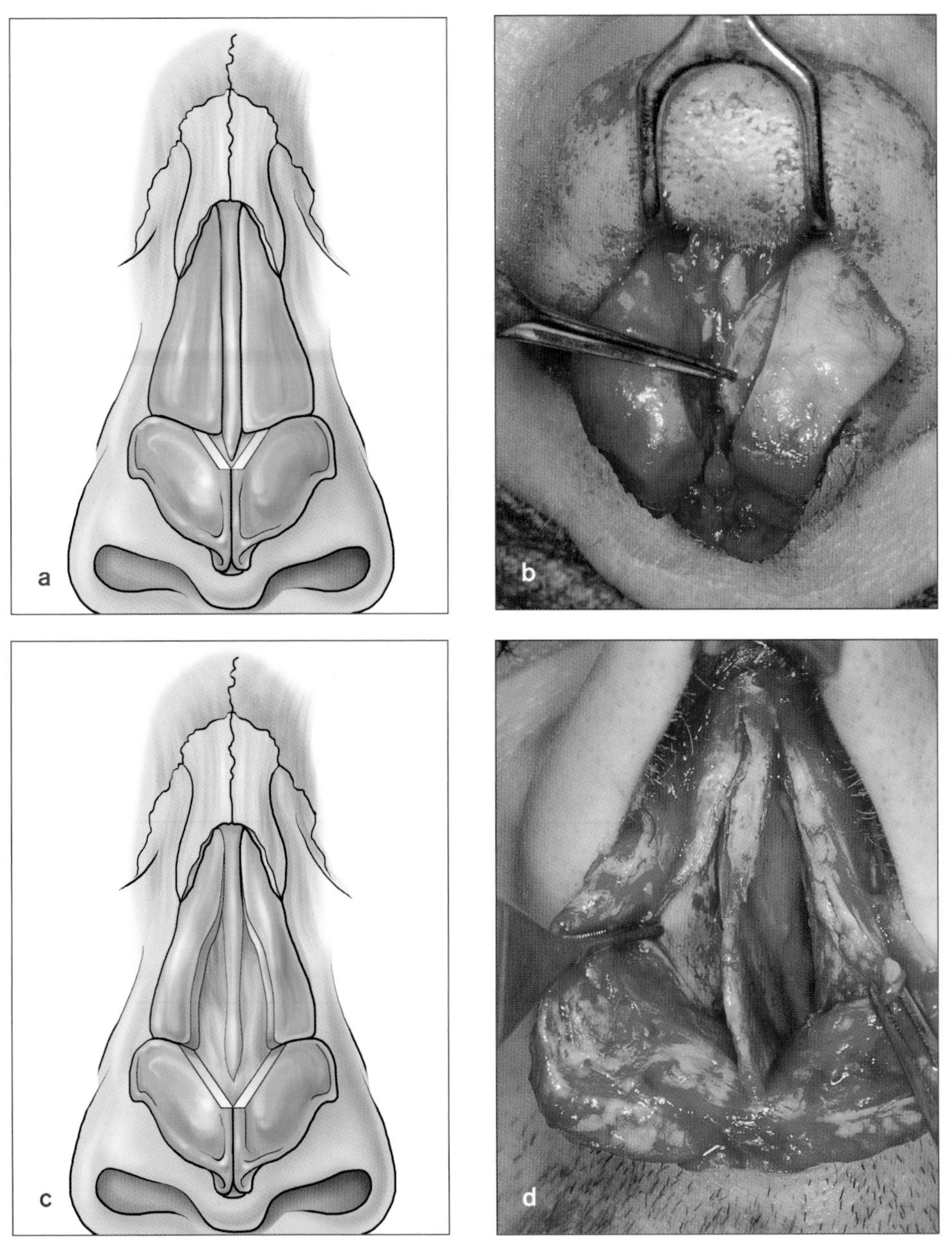

Fig 1-14 Wide release of deforming mucoperichondrial attachments. *(a and b)* Cephalic trim is performed to release the lower lateral cartilages from the upper lateral cartilages. *(c and d)* The upper lateral cartilages are released from the dorsal septum. An open approach to the septum provides improved access to manage septal deviations, especially anterior/dorsal or more severe deviations.

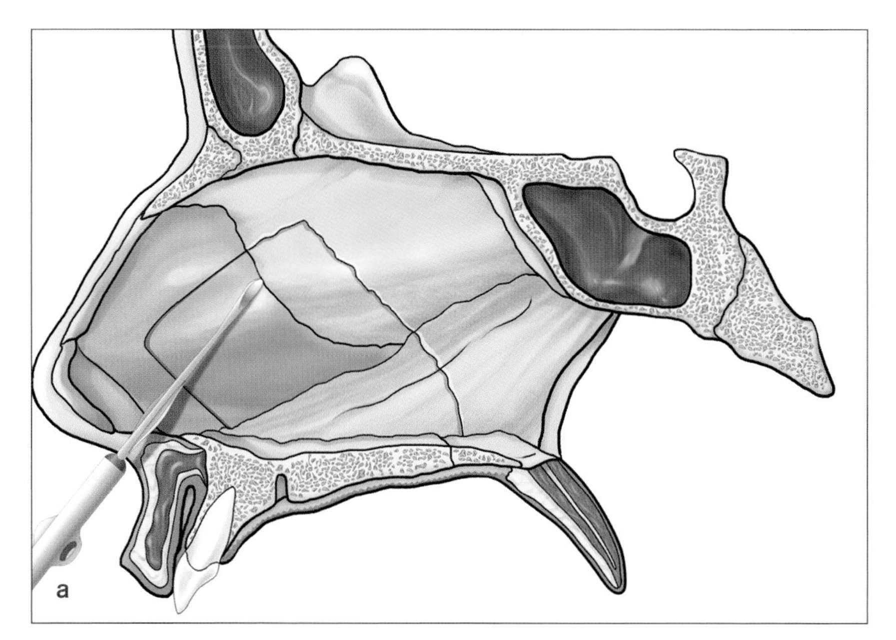

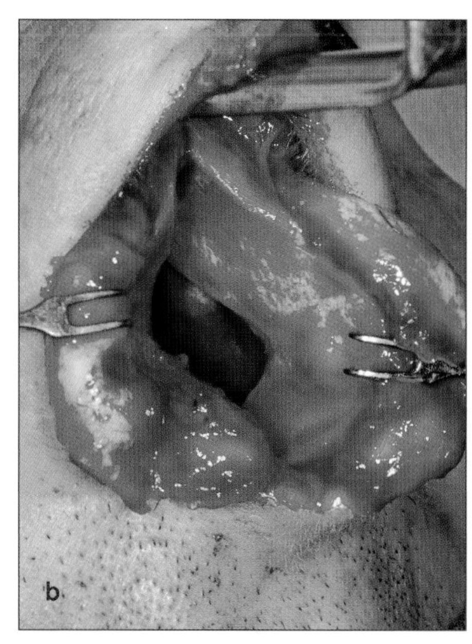

Fig 1-15 **Septoplasty.** ***(a)*** **Removal of portions of the quadrangular cartilage, perpendicular plate of the ethmoid, and vomer.** ***(b)*** **The L-strut of the dorsal and caudal septum should be preserved to maintain septal support to the external nose. Osteotomies of the bony septum should be performed as needed to eliminate intrinsic deforming forces that can lead to residual long-term nasal deviation.**

Septoplasty for graft harvest and straightening the deviated septum

Septoplasty is undertaken to help straighten the septum and harvest cartilage and bone for structural grafting. In so doing, it is important to maximize residual dorsal nasal support. Septal tilt and C-shaped and S-shaped deviations are corrected by first removing the posterior portion of the septum. The resection may include the perpendicular plate of the ethmoid bone, vomer, maxillary crest, and bone spurs in addition to cartilage. At least an 8- to 10-mm dorsal and caudal L-strut of septal cartilage should be maintained so as to provide residual septal support to the external nose. Care should be taken to maintain the attachment of the L-strut to the perpendicular plate of the ethmoid bone at the keystone area and the anterior nasal spine (Fig 1-15).

If there is a high septal deviation involving the perpendicular plate of the ethmoid bone, septal scissors are used to incise the ethmoid bone beyond the dorsal incision in cartilage. This helps weaken deforming forces in the bony septum and permits resection of the bone if necessary. If the anterior nasal spine or residual vomer is malpositioned, an osteotomy along the nasal floor can be performed to straighten the bony segment (see Fig 1-15).

If a dorsal hump and/or caudal septum reduction is needed, this should be done before septoplasty to maintain the proper width of residual L-strut of cartilage. The authors of this chapter prefer the component dorsal hump reduction technique advocated by Rohrich et al[18] to minimize potential untoward sequelae that can occur, such as middle nasal vault collapse and nasal valve dysfunction.

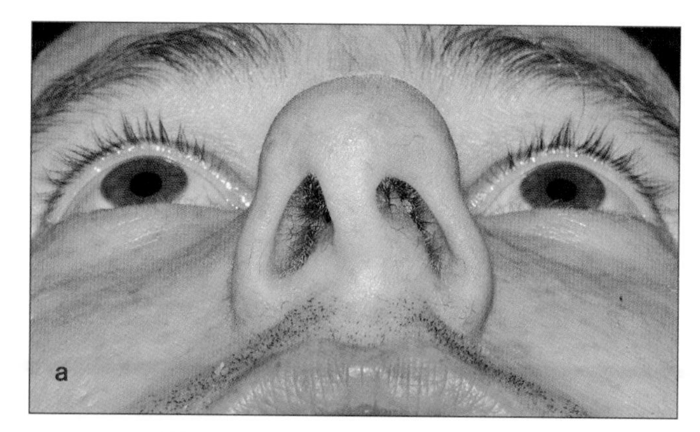

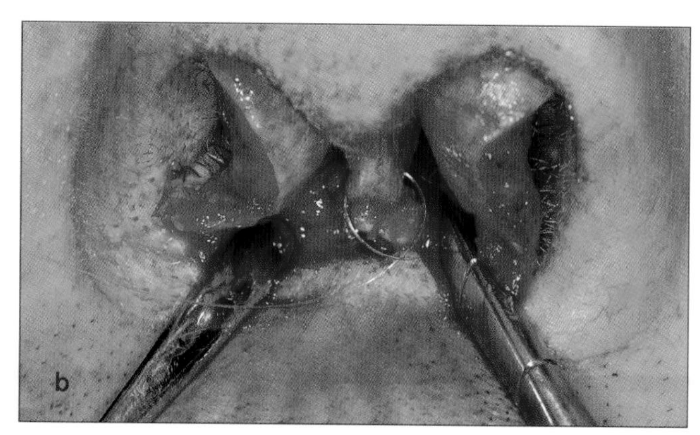

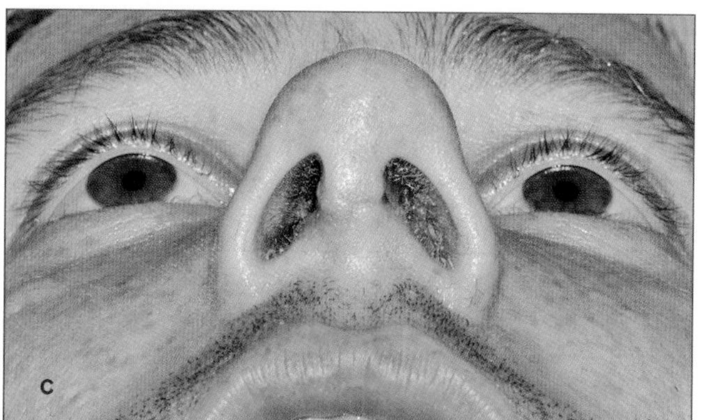

Fig 1-16 *(a)* Preoperative view showing a dislocated caudal septum that is contributing to obstruction of the patient's left nasal passage. *(b)* During an open rhinoplasty, a small strip of septum along the floor was resected to help reposition the septum to midline. A figure-of-eight suture is used to secure the caudal septum to the anterior nasal spine after a purchase hole is placed with a wire-passing drill. *(c)* Postoperative view shows the caudal septum midline. Note that the boxy tip was managed with cephalic trim of the lower lateral cartilages and transdomal sutures.

If the caudal septum is dislocated off the nasal spine (Fig 1-16), it must be freely mobilized and passively stabilized to the anterior nasal spine with a figure-of-eight suture. If the caudal septum is still deviated to one side, a "swinging door" flap with vertical wedge sectioning of the septum at the point of deviation can be performed.

Intrinsic deforming forces that remain in patients having C-shaped or S-shaped deviations can be overcome by scoring the cartilage along the concave side of the deviation (Fig 1-17). Guyuron[14] advocates using bilateral extramucosal stents fixed in position with through-and-through sutures after the cartilage is scored. The stents are kept in place for 3 weeks and the patient maintained on oral antibiotics.[14] Cartilage batten grafts are another means of overcoming residual septal deviations. A batten graft can be suture stabilized to the caudal septum. Bilateral spreader grafts can straighten residual deviation of the dorsal septum in addition to restoring support and dorsal esthetic lines (discussed later).

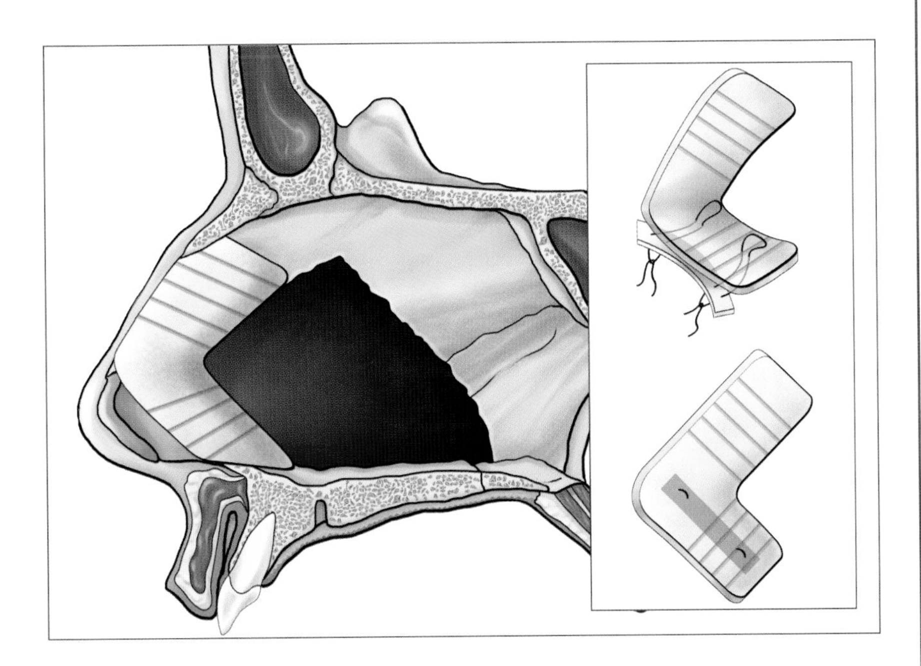

Fig 1-17 Scoring the L-strut of cartilage along the concave side of the deviation can decrease intrinsic deforming forces. A cartilage batten graft can be suture stabilized to the caudal septum to overcome residual deviation (see inset).

Reduction of hypertrophied turbinates

If the deviated septum is surgically corrected to the midline and compensatory inferior turbinate hypertrophy is present, the enlarged turbinate can increase obstruction. It can also prevent the septum from being repositioned to the midline.[19,20] For this reason, the authors of this chapter prefer to perform partial inferior turbinectomy at this point, if needed. The anteroinferior turbinate soft tissue and bone are resected, followed by electrocauterization of the base. Overaggressive resection is avoided because of potential complications such as bleeding and nasal dryness.

Osteotomies of the bony pyramid

A deviated nasal bony pyramid and central complex are extrinsic deforming forces. The authors of this chapter prefer to perform osteotomies and fracture of the central complex, if indicated to eliminate their effect before performing any grafting to reestablish structural support to the nose.

If a dorsal hump is present, it must be reduced before osteotomies are performed, while the bony pyramid and dorsum are still stable. If the nasal bones are asymmetric, less bone should be excised from the side that is more vertically oriented. This prevents excessive reduction in nasal bone height on that side after the bony complex is reduced.

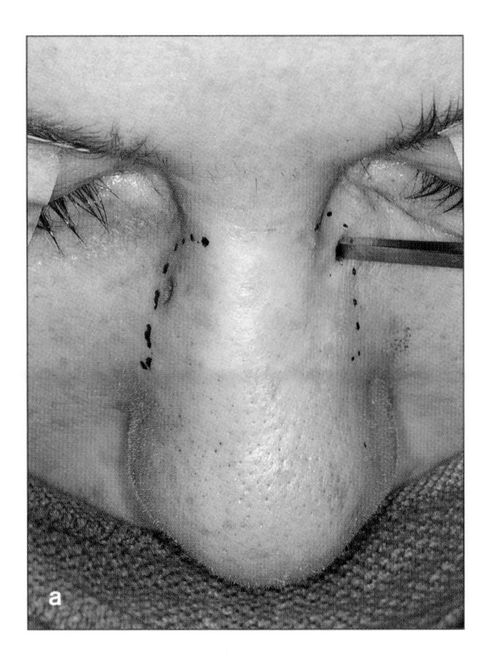

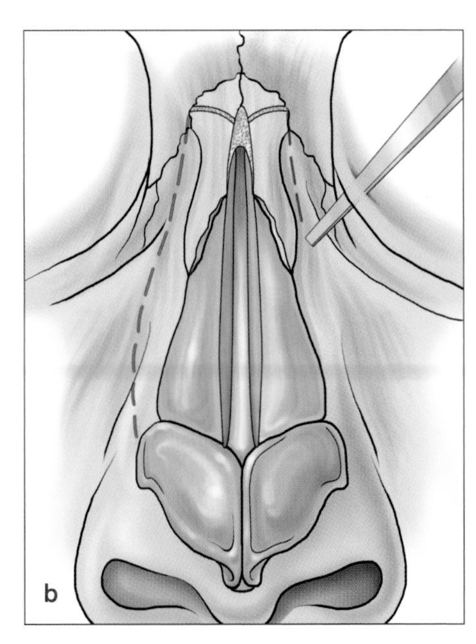

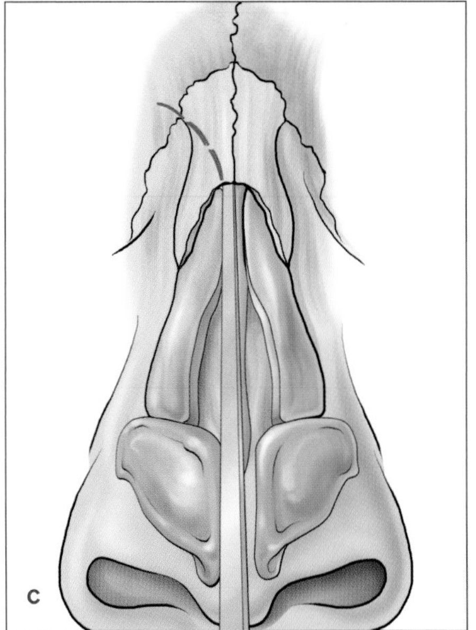

Fig 1-18 *(a and b)* **Percutaneous lateral osteotomies are performed with a 2-mm straight osteotomy.** *(c)* **Fading medial osteotomies are carried out first if there is any significant degree of bony asymmetry. Osteotomies must allow passive resetting of the bony pyramid to prevent redeviation postoperatively.**

Lateral osteotomies alone are indicated if the nasal bones are deviated but symmetric. The authors of this chapter prefer performing these percutaneously with a 2-mm osteotome. Medial osteotomies are required if there are nasal bone asymmetries to allow independent movement of each nasal bone (Fig 1-18). They must be performed before the lateral osteotomies, while the bony pyramid is stable. Intermediate-level osteotomies are needed to manage nasal bone convexity. Care should be taken to minimize periosteal release from the nasal bones to help in stabilization of fragments, especially if there is comminution from multiple osteotomies. Adequate osteotomies must be performed that allow full mobility and passive resetting of the bony pyramid (Fig 1-19). Otherwise, redeviation may occur postoperatively because of tissue memory.

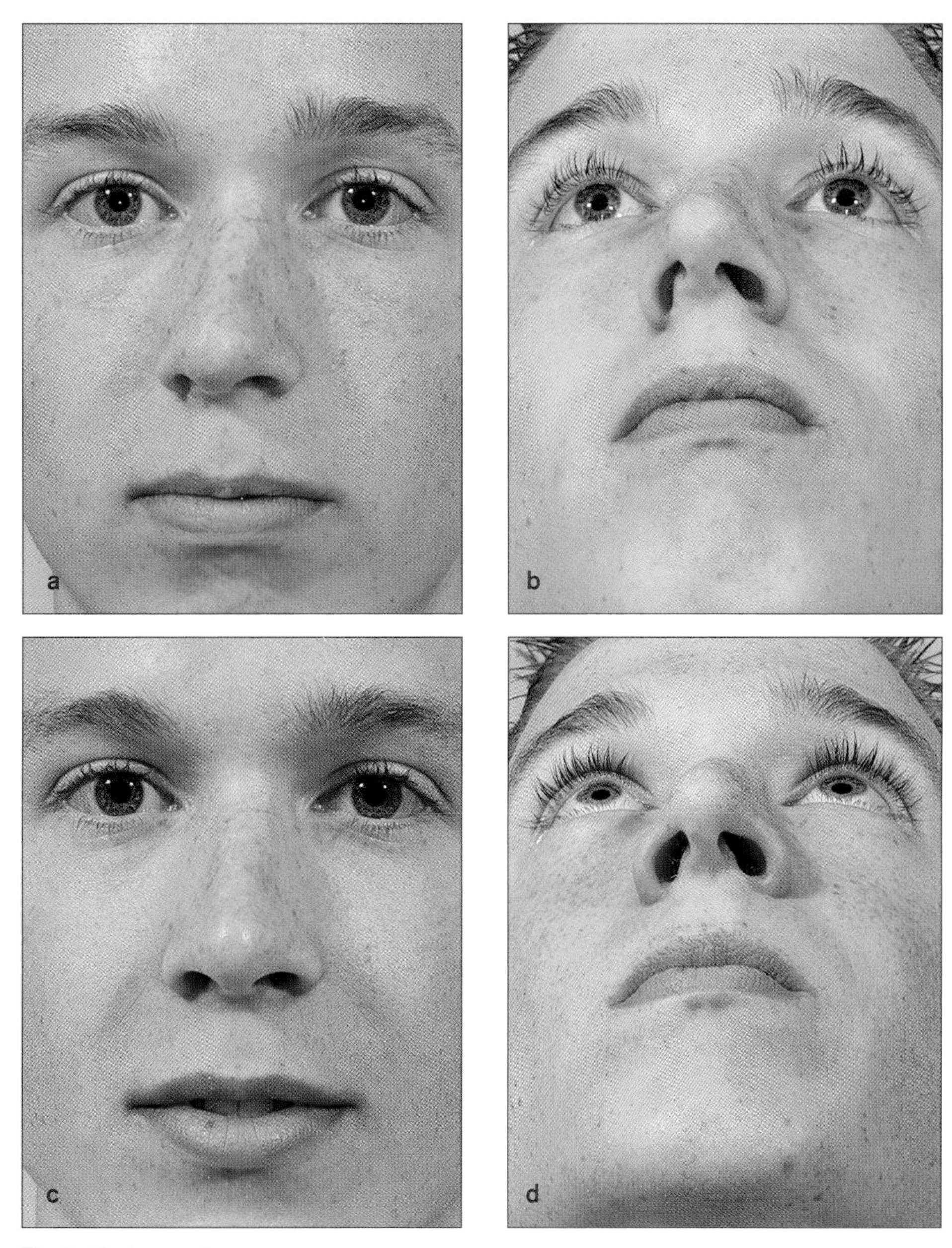

Fig 1-19 *(a and b)* Preoperative views of a patient with a deviated nose classified as a septal tilt. He sustained nasal trauma in an all-terrain vehicle accident. *(c and d)* Twelve-month postoperative views, after bilateral osteotomies were performed in conjunction with a Le Fort I osteotomy to manage his dentofacial deformity. In addition to the lateral osteotomies, the only other maneuver performed was the complete freeing of the nasal septum from the maxillary crest. This outcome highlights the importance of eliminating septal deforming forces to straighten the nose.

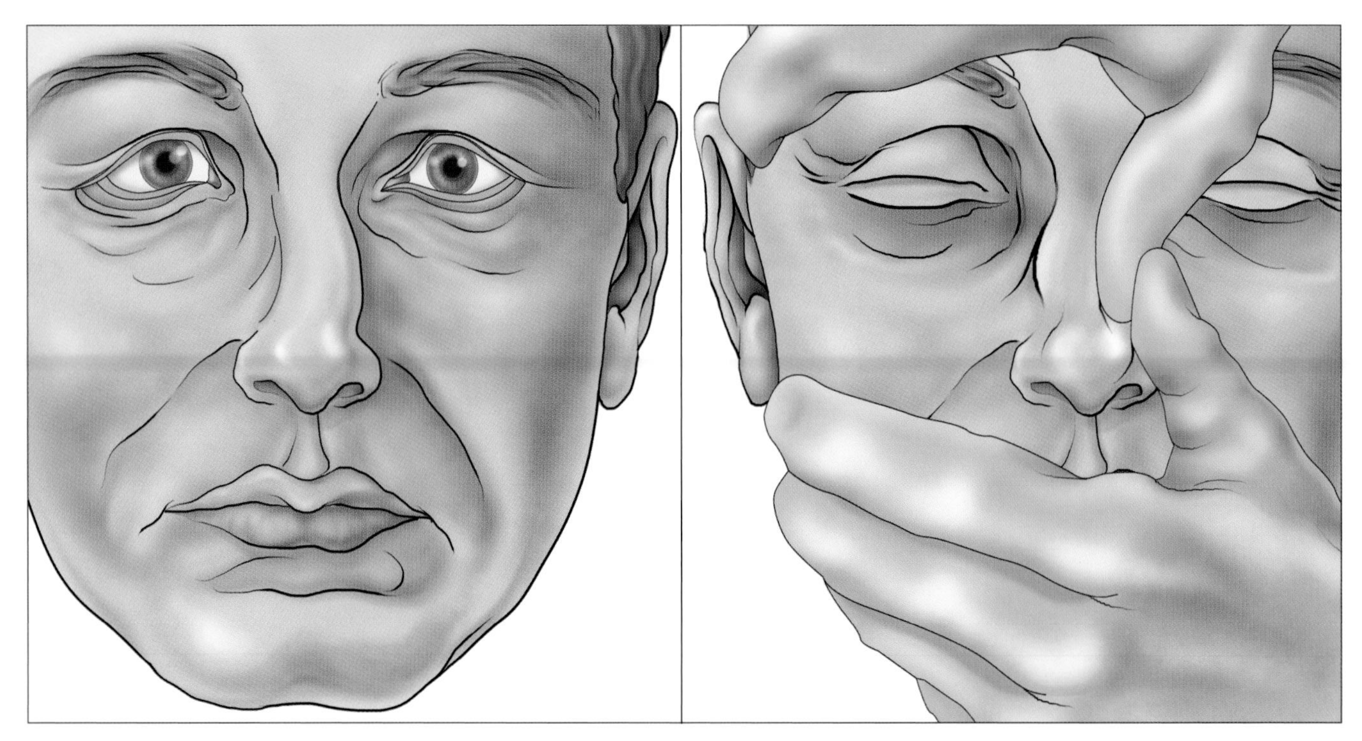

Fig 1-20 Digital fracture of the central complex is sometimes necessary as a final step to eliminate deforming forces and straighten the external nose.

Digital fracture of the central complex

After release of the upper lateral cartilages from the septum, septoplasty, and osteotomies, the nose is usually straight. On occasion, however, the central complex, which is the extension of the perpendicular plate of the ethmoid bone underneath the nasal bones, remains crooked and causes residual deviation to the bony pyramid. If so, digital fracture of the central complex must be carried out to eliminate this extrinsic deforming force (Fig 1-20).

Restoration of dorsal septal support

After the deforming forces are removed, the residual L-strut of septal cartilage is left weakened. The septum must be strengthened to maintain long-term support to the external nose. If a significant dorsal hump is reduced, an open-roof deformity may exist. Internal nasal valve function and dorsal esthetic lines may need to be maintained or restored. Spreader grafts are the primary means of achieving these goals[21] (Fig 1-21).

Septal cartilage is the best donor source for spreader grafts. Grafts are typically 4 to 5 mm wide and 25 to 30 mm long. They are tucked beneath the nasal bones and extend the full length of the dorsal septum to the anterior septal angle. They are usually placed bilaterally. On occasion, a graft is placed unilaterally to camouflage a dorsal septal deviation. It can significantly broaden the middle nasal vault if placed even

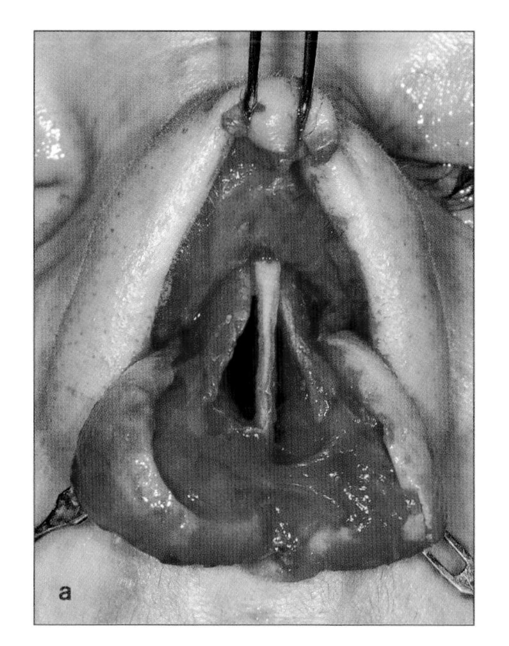

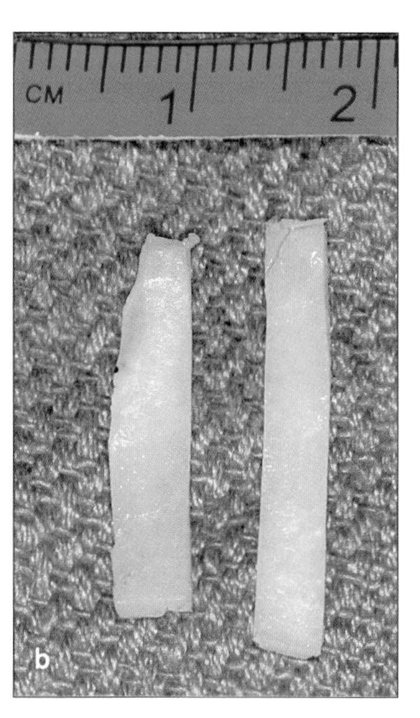

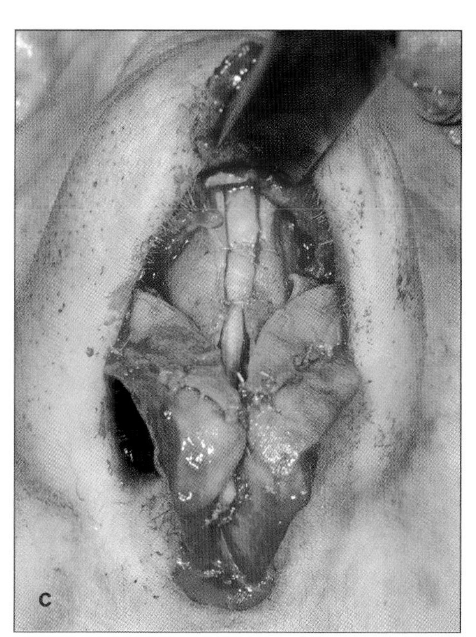

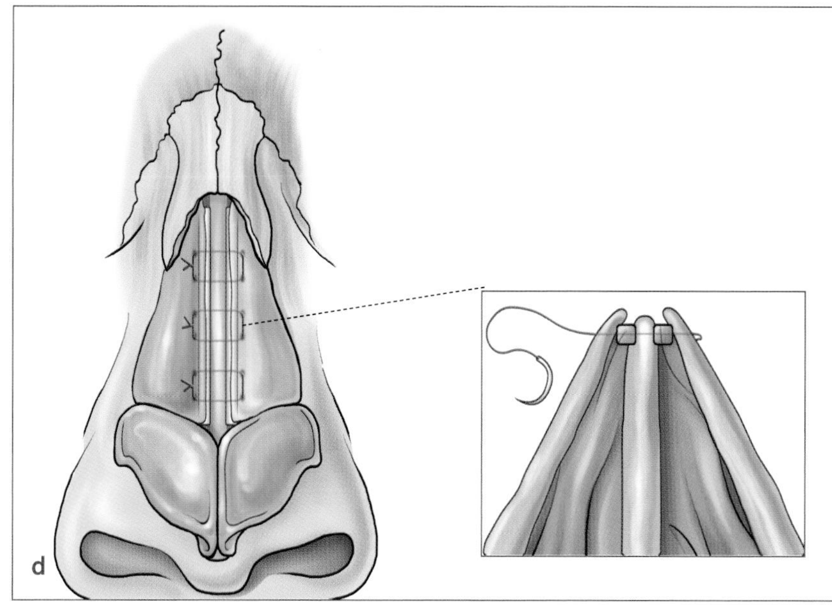

Fig 1-21 Spreader grafts. *(a)* The upper lateral cartilages are shown released from the septum. *(b)* Spreader grafts are carved from septal cartilage. They are typically 4 to 5 mm wide and 25 to 30 mm long and extend the full length of the dorsal septum. *(c)* The spreader grafts in this instance were placed slightly below the dorsal septum so as not to widen the middle nasal vault. The upper lateral cartilages are resuspended to the dorsal septum. Note that one spreader graft is serving as a caudal extension graft. The middle crura are resuspended to it to increase tip projection. Also, lateral crural turnover grafts have been performed. *(d)* Illustration of bilateral spreader grafts sutured in place.

with the dorsal septum. If this is esthetically undesirable, the graft can be secured slightly below the dorsal septum. It is important to resuspend and resecure released upper lateral cartilages to the spreader graft/dorsal septal complex. The upper lateral cartilage and spreader graft on each side can be secured together to the septum with two or three horizontal mattress or single interrupted sutures of 5-0 polydioxanone suture (PDS, Ethicon). Single interrupted sutures are easier to throw, but the disadvantage is that subsequent dorsal reduction cannot be done without cutting loose the sutures.

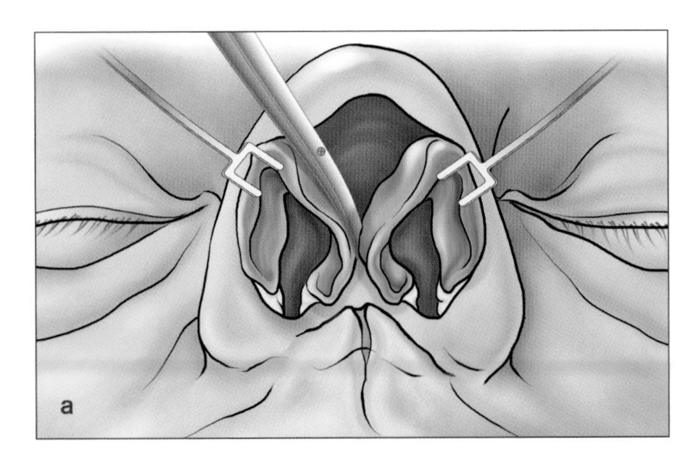

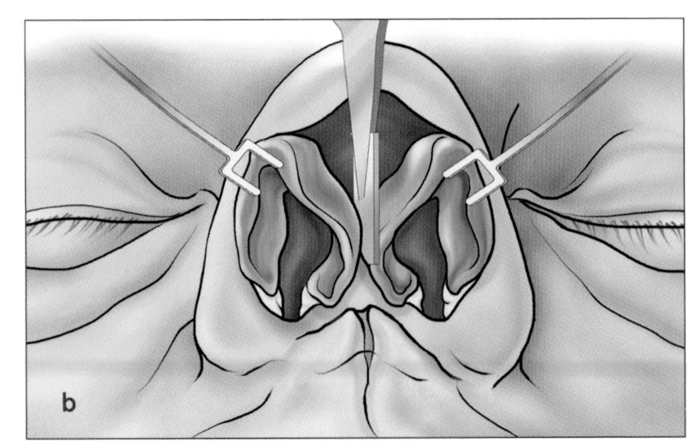

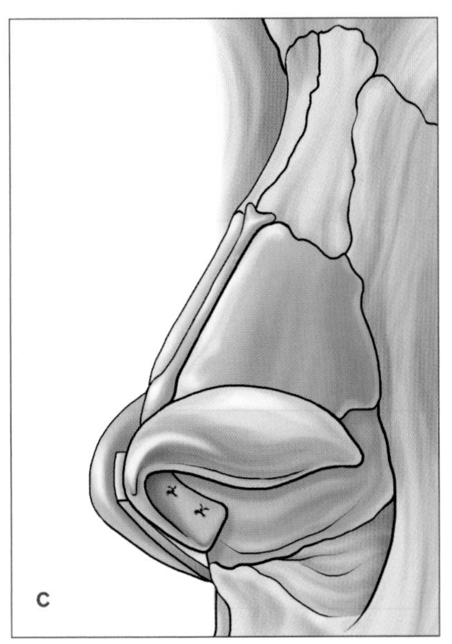

Fig 1-22 Columellar strut graft can be used to increase tip projection and stabilize the nasal base. Septal cartilage is preferred. *(a)* A pocket is created between the medial crura. *(b and c)* The columellar strut graft is placed in the pocket and secured.

Stabilization of the nasal base

Nasal tip support is left significantly compromised after the wide release of deforming mucoperichondrial attachments and must be restored. Various cartilage grafting maneuvers can be employed to restore tip projection and stabilize the nasal base to maintain long-term tip support. A columellar strut graft is frequently used to accomplish this. Septal cartilage is the preferred graft material, although costal cartilage is used when a stronger strut and projection are desired. A pocket is created between the medial crura for placement of the graft (Figs 1-22a and 1-22b). The soft tissue in front of the nasal spine is preserved to prevent graft displacement. Horizontal mattress sutures of 5-0 PDS secure the strut to the cephalic aspect of the medial crura (Fig 1-22c). A septal or caudal extension graft or suturing of the medial crura to an overly long/plunging caudal septum is also effective at stabilizing the nasal base. Shield or onlay tip grafting is another means of providing tip support as well as projection and definition.[22]

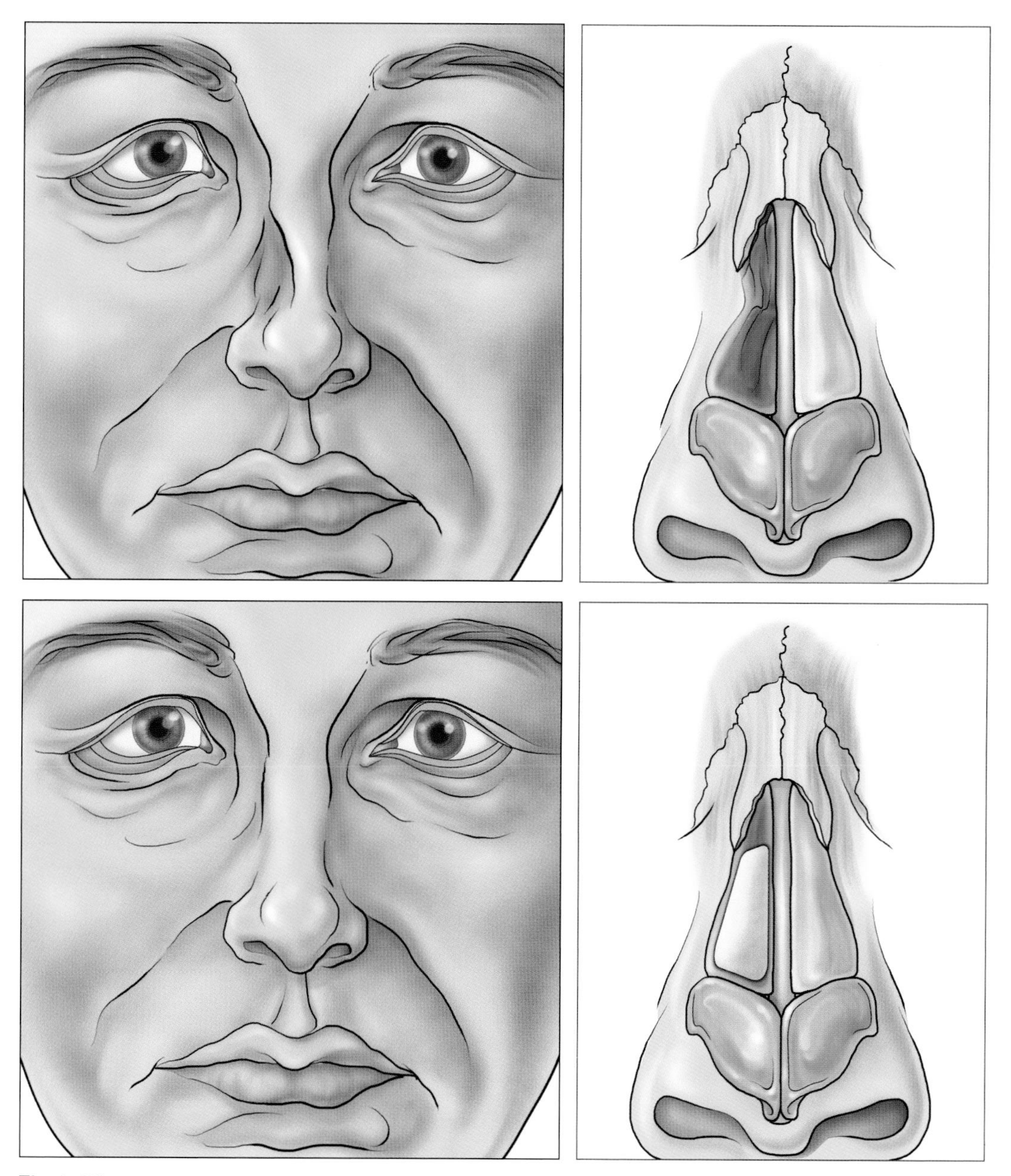

Fig 1-23 **Crushed cartilage graft placed along the nasal sidewall can camouflage a mild depression that exists after performing other maneuvers to straighten the nose.**

Camouflaging crushed cartilage grafting of nasal sidewalls

At times, residual asymmetry along the nasal sidewall may remain after osteotomies. This may be related to a disarticulated upper lateral cartilage from the nasal bone or an inability to completely outfracture a medially shifted nasal bone. In either situation, a crushed cartilage graft placed along the sidewall can camouflage a mild irregularity and improve symmetry (Fig 1-23).

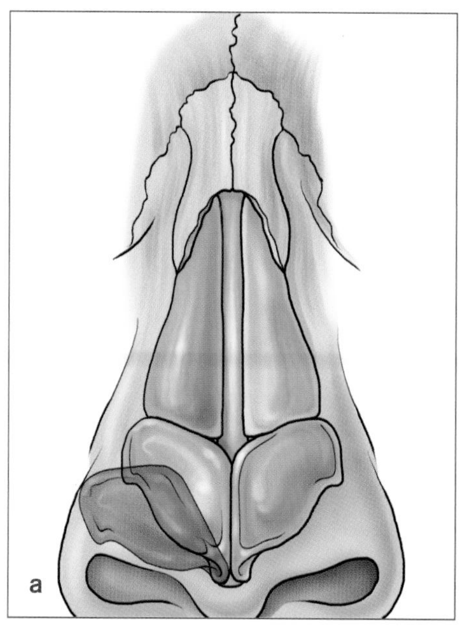

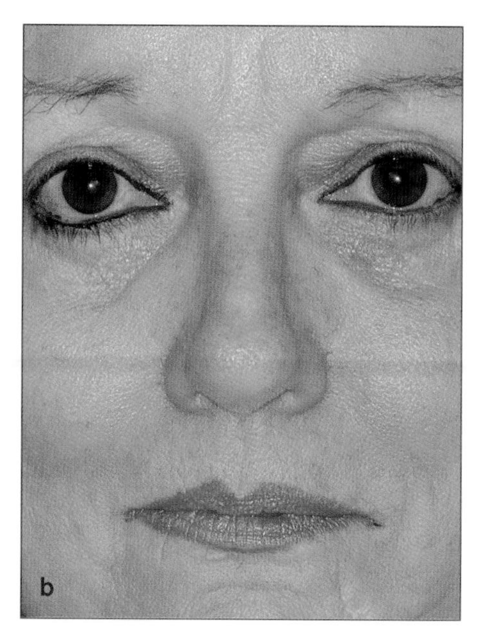

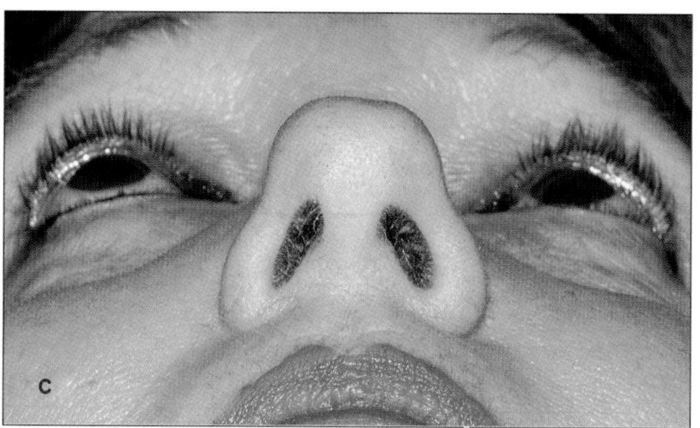

Fig 1-24 *(a to c)* Cephalic malposition of the lower lateral cartilages can cause a boxy tip and contribute to external nasal valve dysfunction. Note that the patient pictured in Figs 1-24b and 1-24c was pictured in Fig 1-9 to illustrate external nasal valve dysfunction on deep inspiration.

Structural alar grafting and tip refinement

The purpose of structural alar grafting is to enhance support to the external nasal valves and improve the esthetics of the tip region. The strength and anatomical position of the lateral crura affect the location, contour, and functional stability of the alae. Cephalically malpositioned lower lateral cartilages demonstrate this. Cephalic rotation of the lateral crura toward the nasal dorsum leaves the alae devoid of cartilage support and prone to external nasal valve collapse on deep inspiration. The overlying tip contour can take on a boxy shape or parenthesis deformity (Fig 1-24). Cephalic malposition can also cause alar retraction with resultant increased columellar show.[23,24]

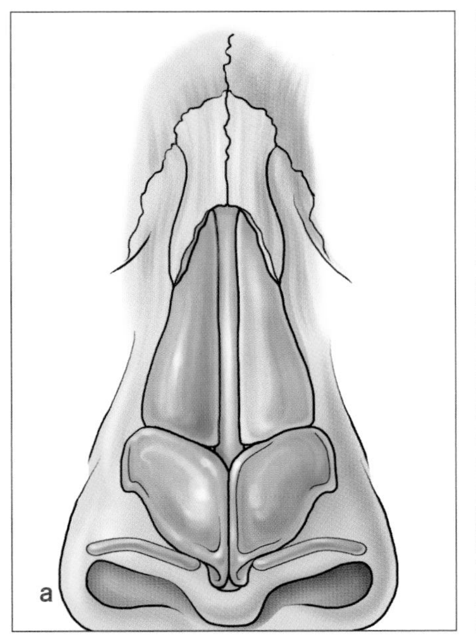

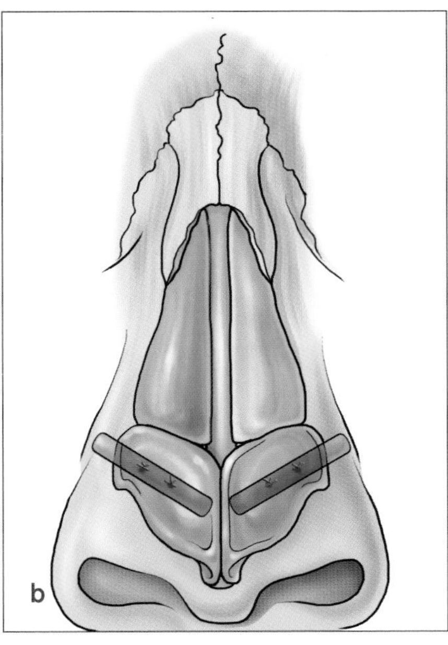

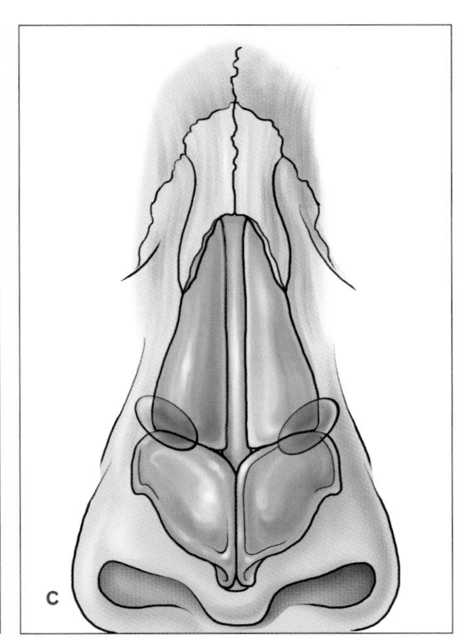

Fig 1-25 *(a)* **Alar contour grafts.** *(b)* **Lateral crura strut grafts.** *(c)* **Alar batten grafts.**

Rohrich et al[23] introduced the alar contour graft to correct alar rim cosmetic deformities and external nasal valve collapse (Fig 1-25a). Their technique involves nonanatomical insertion of an autogenous cartilage strip into an alar-vestibular pocket via an open approach. Septal cartilage is the graft material of choice, but ear cartilage can be used if septal cartilage is unavailable. The exact length and width of the graft is dependent on the amount needed to span the notched alar rim area with a straight piece of cartilage. It must fit snugly into a pocket that is carefully dissected below the infracartilaginous/marginal incision.

Gunter and Friedman[25] introduced the lateral crura strut graft to support the incompetent external nasal valve due to cephalically malpositioned lateral crura (Fig 1-25b). Lateral crura struts are useful in the correction of the boxy nasal tip, alar rim retraction, alar rim collapse, and concave lateral crura. Strips of autogenous cartilage are sutured to the deep surface of the lateral crura to reshape, reposition, or reconstruct them and strengthen the alar sidewall.

Alar batten grafts have been popularized by Toriumi et al.[26] They are rectangular cartilage grafts that are placed into a precise subcutaneous pocket at the point of maximal lateral wall collapse or supra-alar pinching (Fig 1-25c). They can be placed via a closed or open rhinoplasty approach. These grafts can be used for correction of internal or external nasal valve collapse, depending on where they are placed. The grafts span from the pyriform aperture to the junction between the middle and lateral third of the lateral crura. In most cases, the grafts measure 10 to 15 mm in length and 4 to 8 mm in width. If there is a convex surface to the grafts, it is oriented laterally to provide support for the collapsed region of the lateral nasal wall.

A bulbous or amorphous tip is typically managed with a cephalic trim of the lateral crura and/or suturing techniques of the domes to improve tip definition (Fig 1-26). When performing a cephalic trim, at least 6 mm of the lateral crura should be maintained. This makes suture manipulation easier and preserves the integrity of the

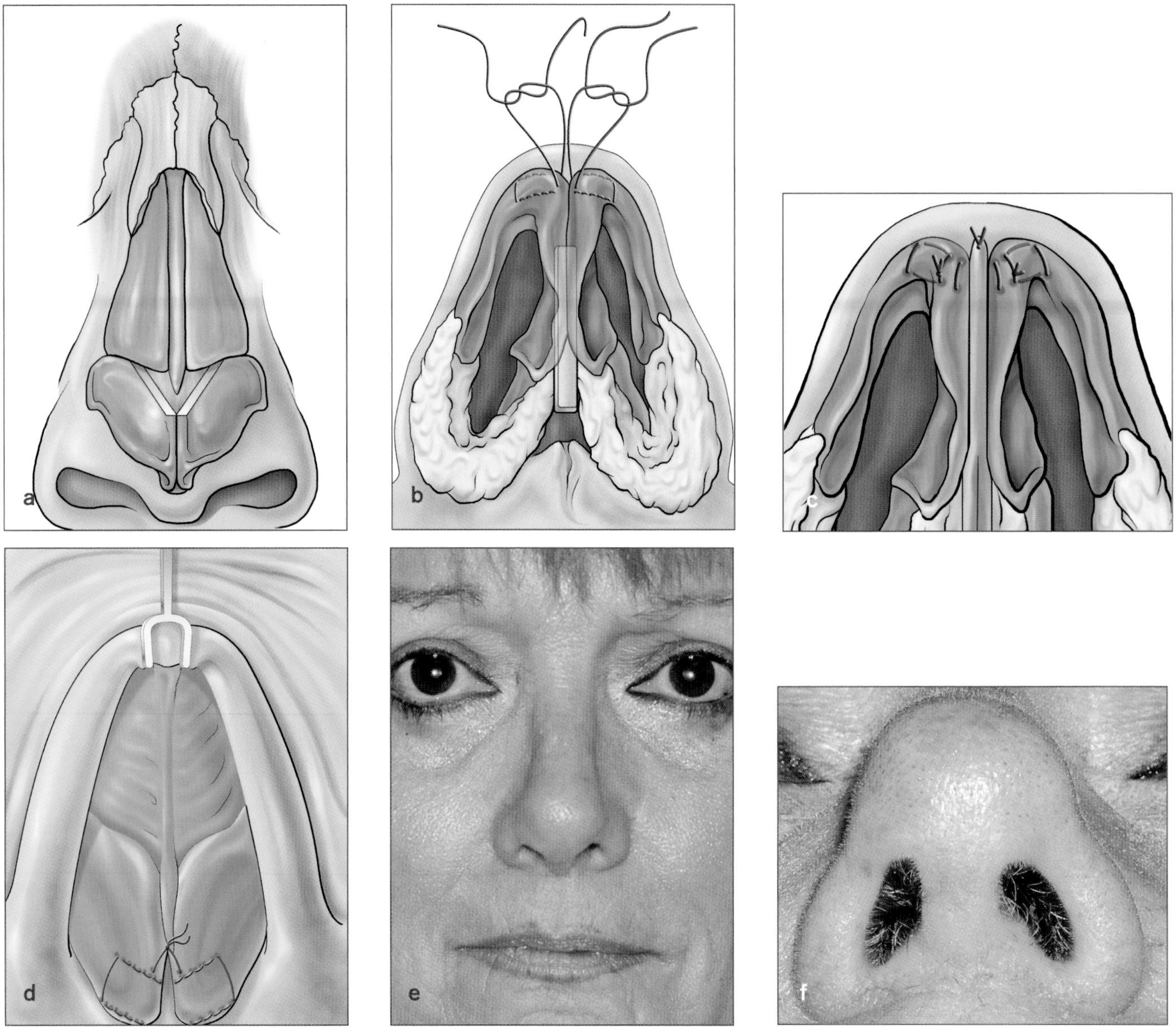

Fig 1-26 *(a to d)* **Cephalic trim and transdomal and interdomal suturing are performed to improve tip definition.** *(e and f)* **Postoperative view at the 3.5-month appointment following a cephalic trim and placement of interdomal and transdomal sutures to manage a boxy tip. The patient has also had alar batten and spreader grafts placed to manage valve dysfunction. Note that this same patient was pictured preoperatively in Figs 1-9 and 1-24.**

cartilage for structural support. Care should be taken to preserve as much of the scroll as possible laterally. Dome division is avoided because of potential negative long-term esthetic and functional sequelae. *Transdomal sutures* narrow the dome. A 5-0 PDS mattress suture is applied with the knot placed on the medial side of the dome. Care is taken not to penetrate the vestibular skin. *Interdomal sutures* reduce interdomal width, manage asymmetry between dome heights, and can unite the domes and strengthen the tip cartilages. A 5-0 PDS suture is used to approximate the middle crura at a level 3 to 4 mm posterior to the domes so that their normal separation is maintained.[27]

Complications

Complications following rhinoplasty can be numerous and have been reported in as many as 10% of cases.[28,29] Approximately 8% to 15% of patients who undergo primary rhinoplasty undertake some type of revision procedure.[29,30] Most complications arise as a result of overresecting, underresecting, or asymmetric changes[31] and include internal and external nasal valve collapse, nasal tip deformities, pollybeak deformity, saddle nose deformity, inverted V deformity, and rocker deformity. Other complications include persistent swelling, ecchymosis, and discoloration of the nasal skin.[29]

Internal nasal valve collapse occurs as a result of weakness at the junction of the caudal margin of the upper lateral cartilage and the nasal septum, which is where the internal nasal valve is located. The collapse is apparent on inspiration and results in nasal obstruction. External nasal valve collapse occurs as a result of weakness of the skeletal support of the nasal alar wall and is also evident on inspiration. It is important to maintain the support of the caudal aspect of the upper lateral cartilage at the dorsal septum and prevent overresecting the lateral crura in order to preserve valve function.[31] Treatment of internal nasal valve dysfunction is best performed with spreader grafts, which can correct a collapsed or excessively narrow internal nasal valve. Alar batten grafts can be used to treat external nasal valve collapse.

Nasal tip deformities result from underresection, overresection, or asymmetric resection of cartilage at the nasal tip. Tip imperfections can be problematic in a patient with a thin skin drape because irregularity of the underlying lower lateral cartilages is readily evident. The ptotic tip results from a loss of tip support and leads to the droopy, underprojected nose. Correction of this deformity requires reestablishment of tip support and projection.

Overresecting the caudal septum can lead to overrotation of the tip, which can lead in turn to an excessively obtuse nasolabial angle and a foreshortened nose. Correction requires nasal-lengthening procedures as well as techniques to counterrotate the tip to the desired location.

The pollybeak deformity can result from inadequate cartilaginous dorsal hump removal or loss of tip support. It presents as fullness at the supratip break and an abnormal tip-supratip junction.[31] It is important to either reestablish nasal tip support or remove additional cartilaginous dorsal hump to correct this deformity.

Overresection of the nasal septum can lead to loss of nasal dorsum support and result in a saddle nose deformity. Generally, this deformity stems from a failure to maintain an adequate amount of septal cartilage (10 to 15 mm) when reducing the dorsal hump. It can also occur secondary to septal hematoma that results in cartilage resorption.[31] Intranasal splints should be placed after septoplasty to prevent a septal hematoma. Correction of the saddle nose can be achieved with onlay grafting procedures using autogenous auricular or costochondral cartilage or an allograft such as Alloderm (LifeCell).

An open roof deformity can occur after dorsal hump removal. This can be avoided by performing adequate lateral nasal osteotomies and resuspending the upper lateral cartilages to the dorsal septum to prevent collapse of the middle nasal vault. Spreader grafts can also be used, where appropriate, to reconstruct the middle nasal vault. If the open roof deformity is not properly managed, over time the caudal edges of the nasal bones will be able to be palpated through the skin as the upper lateral cartilages collapse and a long-term inverted V deformity develops.

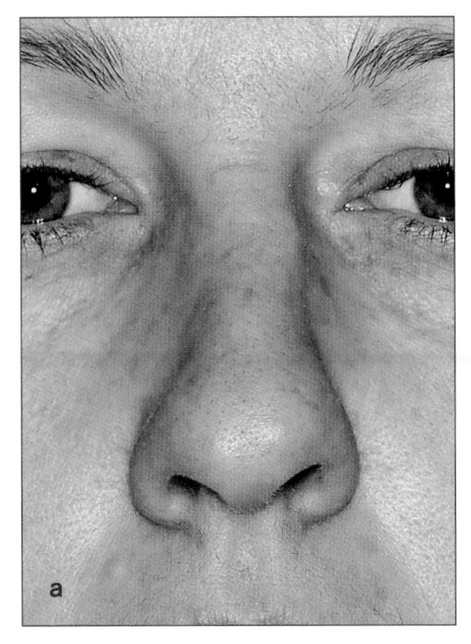

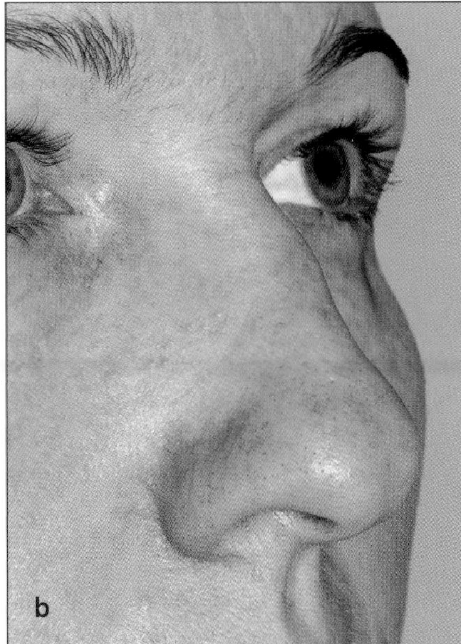

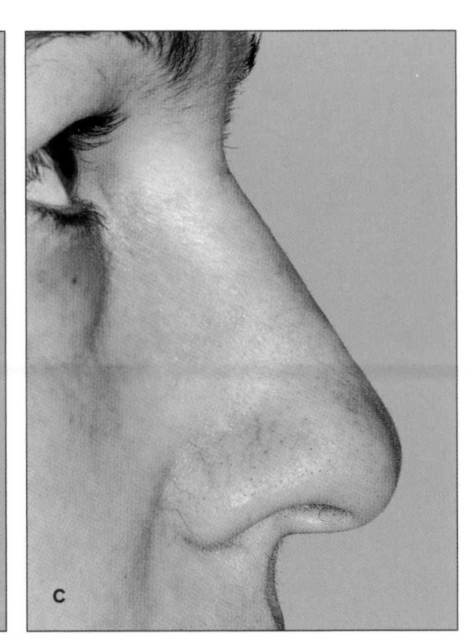

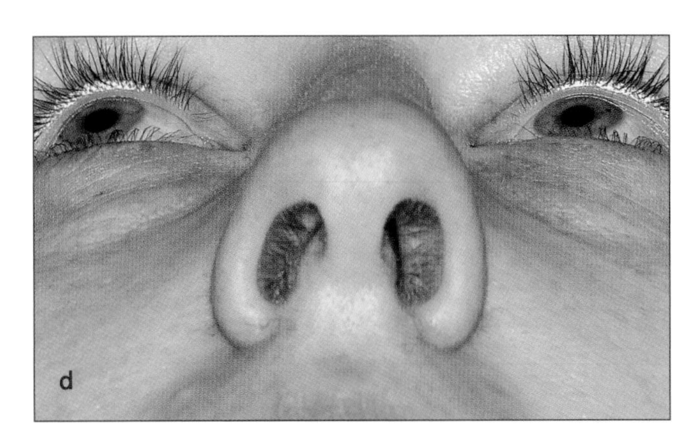

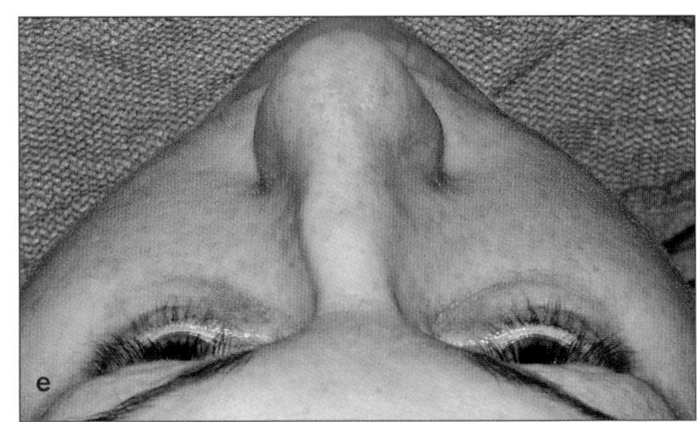

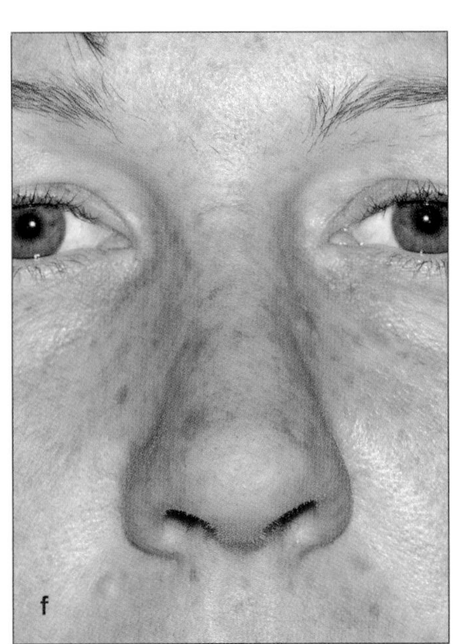

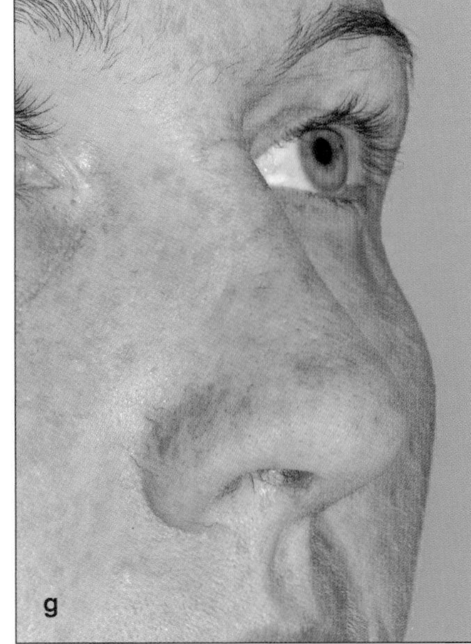

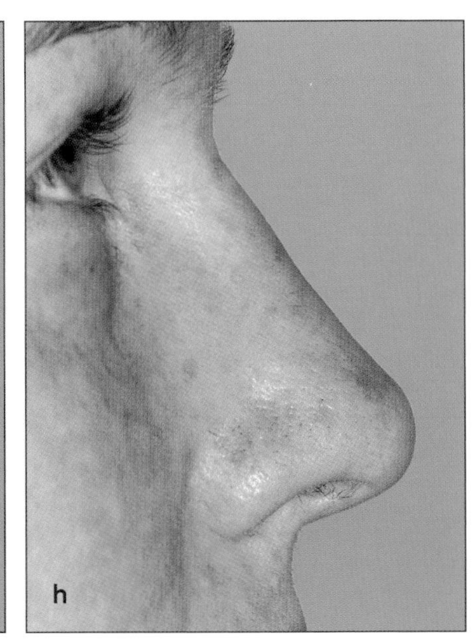

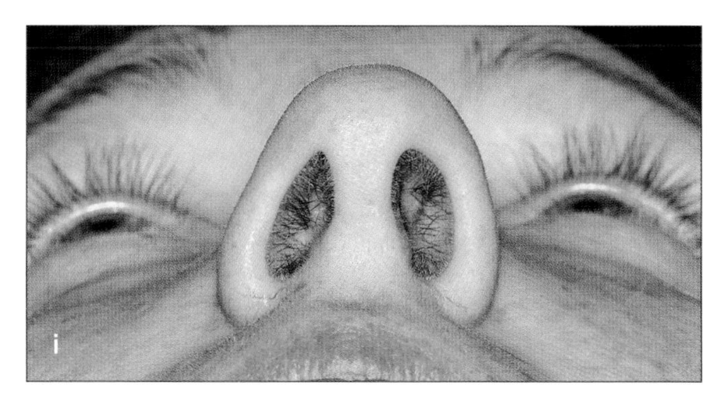

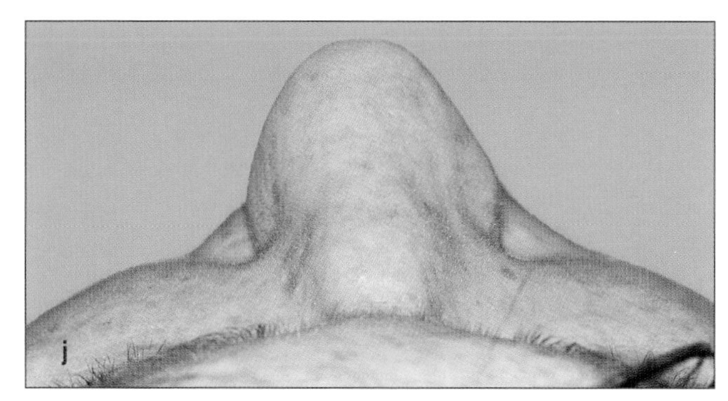

Fig 1-27 *(a to e)* **Preoperative clinical situation. The patient has a reverse C-shaped nasal deformity with disruption of her dorsal esthetic lines. She also has an overly projected nasal dorsum, tip ptosis, and dome asymmetry.** *(f to j)* **At 4 months postoperatively, there is improvement in the nasal deviation and dorsal esthetic lines. The patient has increased tip projection and a more esthetic dorsal-tip relationship. Her tip has improved definition and dome symmetry.**

Rocker deformity is a result of lateral nasal bone osteotomies being taken too high into the frontal bone. The superior portion of the osteotomy may rock laterally or project outward after infracturing the nasal bones. Correction may be achieved percutaneously with a small osteotome directed superiorly to create an improved fracture line.[31]

Case Report

This 36-year-old woman presented with a reverse C-shaped deformity (Fig 1-27a to 1-27e). Her dorsal esthetic lines were disrupted due to infracture of the right nasal bone and lateral displacement of the left nasal bone and left upper lateral cartilage at the keystone area. She had an overly projected nasal dorsum. Her nasal tip was ptotic and bulbous with asymmetry in the domes. Intranasal examination revealed a deviated nasal septum with a bone spur on the floor. She also had mucosal edema indicative of rhinitis.

The patient underwent an open rhinoplasty with a stairstep transcolumellar incision. The lower lateral cartilages were released from the upper lateral cartilages at the scroll, the upper lateral cartilages were released from the dorsal septum, and mucoperichondrial flaps were reflected to widely expose the deviated nasal septum. A component dorsal hump reduction of the cartilaginous and bony septum was performed before septoplasty. The displaced portion of left upper lateral cartilage at the keystone area was excised. A septoplasty was performed with care to leave a 1-cm L-strut. The bone spur was excised from the nasal floor. Bilateral lateral osteotomies were performed. Bilateral spreader grafts formed from septal cartilage were placed to restore dorsal septal support and straighten the septum. They were placed slightly below the dorsal septum to avoid excessively widening the middle nasal vault. One of the spreader grafts extended beyond the anterior septal angle to serve as a septal extension graft for control of tip projection. Lateral crural turnover grafts were performed—the cephalic portions of the lateral crura were undermined, partially incised, and turned into the caudal segments of the crura. This was done to improve tip definition and increase the strength of the crura.[22] The middle crura were then sutured to the septal extension (spreader) graft to increase tip projection. Additionally, interdomal sutures were placed to unite the domes and manage the asymmetry (Figs 1-27f to 1-27j).

Summary

- The deviated nose is a challenge because of complex esthetic and functional problems that typically coexist. A major septal deformity is almost always a component of a nose with significant dorsal deviation.
- It is important to understand the functional components of the airway because nasal deviation usually causes some level of airway compromise that should be addressed. If the structural integrity of the internal and/or external nasal valve framework is compromised, it must be corrected.
- Intrinsic and extrinsic forces lead to nasal deviation. These forces result in septal deviation responsible for the esthetic and functional deformity.
- Clinical analysis is important in planning surgery. Visual inspection, palpation, and anterior rhinoscopy are key components of the examination. Defining the type of septal deviation and external nasal deformity helps with treatment planning.
- Esthetic goals include straightening the bony pyramid and dorsum to improve dorsal esthetic lines and defining the tip to enhance tip esthetics. It is important to have a straight nose at the end of surgery.
- Functional goals aim to improve the nasal airway, including straightening the septum, restoring nasal valve integrity, and correcting (compensatory) inferior turbinate hypertrophy.
- A treatment algorithm is followed that has two primary components: *(1)* elimination of extrinsic and intrinsic deforming forces and *(2)* reestablishment of structural support. All structures that are malpositioned must be freely mobilized of all attachments and placed into their correct anatomical positions. Structural grafting is performed to remove residual septal deviation and reestablish skeletal support.
- Patients should never be guaranteed an absolutely straight nose. By adhering to sound treatment principles and with use of good surgical technique, improvement—though not perfection—can be predictably achieved.

Rhinoplasty Tray

- Adson-Brown forceps, two (KLS-Martin)
- Knife handle, four (Snowden-Pencer)
- Nasal speculum cottle long (KLS-Martin)
- Nasal speculum cottle short (Snowden-Pencer)
- Fomon double ball-end retractor (Snowden-Pencer)
- Gutherie double hook (Snowden-Pencer)
- Single skin hook (Snowden-Pencer)
- Dental amalgam plugger (Henry Schein)
- Killian nasal forceps (KLS-Martin)
- Hartman nasal forceps (KLS-Martin)
- Takahashi ethmoid bone forceps (KLS-Martin)
- Jansen Middleton septum forceps (KLS-Martin)
- Caplan septum scissors (KLS-Martin)
- Fomon nasal scissors (KLS-Martin)
- Metzenbaum-Nelson scissors (KLS-Martin)
- Buck suture scissors (KLS-Martin)
- Cottle nasal skin hook (KLS-Martin)
- Converse angled scissors (KLS-Martin)

- Converse angled scissors (Snowden-Pencer)
- Aufricht retractor (KLS-Martin)
- Converse nasal retractor (KLS-Martin)
- Maltz nasal rasp (KLS-Martin)
- Fomon nasal rasp (KLS-Martin)
- Cottle osteotome (KLS-Martin)
- Neivert-Anderson osteotome (KLS-Martin)
- Sheehan osteotome, 3 mm straight (KLS-Martin)
- Nasal freer, two (KLS-Martin)
- Molt no. 9 periosteal elevator, two (KLS-Martin)
- Micro-Webster needle holder, two (KLS-Martin)
- Mallet (KLS-Martin)
- Syringe (KLS-Martin)
- Frazier-tip suction (KLS-Martin)
- Obwegeser nasal saddle punch (KLS-Martin)
- Iodine cup (Biomet)
- Mayo scissors (Snowden-Pencer)
- Fomon lower lateral scissors (Snowden-Pencer)
- Webster glabella rasp (Snowden-Pencer)
- Rubin osteotome (Snowden-Pencer)
- Tebbetts dorsum osteotome (Snowden-Pencer)
- Mosquito hemostat, four (Snowden-Pencer)

References

1. Rohrich RJ, Gunter JP, Deuber MA, Adams WP. Management of the deviated nose. In: Gunter JP, Rohrich RJ, Adams WP (eds). Dallas Rhinoplasty: Nasal Surgery by the Masters, ed 2. St Louis: Quality Medical, 2007:973–998.
2. Staffel JG. The crooked nose. In: Staffel JG (ed). Basic Principles of Rhinoplasty. Alexandria, VA: Education and Research Foundation for the American Academy of Facial Plastic and Reconstructive Surgery, 1996:40–44.
3. Beeson WH. The nasal septum. Otolaryngol Clin North Am 1987;20:743–767.
4. Chand MS, Toriumi DM. Nasal physiology and management of the nasal airway. In: Gunter JP, Rohrich RJ, Adams WP (eds). Dallas Rhinoplasty: Nasal Surgery by the Masters, ed 2. St Louis: Quality Medical, 2007:643–661.
5. Bridger GP. Physiology of the nasal valve. Arch Otolaryngol 1970;92:543–553.
6. Constantian MB. The incompetent external nasal valve: Pathophysiology and treatment in primary and secondary rhinoplasty. Plast Reconstr Surg 1994;93:919–931.
7. Haight JS, Cole P. The site and function of the nasal valve. Laryngoscope 1983;93:49–55.
8. Byrd HS, Salomon J, Flood J. Correction of the crooked nose. Plast Reconstr Surg 1998;102:2148–2157.
9. Murray JA, Maran AG, MacKenzie J, Raab G. Open versus closed reduction of the fractured nose. Arch Otolaryngol 1984;110:797–802.
10. Verwoerd CD. Present day treatment of nasal fractures: Closed versus open reduction. Facial Plast Surg 1992;8:220–223.
11. Rohrich RJ, Adams WP, Gunter JP. Advanced rhinoplasty anatomy. In: Gunter JP, Rohrich RJ, Adams WP (eds). Dallas Rhinoplasty: Nasal Surgery by the Masters, ed 2. St Louis: Quality Medical, 2007:11–27.
12. Khosh MM, Jen A, Honrado C, Pearlman SJ. Nasal valve reconstruction: Experience in 53 consecutive patients. Arch Facial Plast Surg 2004;6:167–171
13. Park SS. Treatment of the internal nasal valve. Otolaryngol Clin North Am 2001;34:805–821.
14. Guyuron B. Classification of septal deviation and reconstructive technique. In: Gunter JP, Rohrich RJ, Adams WP (eds). Dallas Rhinoplasty; Nasal Surgery by the Masters, ed 2. St Louis: Quality Medical,2007:929–938.
15. Guyuron B, Uzzo CD, Scull H. A practical classification of septonasal deviation and an effective guide to septal surgery. Plast Reconstr Surg 1999;104:2202–2209.
16. Gunter JP, Rohrich RJ. Management of the deviated nose: The importance of septal reconstruction. Clin Plast Surg 1988;15:43–55.
17. Rohrich RJ. In discussion of: Guyuron B, Uzzo CD, Scull H. A practical classification of septonasal deviation and an effective guide to septal surgery. Plast Reconstr Surg 1999;104:2210–2212.
18. Rohrich RJ, Muzaffar AR, Janis JE. Component dorsal hump reduction: The importance of maintaining dorsal aesthetic lines in rhinoplasty. Plast Reconstr Surg 2004;114:1298–1308.
19. Jackson LE, Koch RJ. Controversies in the management of inferior turbinate hypertrophy: A comprehensive review. Plast Reconstr Surg 1999;103:300–312.
20. Toriumi DM. In discussion of: Constantian MB, Clardy RB. The relative importance of septal and nasal valvular surgery in correcting airway obstruction in primary and secondary rhinoplasty. Plast Reconstr Surg 1996;98:55–58.
21. Rohrich RJ, Hollier LH. Use of spreader grafts in the external approach to rhinoplasty. Clin Plast Surg 1996;23:255–262.

22. Gunter JP, Landecker A, Cochran CS. Frequently used grafts in rhinoplasty: Nomenclature and analysis. Plast Reconstr Surg 2006;118:14e–29e.
23. Rohrich RJ, Raniere J Jr, Ha RY. The alar contour graft: Correction and prevention of alar rim deformities in rhinoplasty. Plast Reconstr Surg 2002; 109:2495–2505.
24. Sheen JH. Aesthetic Rhinoplasty. St Louis: Mosby, 1978.
25. Gunter JP, Friedman RM. Lateral crura strut graft: Technique and clinical applications in rhinoplasty. Plast Reconstr Surg 1997;99:943–952.
26. Toriumi DM, Josen J, Weinberger M, Tardy ME Jr. Use of alar batten grafts for correction of nasal valve collapse. Arch Otolaryngol Head Neck Surg 1997;123:802–808.
27. Gruber RP, Bates SJ, Le FL. Advanced suture techniques in rhinoplasty. In: Gunter JP, Rohrich RJ, Adams WP (eds). Dallas Rhinoplasty: Nasal Surgery by the Masters, ed 2. St Louis: Quality Medical, 2007:411–446.
28. Weimert TA, Yoder MG. Antibiotics and nasal surgery. Laryngoscope 1980;90:667–672.
29. Greene RM, Toriumi DM. Rhinoplasty in the aging patient. In: Azizzadeh B, Murphy MR, Johnson CM Jr (eds). Master Techniques in Facial Rejuvenation. Philadelphia: Saunders, 2007:285–302.
30. Byrd HS, Hobar PC. Rhinoplasty: A practical guide for surgical planning. Plast Reconstr Surg 1993; 91:642–656.
31. Becker DG. Complications of rhinoplasty. In: Papel I (ed). Facial Plastic and Reconstructive Surgery. New York: Thieme, 2002:452–459.

2

OTOPLASTY

JOHN E. GRIFFIN, DMD
KING KIM, DMD

Techniques to repair congenitally hypoplastic, hyperplastic, malformed, or misshapen ears are described well in the literature. This chapter addresses a very effective, straightforward approach for the patient with conchal hyperplasia and/or absent or hypoplastic antihelical folds. In the authors' experience, the Davis[1] and Mustarde[2] techniques have led to excellent results with virtually no relapse. These procedures may be used independently or in conjunction with each other, depending on the patient's presentation. The surgical technique described later in this chapter addresses the patient with both conchal hyperplasia and lack of an antihelical fold.

Applied Anatomy

Normal ear anatomy can be analyzed with certain objective measurements. The long axis is approximately 20 degrees from the vertical axis of the skull. The angle of protrusion, measured as the *auriculomastoid angle*, is from 15 to 30 degrees. The width of the ear is roughly half the length.[3]

The ear consists of one sheet of elastic fibrocartilage possessing a concave anterior side with multiple elevations and depressions and a convex posterior side. Both anterior and posterior surfaces are covered with perichondrium. The skin overlying the anterior surface is thin and adheres intimately to the perichondrium. There is virtually no subcutaneous fat found anteriorly, but a subdermal vascular plexus is present. By contrast, the skin covering the posterior surface is less adherent. The posterior surface also has two layers of subcutaneous fat and a subdermal plexus of arteries, veins, and nerves.[4] In addition, the fibrocartilage of the ear attaches to itself and the external auditory meatus by means of intrinsic ligaments. The extrinsic ligaments of the ear attach the auricle itself to the side of the scalp.[3]

The outer rim of the ear consists of an important structure known as the *helix*. Anterior to the helix is the *antihelix*, which runs parallel to the helix. Between the helix and the antihelix is the *scaphoid fossa*. The antihelix continues inferiorly where it divides into the *superior* and *inferior crura*, which both surround the *triangular fossa*. The antihelix also surrounds a depression in the ear known as the *concha*. The concha is further separated into a superior cavity called the *cymba concha* and an inferior cavity called the *cavum concha*. The *tragus* is a prominent structure that lies anterior to the external auditory meatus. The *antitragus* is located posterior and inferior to the tragus. Below the antitragus lies the *lobule*, which is composed primarily of fat and areolar tissue.[1,5,6] Please refer to Fig 2-1 for key anatomical points.

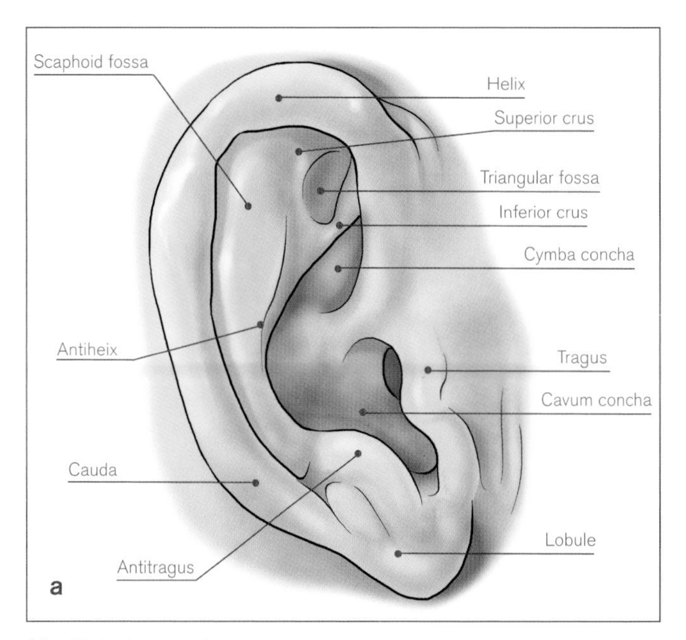

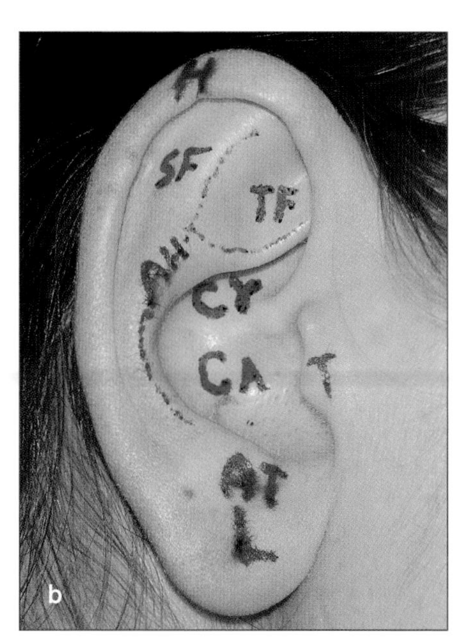

Fig 2-1 *(a and b)* **Surface anatomy of the ear. AH–antihelix; AT–antitragus; CA–cavum concha; CY–cymba concha; H–helix; L–lobule; SF–scaphoid fossa; T–tragus; TF–triangular fossa.**

The blood supply to the ear comes from two main sources (Fig 2-2): *(1)* the superficial temporal artery and *(2)* the posterior auricular artery. The superficial temporal artery exits the parotid capsule approximately 1 cm anterior to the tragus and divides into superior, middle, and inferior branches that supply the lateral and anterior ear. The posterior auricular artery parallels the posterior auricular crease and passes below the greater auricular nerve and underneath the posterior auricular muscle. Venous drainage is directed inferiorly to the external jugular vein. Lymphatic channels in three surrounding areas of the ear drain the lymphatic fluid.[4]

Sensory innervation to the ear is via anterior and posterior branches of the greater auricular nerve, the auriculotemporal nerve, and a branch of the vagus nerve. The greater auricular nerve travels over the sternocleidomastoid muscle upward approximately 8 mm posterior to the posterior auricular crease, making it susceptible to injury during otoplasty. The auriculotemporal nerve provides sensory input to the anterior surface of the ear (Fig 2-3). The nerve of Arnold is a branch of the vagus nerve that innervates the posterior aspect of the external auditory meatus.[4] The temporal branch of the facial nerve provides branches that stimulate motor innervation to the anterior and superior auricularis muscles surrounding the ear.

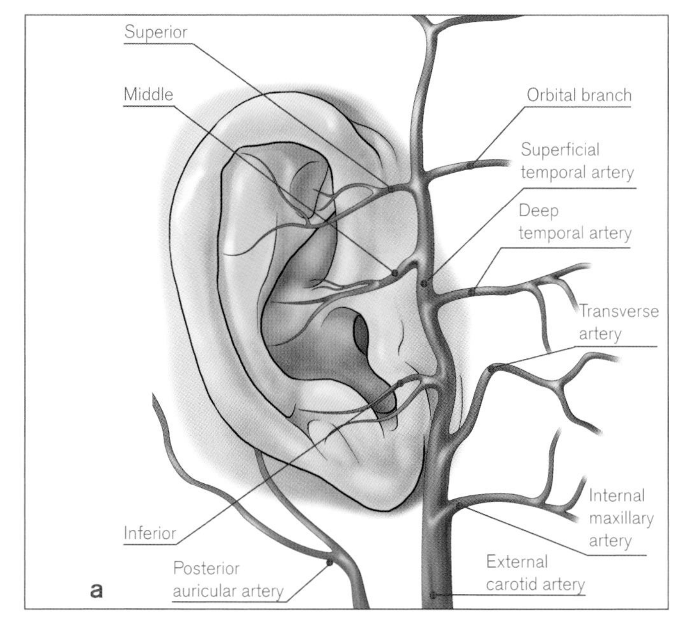

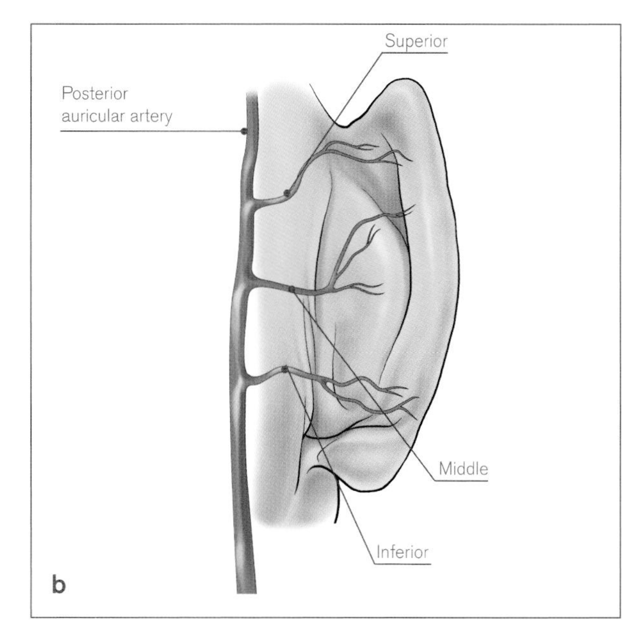

Fig 2-2 Arterial blood supply to the ear: *(a)* anterior ear and *(b)* posterior ear.

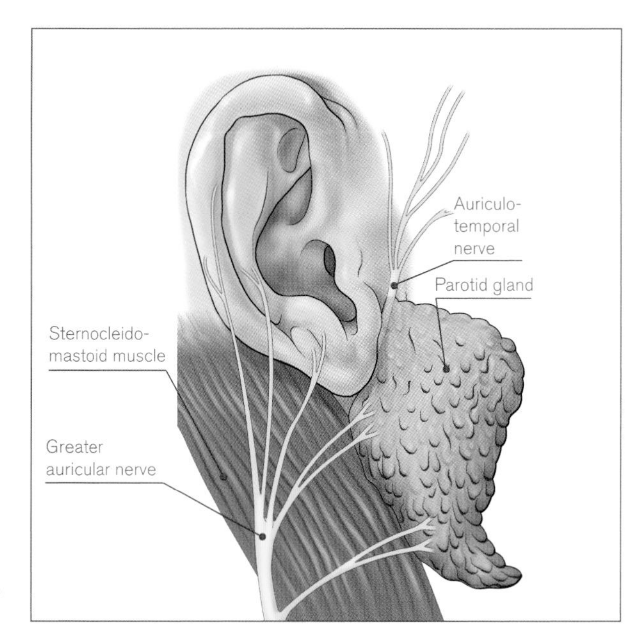

Fig 2-3 Sensory innervation to the ear.

Preoperative Evaluation

It is crucial when evaluating a patient with a chief complaint of misshapen ears that the correct diagnosis of protruding ears can be made. In many instances, the posterior conchal wall is especially hyperplastic, leading to the protrusion of the ears. In the normal ear, the development of the antihelix brings the ear closer to the scalp. In about 67% of patients with protruding ears, the presentation is lack of development of the antihelix. In about 33%, the problem is caused by overly developed conchal walls.[3] Subjectively, the practitioner can see ears that excessively extend outward from the skull base. Much of the inner aspect of the auricles, including the lack of an antihelical fold, helix, and scaphoid fossa, can be seen when looking at the patient

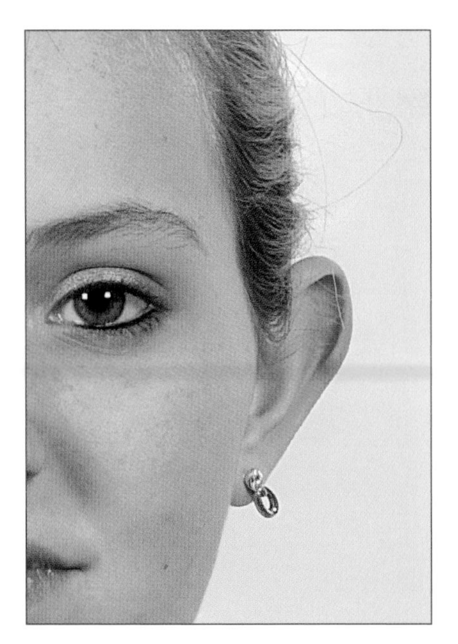

Fig 2-4a Frontal view of ear with conchal hyperplasia.

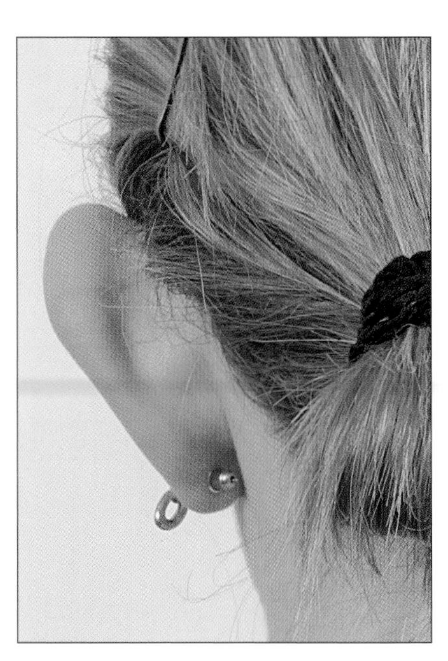

Fig 2-4b Rear view of ear with conchal hyperplasia.

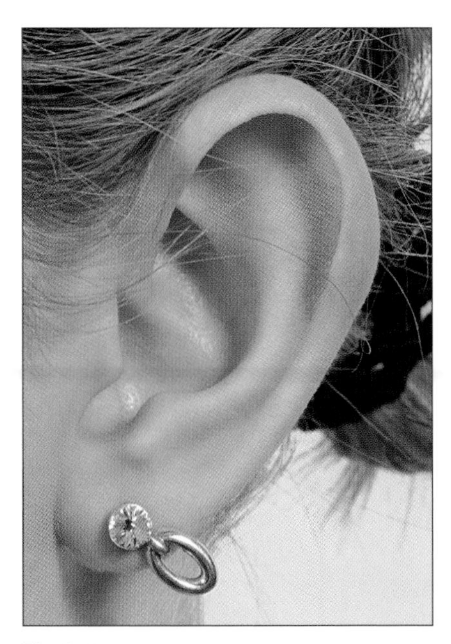

Fig 2-4c Lateral view of ear with slight appearance of antihelical fold.

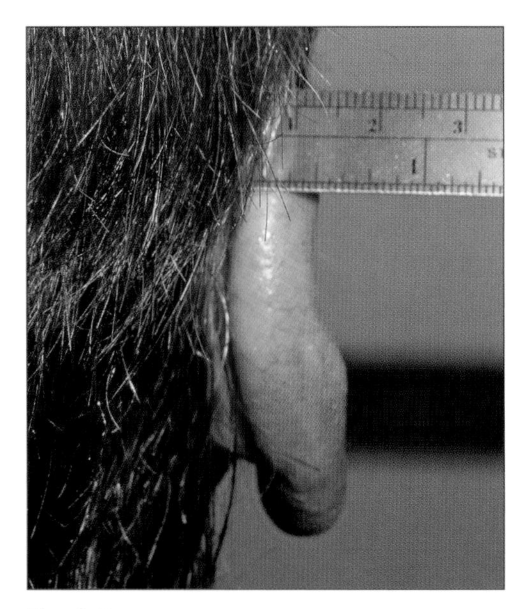

Fig 2-5a Measurement at superior auricle from outer rim of ear to skull base.

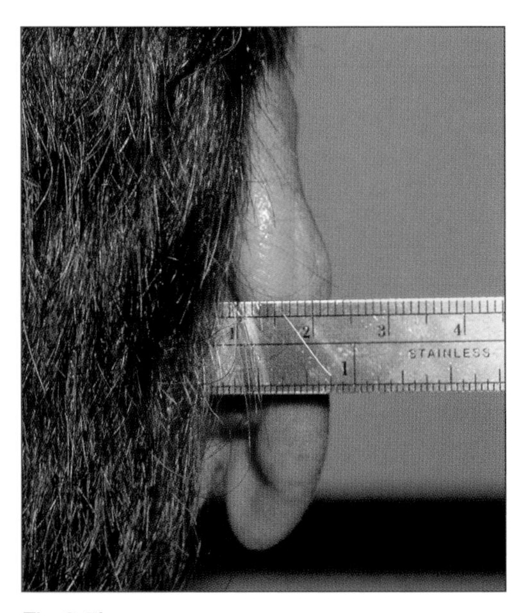

Fig 2-5b Measurement at middle auricle from outer rim of ear to skull base.

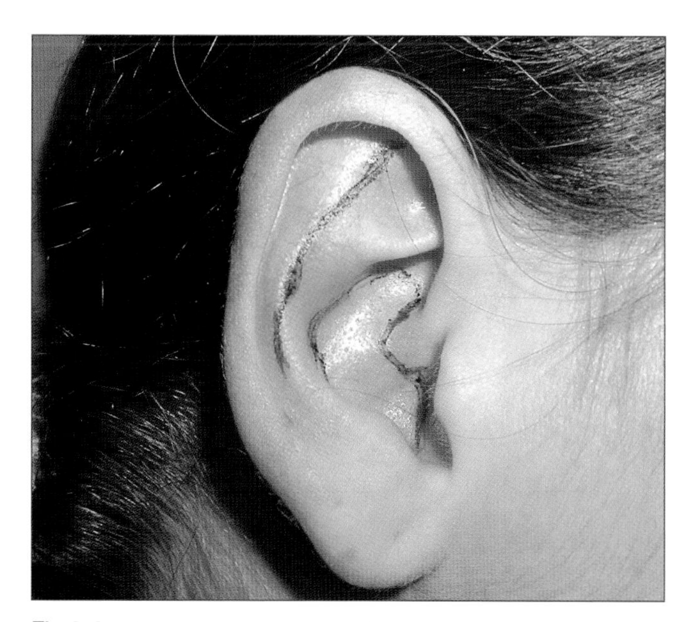

Fig 2-6a Proposed incision for conchal bowl resection and delineation for antihelical fold.

from the front (Fig 2-4a). The amount that the auricles protrude from the skull base can be seen equally well from behind (Fig 2-4b). In addition, viewing the auricle directly from the side can reveal the complete absence of or very slight appearance of an antihelical fold (Fig 2-4c). Objectively, a millimeter ruler can be used to measure the superior and middle aspects of the helical rim. The measurement at midhelix should be superior to the lobule. When taking the measurement from the skull base (mastoid area) to the outer helical rim, the superior aspect should measure 10 mm (Fig 2-5a), while the middle portion should measure 20 mm (Fig 2-5b).

It has been advocated that patients with protruding ears undergo surgery at age 4 to 6 years. The reason for this is that the ears typically are fully developed by age 8 years and 85% developed by age 3 years. Therefore, it is in the 4- to 6-year-old age range that the ears are nearly fully grown and patients are thought able to participate in postoperative care. In addition, patients in this age range are usually about to enter school, where social factors and ridicule from peers become concerns. Nevertheless, patients who have developed protruding ears can have corrective surgery at any age on into adulthood.

Surgical Procedures

Markings and incision design

After preparing and draping the patient, a kidney bean–shaped marking is drawn on the skin overlying the anterior conchal bowl (Fig 2-6a). This marking outlines the proposed conchal bowl resection, which is described by the Davis technique.[1] Also on the outer auricle is the marking to delineate the proposed antihelical fold. This is done essentially by folding the scapha against the scalp, creating an antihelical fold.[4] The crest of the fold is where the marking should be placed. The Mustarde[2] technique will be used to create this antihelical fold, which is described later.

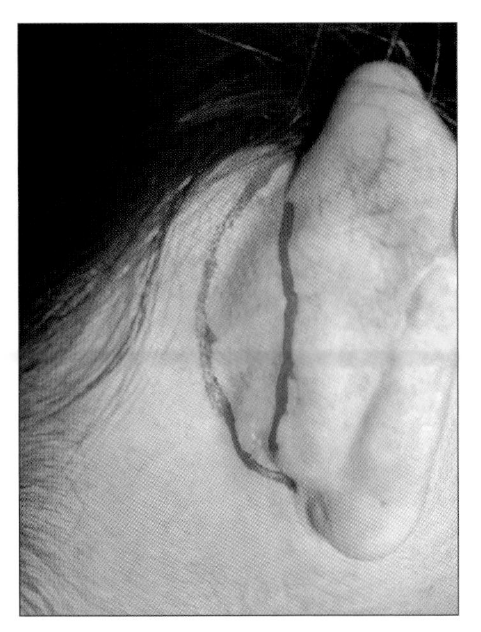

Fig 2-6b Proposed elliptical incision near the posterior auricular crease.

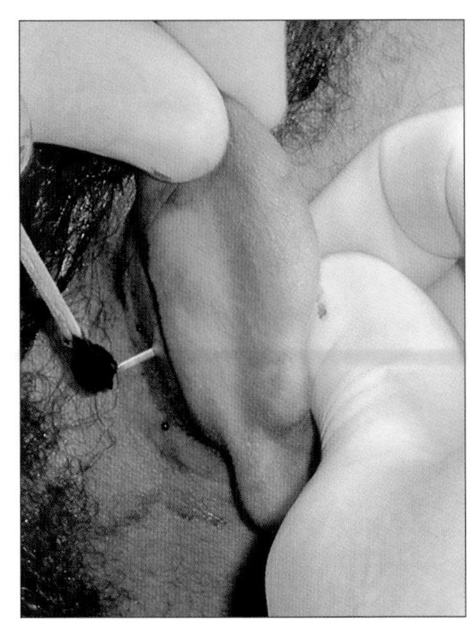

Fig 2-6c Injection of the antihelical fold with methylene blue dye.

A third marking is an incision shape that is drawn on the posterior auricular crease, where the auricle attaches to the skin overlying the mastoid region (Fig 2-6b). This proposed incision is elliptical in shape and is intended to excise excess skin and cartilage to retract the ears closer to the temporal bone. This maneuver is facilitated by the conchal bowl resection, because there will be no cartilaginous tissue to resist the pull.

Surgical technique

Prior to making the first incision, local anesthesia consisting of 2% lidocaine with epinephrine 1:100,000 solution is injected into and around the incison line. Hydrodissection with the same local anesthetic is also performed beneath the skin in the scaphoid fossa and conchal bowl to provide a plane of separation between the skin and cartilage.

Next, a 16-gauge needle is passed through from the proposed antihelical fold on the outer auricle to the posterior side of the ear. The tip of the needle is then swabbed with methylene blue, and the needle is removed along the same path through which it was initially inserted (Fig 2-6c). This maneuver is performed at points along the entire length of the proposed antihelical fold, and the number of passes with the needle is dependent upon the amount of antihelical fold desired. The same maneuver with the 16-gauge needle is also performed at the area of the proposed conchal bowl resection. If these needle passes are performed correctly, methylene

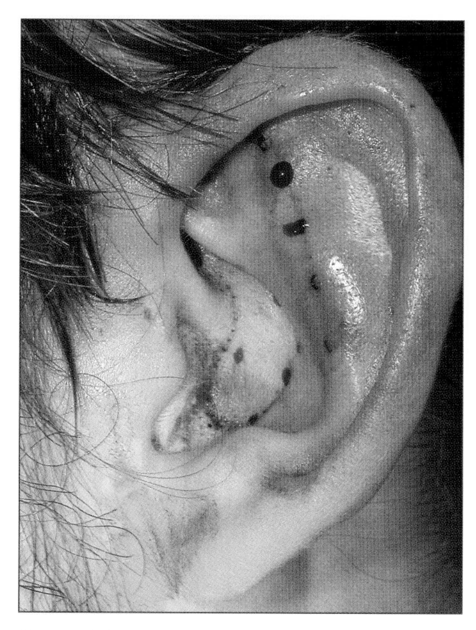

Fig 2-6d Methylene blue markings depicting conchal bowl resection and placement of the antihelical fold.

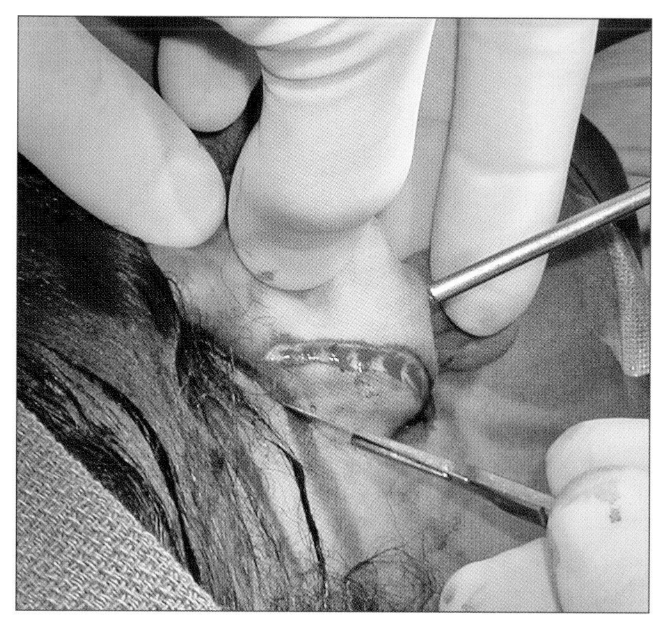

Fig 2-6e Incision through skin only behind the ear near the posterior auricular crease.

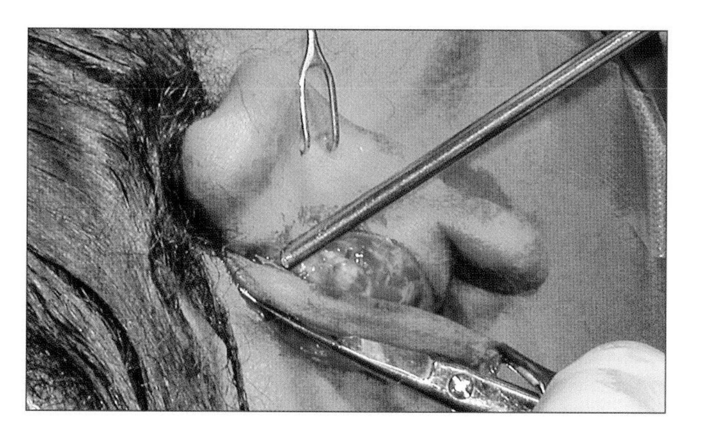

Fig 2-6f Excising the elliptical skin while pulling traction.

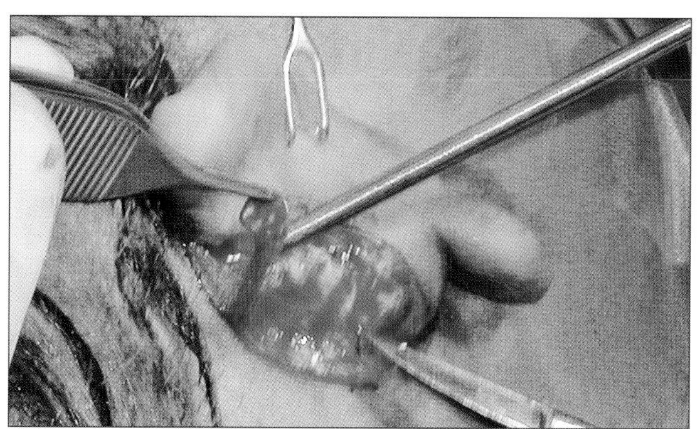

Fig 2-6g Exposure of the underlying conchal cartilage.

blue markings can be observed on the outer auricle (Fig 2-6d). It is important that the markings for the conchal bowl resection reflect a salvaging of approximately 8 mm of posterior conchal cartilage for ear support. Multiple passes with the needle and methylene blue essentially allow visualization of these structures on the posterior conchal and scaphoid cartilage, which will be shown later.

The first incision is made on the posterior aspect of the ear, which is intended to remove skin and excess tissue for adequate retraction of the ears (Fig 2-6e). This incision should be made through skin only. The excision of skin can then be performed using tonotomy scissors while applying traction to the skin (Fig 2-6f). The subcutaneous connective tissue can then be removed with scissors to completely and cleanly expose the underlying cartilage (Fig 2-6g). After adequate removal of connective tissue, the methylene blue markings can be visualized on the cartilage (Fig 2-6h). At this point, the outline that will be used to create the antihelical fold and the outline that will be used to guide the conchal bowl resection can easily be assessed. In Fig 2-6h, the markings on the left delineate the antihelical fold, and the markings on the right signify the conchal bowl resection.

It is important to realize that the incision marking created on skin overlying the anterior conchal bowl at the beginning of the procedure was only made to guide the methylene blue markings that were made on the posterior conchal cartilage. The entire conchal bowl resection is made at the posterior aspect. This is why it is important that the methylene blue markings be accurate. They essentially dictate the conchal bowl resection. In addition, it is important that the resection of the cartilage not be made too deep, because this will result in a perforation through the skin on the anterior side, leading to an unfavorable result. Similarly, the creation of the antihelical fold is guided by the methylene blue markings on the posterior auricular cartilage. These markings allow the surgeon to place the fold in the correct anatomical position, which will be seen on the outer auricle after completion.

The Mustarde[2] technique is performed first. Prior to placing sutures to create the new antihelical fold, it is important to weaken the scaphoid cartilage to facilitate the ease of cartilaginous folding. Weakening the cartilage begins by making a small incision at the base of the proposed antihelical fold. Dissection then proceeds with a Freer elevator to separate the cartilage from the skin on the anterior outer auricle. This pocket created by the Freer elevator now allows the anterior portion of the cartilage to be weakened. A nasal bone rasp can be effectively used to weaken the cartilage. Next, using the methylene blue markings on the posterior scaphoid cartilage as a guide, horizontal mattress sutures consisting of 4-0 polydioxanone suture (PDS, Ethicon) are placed equidistant on both sides of the methylene blue markings perpendicular to the antihelical fold. The sutures pass from the perichondrium on one side of the markings to the perichondrium on the other side and also pass through the cartilage (Figs 2-6i and 2-6j). Placing multiple horizontal mattress sutures in this fashion thereby folds the cartilage and skin into a nice shape resembling the antihelical fold. To assess the accuracy of the placement of the horizontal mattress sutures, the surgeon should check the outer auricle to make sure the skin and cartilage are folded to the desired extent (Fig 2-6k).

The conchal bowl resection, as described by Davis,[1] is performed next. It is started by using a scalpel to sharply dissect the cartilage only while following the methylene blue markings placed on the posterior conchal cartilage (Fig 2-6l). A Freer elevator can then be used to elevate the cartilage planned for resection and gently uncover it from the overlying perichondrium anteriorly (Fig 2-6m). In essence, the posterior and anterior conchal cartilages are resected in a subperichondrial plane, with special attention not to perforate the skin on the anterior outer ear. The entire cartilaginous conchal bowl is then removed, leaving 8 mm of cartilage on the posterior conchal wall for ear support. Once the cartilaginous resection is completed, an outline of the same kidney bean shape should be seen as previously drawn at the beginning of the case (Fig 2-6n). Any connective tissue and muscle attachments can then be removed down to the mastoid fascia to allow the ear to passively adapt against the cranial base.

Fig 2-6h Visualization of the methylene blue markings, which were placed prior to the initial incision.

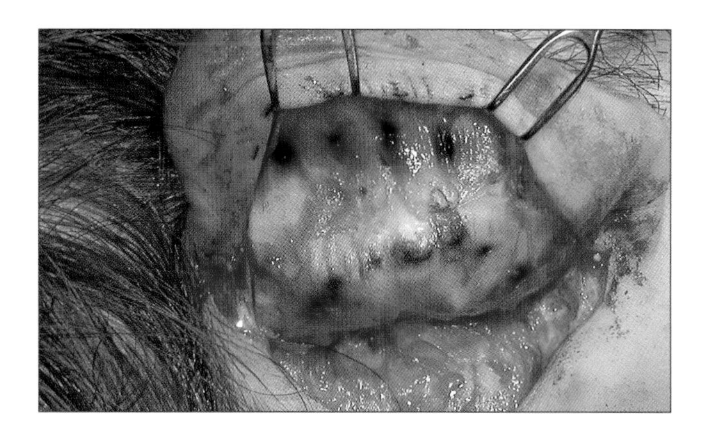

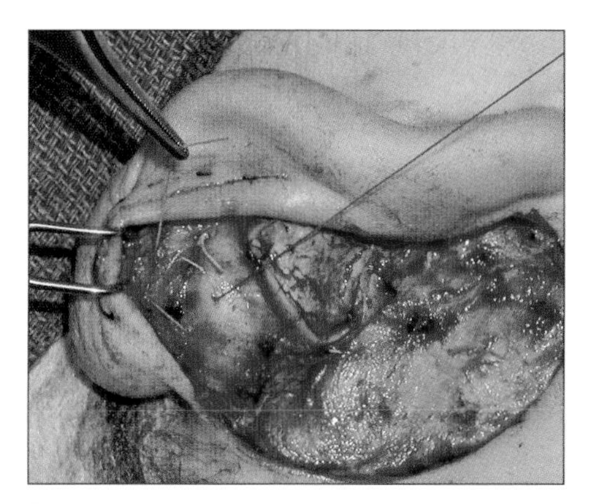

Fig 2-6i Placement of horizontal mattress sutures to create the antihelical fold. (Courtesy of Dr Todd G. Owsley, Greensboro, North Carolina.)

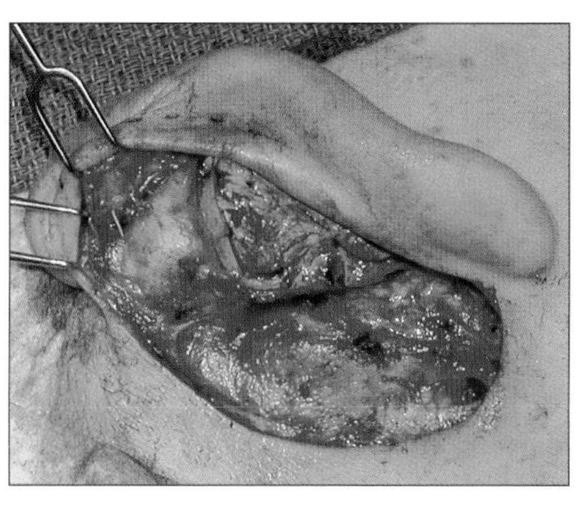

Fig 2-6j Surgical site after creation of the antihelical fold. (Courtesy of Dr Todd G. Owsley, Greensboro, North Carolina.)

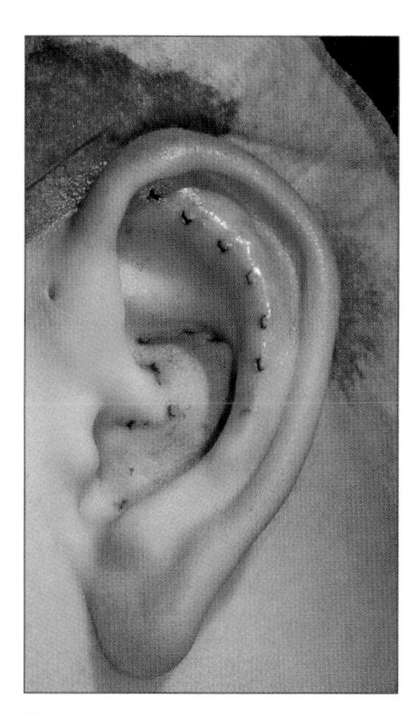

Fig 2-6k External view of ear to assess new antihelical fold. (Courtesy of Dr Todd G. Owsley, Greensboro, North Carolina.)

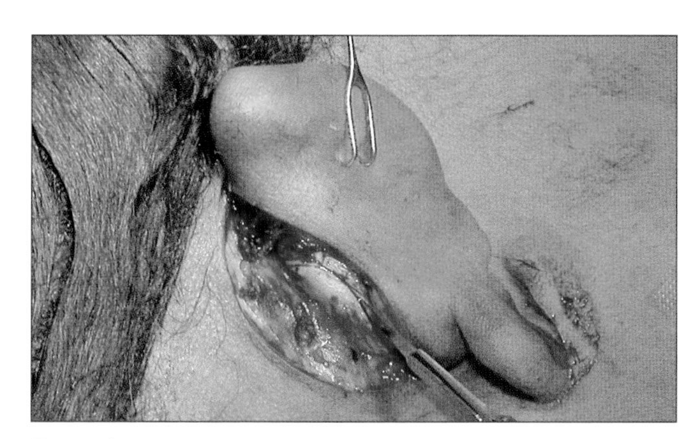

Fig 2-6l Following the methylene blue markings at the posterior conchal bowl; the cartilage resection is started with a no. 15 scalpel.

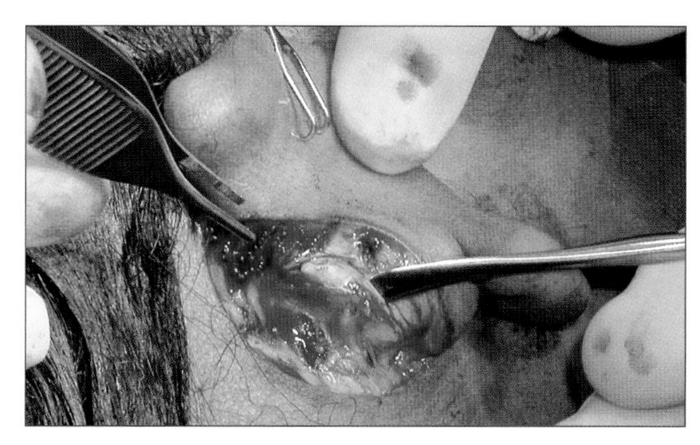

Fig 2-6m A Freer elevator can be used to create a subperichondrial pocket on both the posterior and anterior sides of the conchal cartilage.

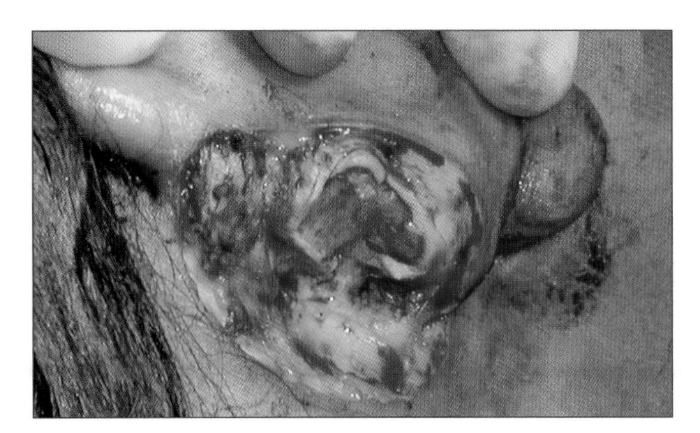

Fig 2-6n Defect created by kidney bean–shaped conchal resection.

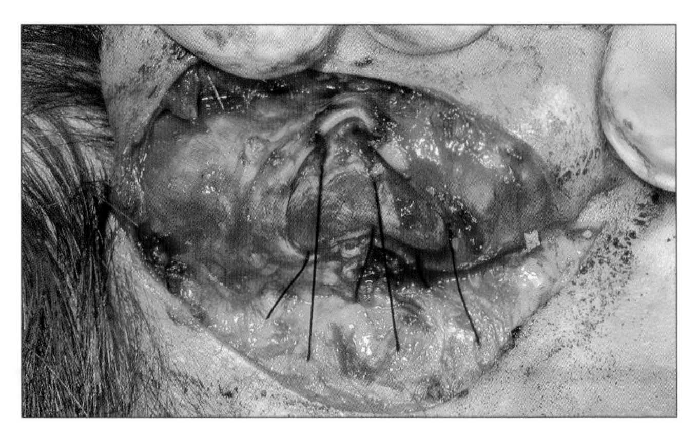

Fig 2-6o View behind the ear of three horizontal mattress sutures placed to essentially retract the protruding ear and pin it down against the cranial base. It is important to grasp a deep bite of mastoid fascia and overlying muscle to facilitate this maneuver.

Once the antihelical fold is created and the conchal bowl has been resected, the ear can be pulled back and secured to the cranial base. This is performed by placing horizontal mattress sutures consisting of 3-0 silk. The first bite of the needle is passed from the skin of the outer auricle along the outer conchal bowl markings made at the beginning of the case. Next, a deep bite consisting of posterior auricular muscle and periosteum overlying the mastoid process is grabbed with one sweep of the needle. The horizontal mattress suture is completed by exiting out the skin of the outer auricle near the first bite of the needle. After the horizontal mattress suture is placed, it is left loose and is not tied down until the bolster dressing is applied. A total of three horizontal mattress sutures are placed in the same fashion, which secure the ear to the cranial base (Fig 2-6o). The horizontal mattress sutures, which were left to hang loosely without being tied, can then be seen on the outer auricle to receive a bolster dressing (Fig 2-6p). A cotton roll is inserted between the loose ends of the mattress sutures and secured firmly to the ear (Fig 2-6q). The cotton roll should rest firmly in the cavum concha and cymba concha. This not only provides compression to reduce dead space and possible hematoma but also allows a manner in which the ear can be fastened very intimately to the cranial base.[4,6] Finally, the incision made at the posterior auricular crease is closed using 6-0 nylon suture in running continuous fashion. Special attention should be given while making a passive closure in this region, because excessive scarring can result if the wound is closed under tension.[4,6] At the conclusion of the case, a compressive head wrap is placed in the form of gauze packs and a Kerlix (Covidien) dressing around the head (Fig 2-6r).

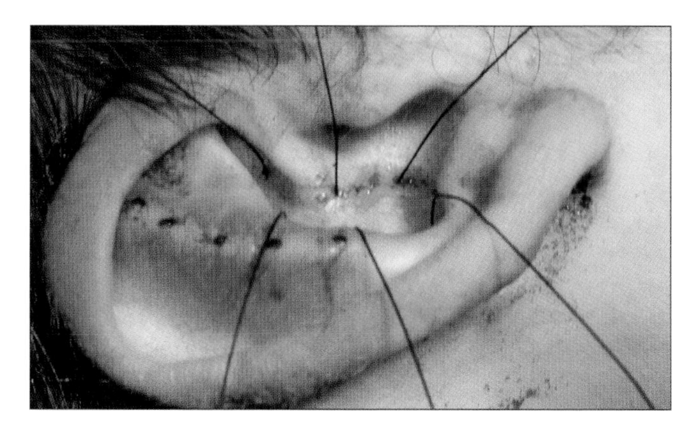

Fig 2-6p View of outer ear with three horizontal mattress sutures. Note that all three sutures are within the anterior conchal bowl.

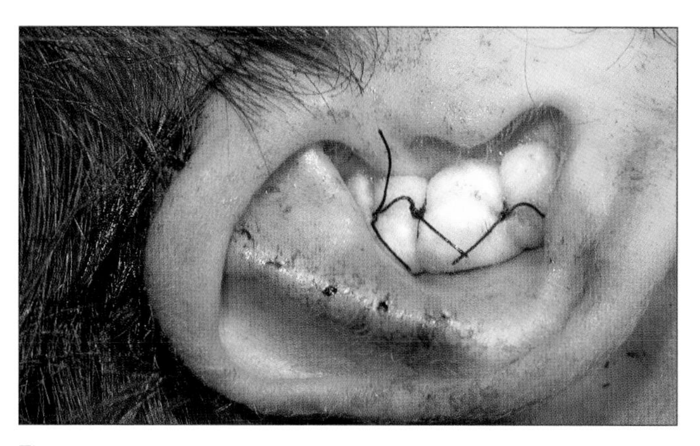

Fig 2-6q Cotton roll placed in the anterior conchal bowl and secured with the three horizontal mattress sutures. This bolster dressing applies favorable compression against the cranial base in addition to preventing hematoma formation.

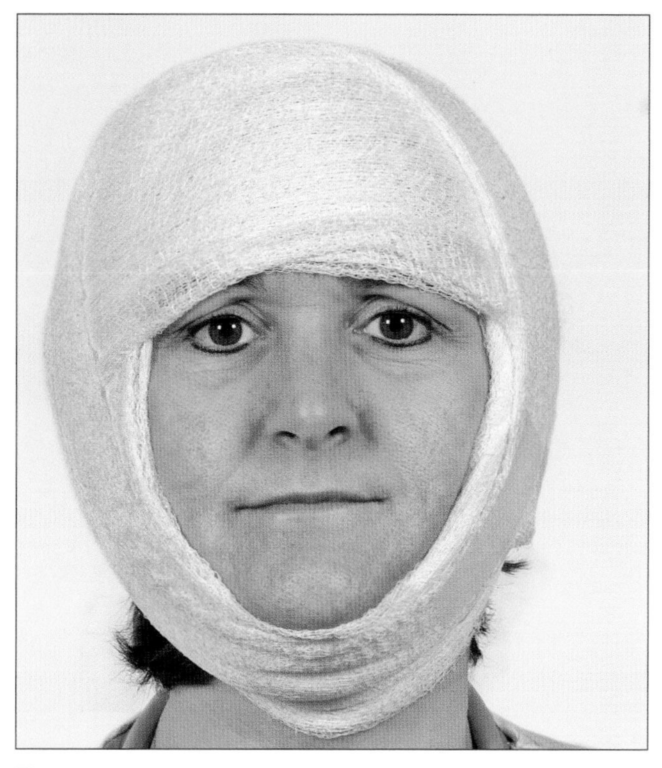

Fig 2-6r Occlusive head wrap placed immediately after surgery.

Postoperative Care

Postoperative care following otoplasty is relatively uncomplicated. The patient is given analgesics and antibiotics and is urged to keep the compressive head wrap on for 2 to 3 days. After removing the head wrap, the patient is instructed to wear a head wrap at nighttime only, prior to sleeping, for an additional 2 weeks. The bolster dressings are removed after 2.5 weeks. Wound care instructions are given to keep the incision clean and prevent infection.

Complications

Early complications after otoplasty can be avoided with sound surgical technique and implementing close follow-up the first week after the procedure. In the early postoperative phase, infection and hematoma are the two most common complications. If hematoma is not managed, pressure necrosis of the auricular cartilage will occur. If infection is not properly controlled, perichondritis may occur. Both may lead to a deformed auricular cartilage and an unesthetic result.

Hematoma can be avoided by using bipolar electrocautery to prevent necrosis of the cartilage; confirming hemostasis; placing a small penrose drain, if deemed necessary; and placing an adequate pressure dressing. Hematoma can be seen by clinical inspection or assumed if the patient complains of unusual pain and discomfort on the affected ear. If a hematoma exists, treatment involves reopening the wound, controlling bleeding, irrigating, and placing another dressing over the ear.

Infection is most common on postoperative day 3 and 4.[7] Erythema with accompanying purulence indicates the need to debride and drain the infection. Systemic antibiotics, which provide coverage for *Pseudomonas aeruginosa* (ciprofloxacin), should be implemented immediately.[4,7] Multiple conservative debridements often are necessary to resolve an infection after otoplasty. Without thorough treatment of infection, cartilage necrosis, perichondritis, or chondritis may occur and may compromise esthetic results.[7]

Late complications following otoplasty include keloid formation, neurosensory deficits, unesthetic ears, and recurrence of ear deformity.[4] Keloid formation can occur if the skin is closed under excess tension. Therefore, it is important to undermine where appropriate in the postauricular area prior to closure. If keloids do develop, treatment options include injections of triamcinolone acetonide 40 mg/mL every 2 to 3 weeks, conservative excision with the carbon dioxide (CO_2) laser, and low-dose radiation therapy.

Summary

The otoplasty procedure as described above is a straightforward cosmetic procedure that can very effectively treat conchal hyperplasia (Figs 2-7 and 2-8). The authors' experience with the technique has led to favorable outcomes, and with practice, it can be added to the oral and maxillofacial surgeon's armamentarium.

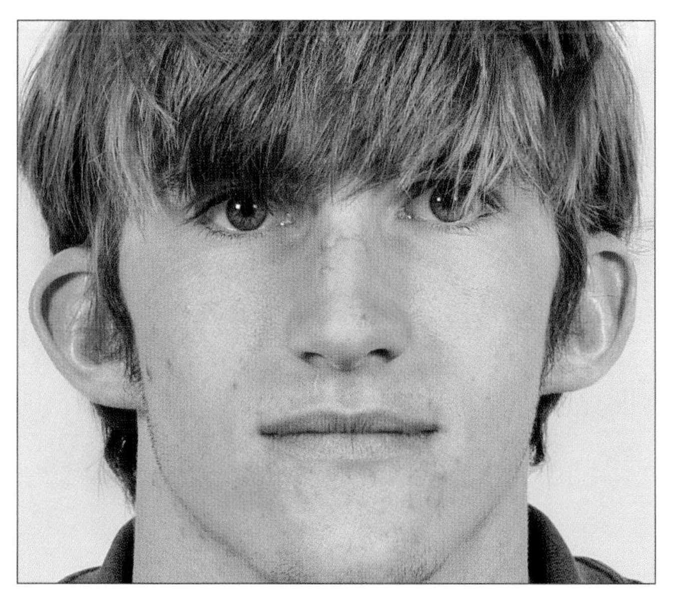

Fig 2-7a Preoperative frontal view of a patient with conchal hyperplasia and hypoplastic antihelical folds.

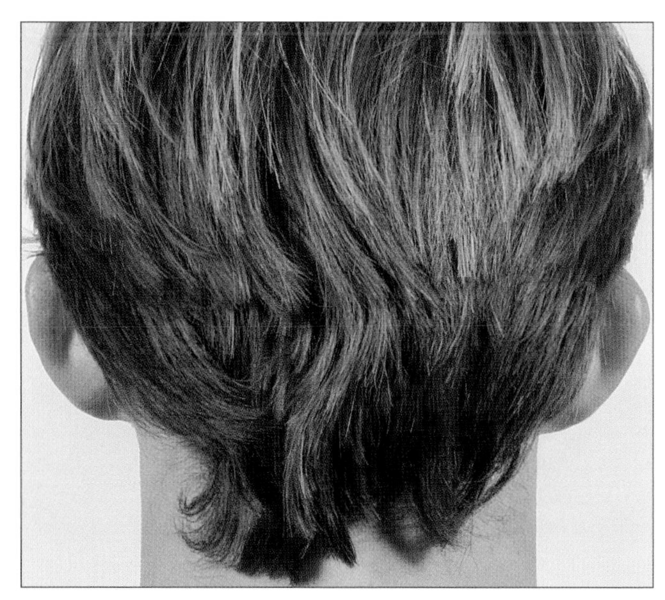

Fig 2-7b Preoperative rear view of the same patient.

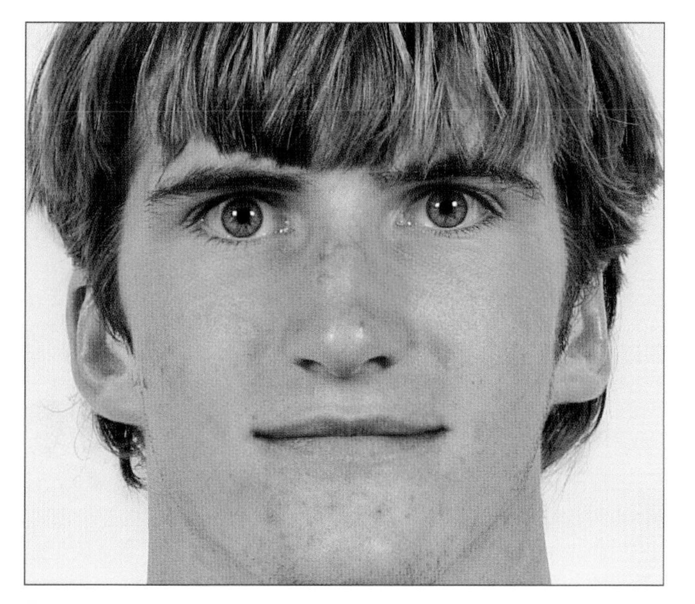

Fig 2-7c Postoperative frontal view.

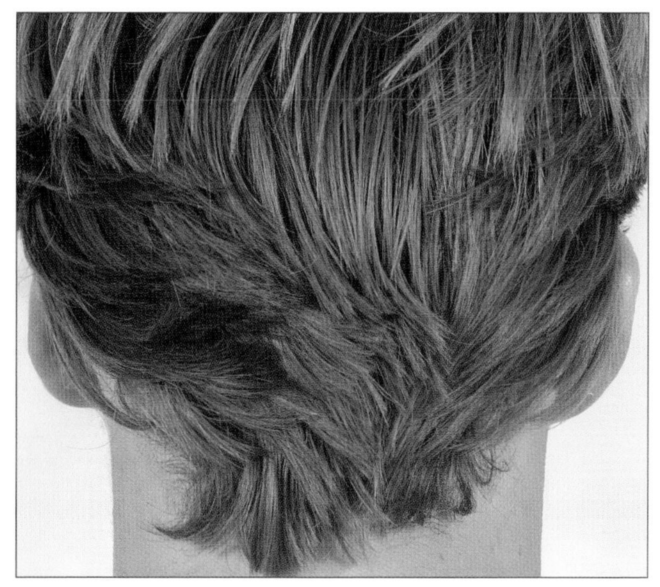

Fig 2-7d Postoperative rear view.

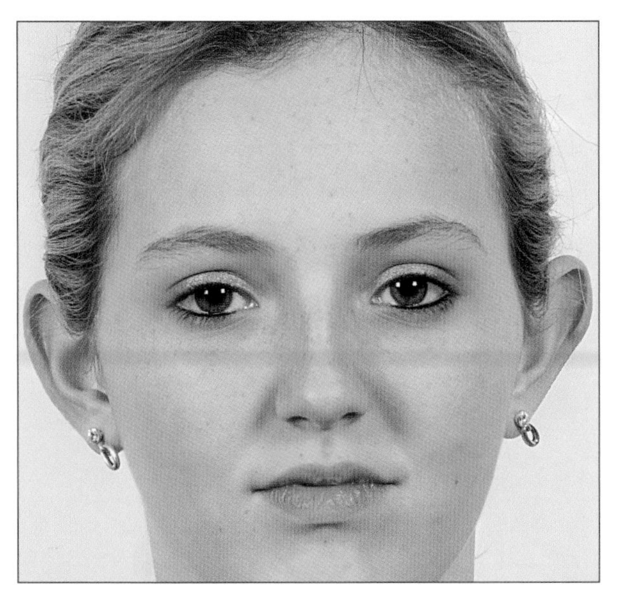

Fig 2-8a Preoperative frontal view of a patient with conchal hyperplasia and hypoplastic antihelical folds.

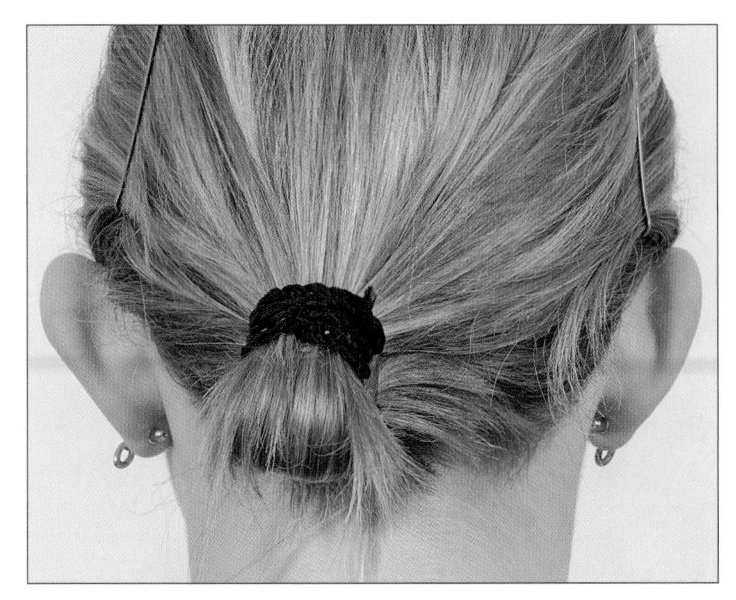

Fig 2-8b Preoperative rear view of the same patient.

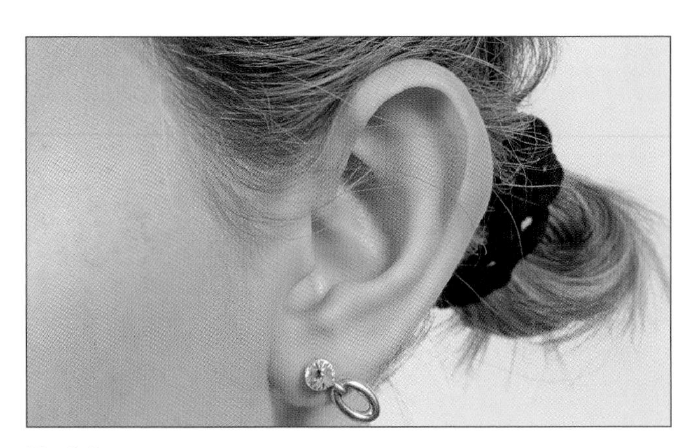

Fig 2-8c Preoperative left lateral view.

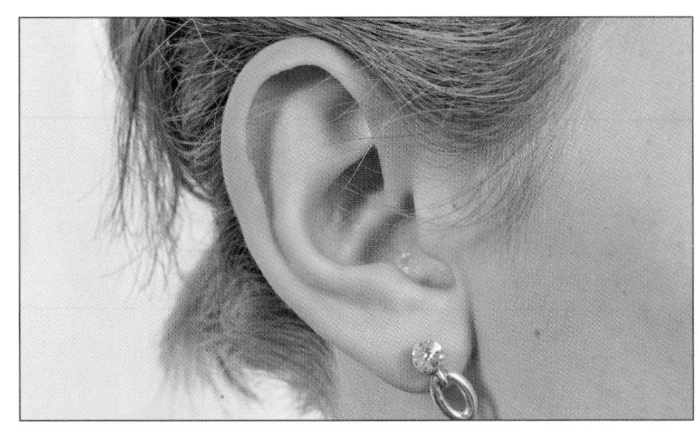

Fig 2-8d Preoperative right lateral view.

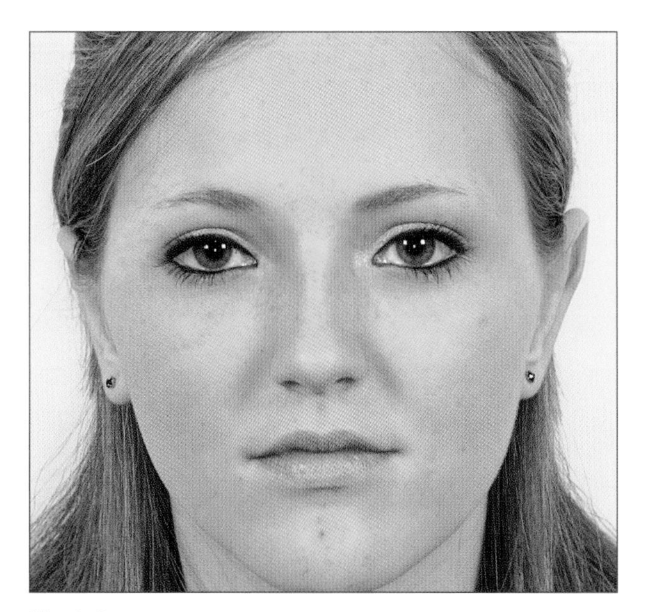

Fig 2-8e Postoperative frontal.

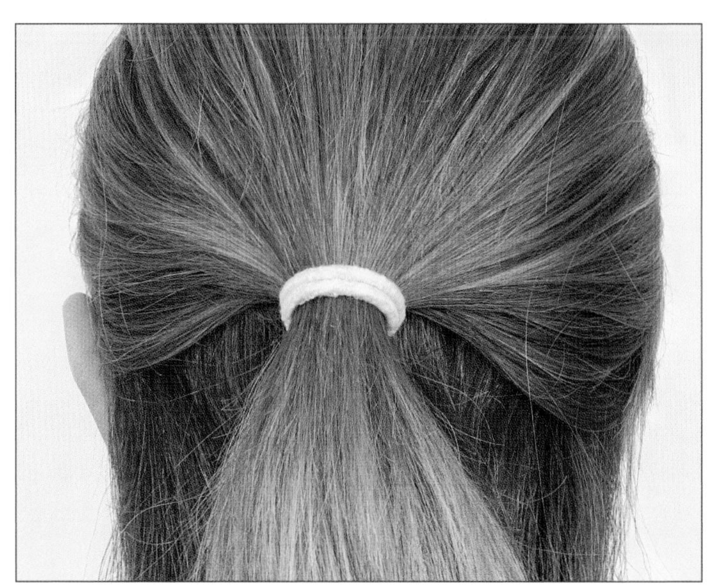

Fig 2-8f Postoperative rear view.

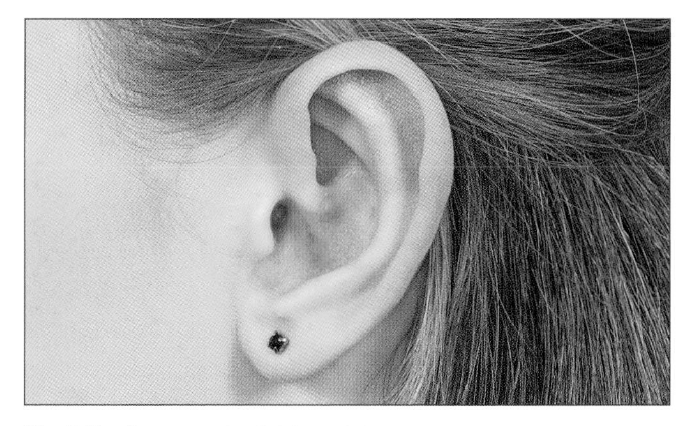

Fig 2-8g Postoperative left lateral view.

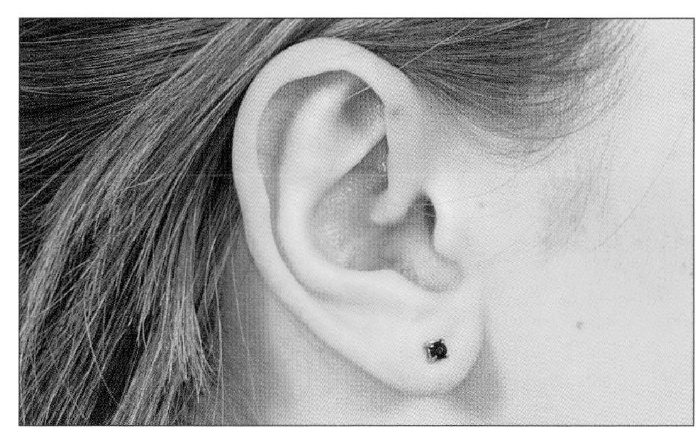

Fig 2-8h Postoperative right lateral view.

Otoplasty Tray

- Scalpel handle, two (KLS-Martin)
- Woodson elevator, two (KLS-Martin)
- Webster needle holder (Snowden-Pencer)
- Mayo scissors (Snowden-Pencer)
- Aspirating syringe (KLS-Martin)
- Freer skin hook (KLS-Martin)
- Joseph skin hook (KLS-Martin)
- Freer elevator (KLS-Martin)
- Adson-Brown forceps (KLS-Martin)
- Frazier-tip suction (KLS-Martin
- Iodine bowl (Biomet)
- Senn retractor, two (Biomet)
- Towel forceps, four (Biomet)
- Mosquito hemostat, four (Snowden-Pencer)

References

1. Davis JE. Aesthetics and Reconstructive Otoplasty. New York: Springer-Verlag, 1987.
2. Mustarde JC. The correction of prominent ears using simple mattress sutures. Br J Plast Surg 1963;16:170–178.
3. Becker DG, Lai SS, Wise JB, Steiger JD. Analysis in otoplasty. Facial Plast Surg Clin North Am 2006;14:63–71.
4. Owsley TG. Otoplastic surgery for the protruding ear. Atlas Oral Maxillofac Surg Clin North Am 2004;12:131–139.
5. Kotler HS, Tardy ME. Reconstruction of the outstanding ear (otoplasty). In: Ballenger JJ, Snow JB (eds). Otorhinolaryngology: Head and Neck Surgery, ed 15. Baltimore: Lippincott Williams & Wilkins, 1996:989–1002.
6. Limandjaja GC, Breugem CC, Mink van der Molen AB, Kon M. Complications of otoplasty: A literature review. J Plast Reconstr Aesthet Surg 2009;62:19–27.
7. Nachlas N. Otoplasty. In: Papel I (ed). Facial Plastic and Reconstructive Surgery. New York: Thieme, 2002:315–321.

3

Forehead and Brow Lifting

DOUGLAS L. JOHNSON, DMD

The orbital and forehead complex is recognized as one of the most important and expressive units of the face.[1–4] The facial cosmetic surgeon must be able to recognize the characteristic patterns of facial aging and be comfortably familiar with all rejuvenation procedures. When properly applied to the forehead-brow complex, even minor surgical procedures can produce a dramatic improvement of facial esthetics.[5] This chapter discusses both forehead and brow lifting rejuvenation procedures. Forehead and brow anatomy are reviewed, as are appropriate patient selection and treatment. Multiple nonsurgical and surgical procedures are discussed to help guide the surgeon through the treatment planning process, meet patients' expectations, and minimize complications.

Pathophysiology of Eyebrow Ptosis

As aging occurs, there is a loss of skin elasticity, reduction of subcutaneous tissue bulk, and increased skull bone resorption.[6,7] Gradual descent of the eyebrow results from the stretching of the soft tissue of the scalp and forehead attributed to gravitational forces, tissue maturation, and the effects of sun exposure. This descent is compounded by the action of the depressors of the eyelids and brow. The descent of the brow is not always uniform. The lateral brow almost always descends earlier and to a greater extent than the medial brow,[7] which leads to upper eyelid pseudodermatochalasis or contributes to dermatochalasis. An analogy of a curtain rod (the brow) with a suspended curtain (the skin of the upper lid) can be used: As the curtain rod lowers, an accumulation of curtain (skin) becomes visible. The resting tone of the frontalis can maintain a chronic contracture state and raise the brow to a false position in an attempt to correct this condition.[5] Chronic contracture usually can be diagnosed by horizontal forehead rhytids. Over time, the vertical distance between the brow and hairline increases, resulting in an elongated appearance of the upper facial third. In addition, the distance between the brow and the eye decreases. Many factors play a role in the ideal forehead and brow position: sex, age, skin quality, hair quality/quantity and pattern, forehead height, eyebrow position and shape, corrugator and procerus muscle balance, motor function, and underlying bony architecture.

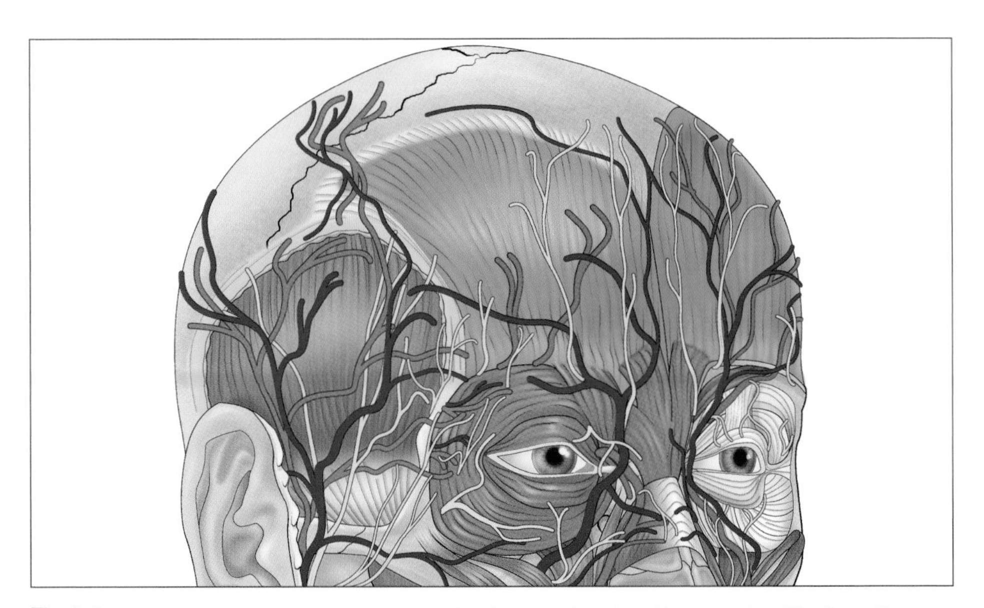

Fig 3-1 Musculature and neurovascular supply of the forehead and brow region. The frontalis muscle *(green)* is the major brow elevator. The brow depressors *(red)* are the midline procerus, orbicularis oculi, and deeper corrugator muscles. Note the line of temporal fusion and orbital ligament *(yellow)*.

Applied Anatomy

Layers of the scalp

It is important to review general anatomy, starting superficially at the skin level and proceeding to the skull base. The mnemonic *SCALP* often is used to generally describe the layers of the scalp: *skin, connective tissue, aponeurosis, loose areolar connective tissue, and periosteum.* The skin on the forehead varies in thickness and quantity of sebaceous glands, depending on age, ethnicity, sex, and intrinsic and extrinsic factors. Subcutaneous fat may be thin and adhere closely to the galea aponeurosis. The aponeurosis covers the frontal-occipital muscular complex and is continuous with the superficial musculoaponeurotic system (SMAS).[8] The three layers of the skin, connective tissue, and aponeurosis tend to move together and allow the skin to glide over the loose tissue plane above the periosteum.

Musculature

The *frontalis*, the "muscle of attention,"[9] and the *corrugator*, the "muscle of pain,"[8] are the elevator muscles of the brow and forehead (Fig 3-1). The frontalis muscle attaches anteriorly to the orbicularis and to the procerus muscles and thus has no direct bony attachment. The frontalis muscle raises the forehead tissue, gives a surprised or scared appearance, and over time, contributes to forehead horizontal rhytids. Laterally, the frontalis muscles may weaken with increasing age, and as they descend, they may contribute to brow ptosis and upper eyelid dermatochalasis, or hooding.[7,10] The lateral extent fuses into the zone of adhesion along the superior temporal line, and its inferior termination point, the orbital ligament, is near the zygomaticofrontal suture.

At the level of the inferior forehead and orbit, the depressor muscles of the forehead are present. The *depressor muscles* are the paired corrugators, the depressor supercilii, the orbicularis oculi, and the midline procerus. The *corrugator supercilii*, the muscle of pain[9] that lies beneath the frontalis and orbicularis muscles, pulls the brows inferiorly and medially, leading to an angry, tired, stern appearance with vertical glabellar rhytid formation. The *procerus*, the "muscle of aggression"[9] that originates on the inferior portion of the nasal bones and inserts in the region between the eyebrows, depresses the central tissue, adding to an angry, stern appearance and giving rise to horizontal rhytids (bunny lines) across the nasal radix.

The *orbicularis oculi*, the "muscle of reflection,"[9] depresses the eyebrow inferiorly. Over time, the fascia may contract and cause permanent skin rhytids even when the muscles are in repose.[1] In the lateral brow, lying superior to the orbicularis, is the orbital fat pad, which can be prominent in some individuals and may atrophy over time. The *periosteum* is confluent laterally with the temporalis fascia directly over the temporalis muscle. At the orbital margin, it is termed the *arcus marginalis*. The periosteum is one of the limiting factors in elevating the brow.

Bony landmarks

The skull in this area is primarily the frontal bone and laterally the parietal bones; inferiorly, the nasal and zygomatic bones are encountered. Important bony landmarks that help guide the extent of dissection are the orbital rim, the nasofrontal suture, the zygomaticofrontal sutures, and the coronal sutures. The thickness of the skull is variable, but in the frontal bone, lateral to the midline venous sinus, the thickness is usually adequate for bony fixation techniques.

Innervation

The major motor nerve is the temporal branch of the facial nerve. This nerve provides motor innervation for the frontalis, corrugator, procerus, and superior orbicularis oculi muscles. The course of this nerve travels through the danger zone of Webster,[4] or the "red zone" as described by Liebman et al.[11] Pitanguy showed that the nerve consistently courses along a line projected from a point 0.5 cm below the tragus to a point 1.5 cm above the lateral aspect of the eyebrow.[7] As the nerve passes from within the parotid gland, the frontal branch lies between the outer layer of the deep temporal fascia and on the deep side of the temporoparietal fascia, which is an extension of the SMAS. The frontal branch proceeds and enters the orbicularis from beneath. Within a 2-cm wide area superolateral to the brow, the surgeon must stay deep to or superficial to the SMAS to avoid potential injury to the frontal branch of the facial nerve.[11]

The *supratrochlear* and *supraorbital* nerves are terminal branches of the ophthalmic division of the trigeminal nerve and are the major sensory nerves to the forehead. The supratrochlear nerve exits the orbit and passes through the corrugator supercilii muscle.[5] The supraorbital nerve exits the orbit by way of a foramen or, more commonly, a notch.[12] It supplies sensation to the greater part of the forehead and scalp. The supraorbital nerve usually has two branches. After exiting the orbit, it divides into a lateral (deep) and a medial (superficial) branch.[5] The deep division may exit its own foramen in 10% of cases and be above the orbital rim by as much as 1.0 cm.[13] Damage to the more consistent deeper branch, which is located more laterally, results in the greatest sequelae.[12] The superficial division of the surpraorbital nerve and the supratrochlear nerve run on top of the frontalis muscle.[5] The deep portion of the supraorbital nerve is under the deep galeal plane.[5] The supratrochlear nerve exits 1.7 cm from the midline and lies 0.8 cm anterior to the supraorbital nerve, which exits 2.7 cm from the midline.[8,14] Cuzalina and Holmes[12] also studied the location of the supraorbital and supratrochlear neurovascular structures as they relate to the medial iris. The researchers found that the surpraorbital neurovascular bundle was 0.56 +/- 0.7 mm from the medial iris. The supratrochlear nerve was located medial to the medial iris by an average of 9.0 +/− 1.0 mm.[12] Smaller sensory nerves exiting the zygoma are the zygomaticofacial and zygomaticotemporal branches. Vascular branches of the occipital, superficial temporal, supraorbital, and supratrochlear vessels form a network of significant anastomoses to give the scalp an excellent blood supply and venous drainage system (see Fig 3-1).

Patient Selection

The primary indication for a forehead or brow lift is ptosis of the eyebrows[15] with concomitant dermatochalasis of the upper eyelids. Secondary indications are for elimination of transverse forehead wrinkles, vertical glabellar frown lines, and transverse wrinkles at the nasal root[6,7] as well as to correct asymmetries[16] and gain an esthetic balance between the upper and middle thirds of the face, especially if facial rhytidectomy is performed.[2]

The aging process of the human face is often first apparent in the upper third. The patient may appear sad, tired, angry, and aged. Evaluating the entire face in a systematic fashion with any of the recognized facial analyses allows the surgeon to appreciate general disharmony (Fig 3-2). A thorough evaluation leads to identification of specific anatomical problems and to selection of the proper surgical procedure. Consideration of individual features, current trends, old pictures, and numeric measurement may help in the evaluation. General evaluation of the face/skin for extrinsic and intrinsic aging factors must be identified. Sun damage, increase in pore size, fine lines, telangiectasia, and irregular texture do not lend well to overall esthetics. The surgeon must be able to identify brow ptosis and distinguish it from conditions that may mimic the effect of brow ptosis on the upper eyelid. The upper facial third is delineated from nasion to trichion. The hairstyle must be recognized, hair quality and quantity must be appreciated, and potential previous scars/incisions should be evaluated. Forehead height relative to facial proportions, skin elasticity and mobility, and eyebrow position and anatomy also must be evaluated. Evidence of static and dynamic forehead rhytids must be recognized. The depth of forehead rhytids can influence the surgical approach. Glabellar rhytids, again in static and dynamic function, should be evaluated. The position of the brow in a truly relaxed state allows the surgeon to evaluate the forehead static tone. This can be appreciated best by having patients close their eyes and then very slowly open them, keeping the brow in its true ptotic position (Fig 3-3).

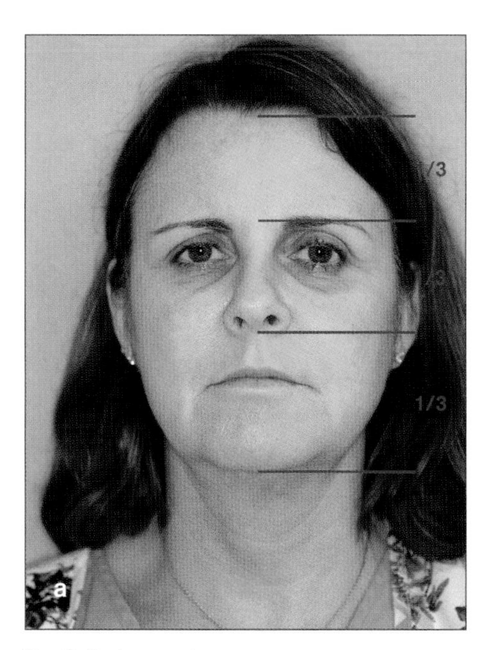

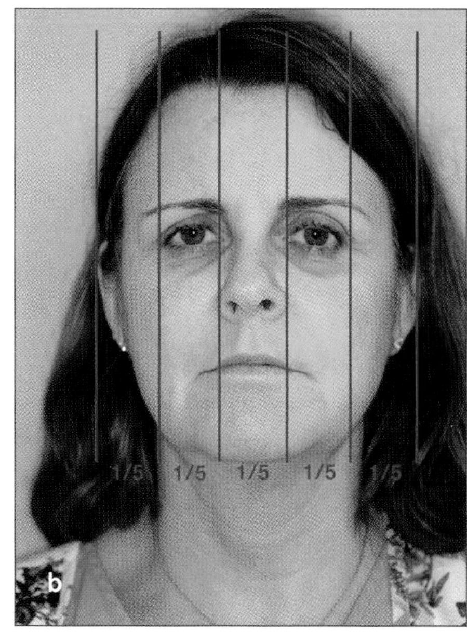

Fig 3-2 *(a and b)* Facial evaluation should help reveal asymmetries and esthetic proportions.

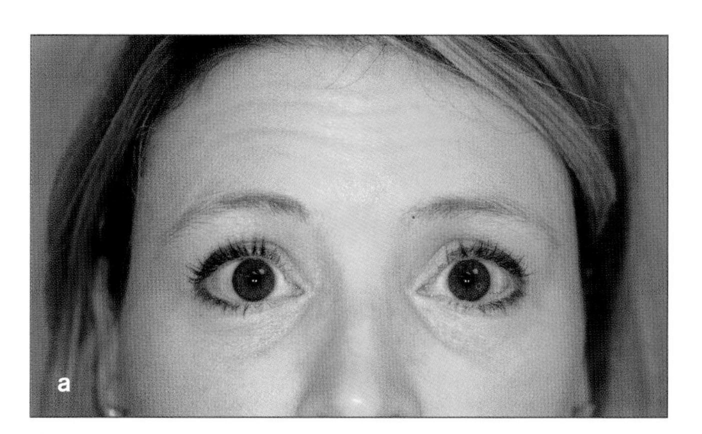

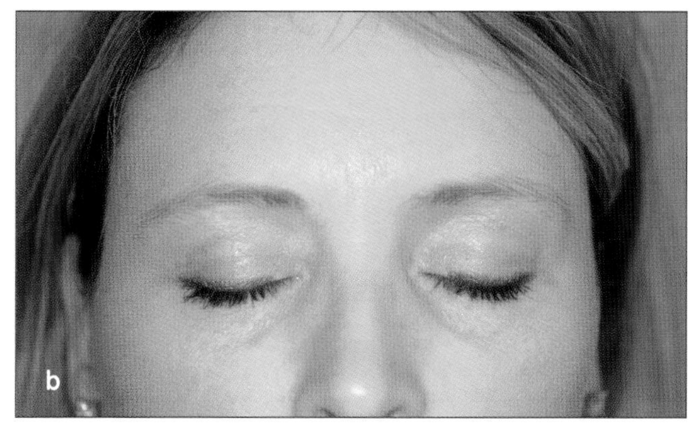

Fig 3-3 *(a)* Patient shown with active frontalis muscle. *(b and c)* Patient closes eyes to relax the frontalis muscle and slowly opens eyes, keeping the frontalis muscle relaxed, to reveal the true brow position.

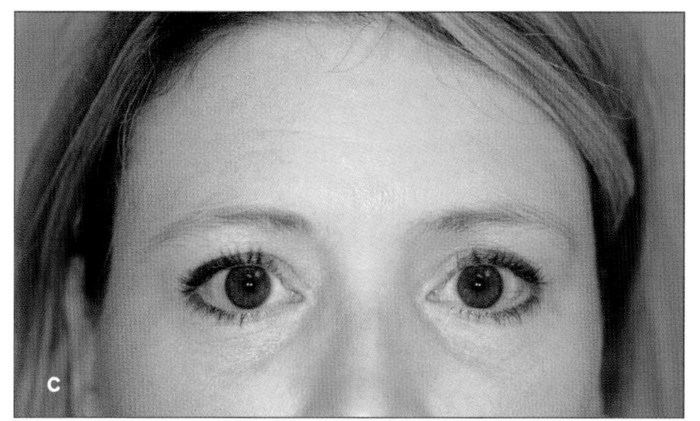

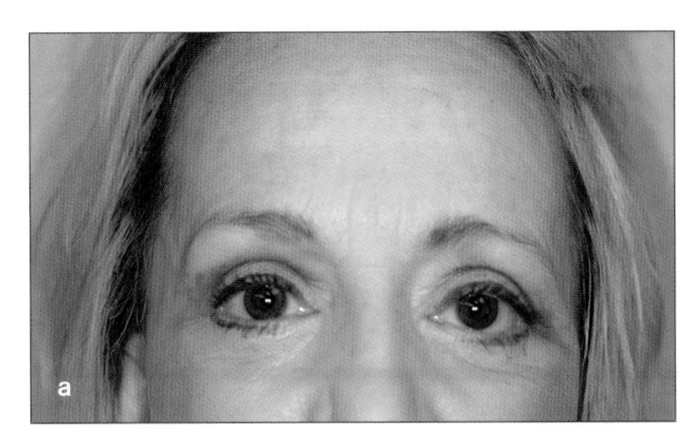

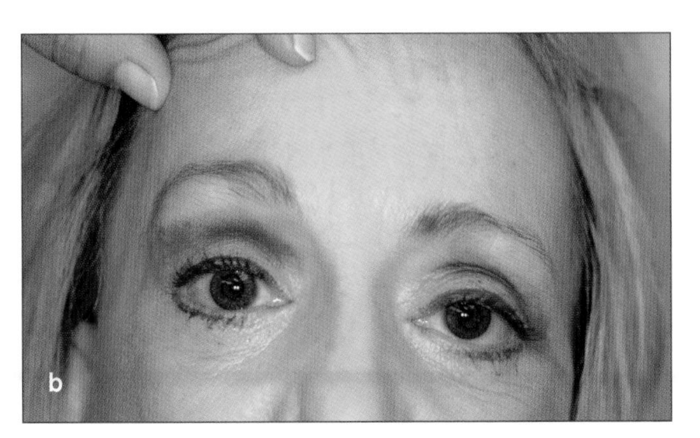

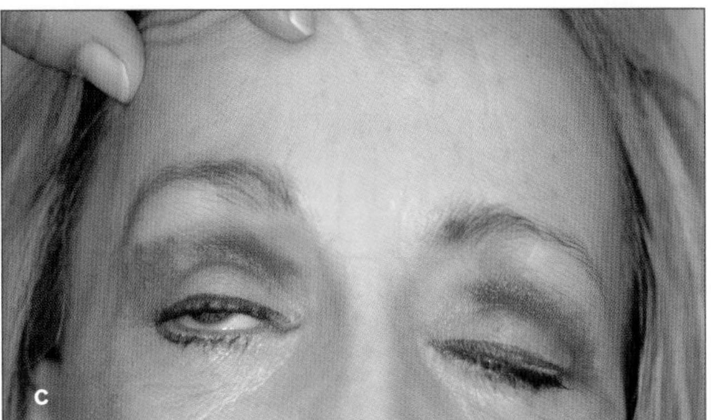

Fig 3-4 *(a)* **Patient with previous aggressive upper eyelid blepharoplasty, now desiring a brow lift.** *(b and c)* **When holding the brow in a more desired position, lagophthalmos occurs and appropriate brow positioning is unattainable.**

Many times a patient expresses interest in an upper eyelid blepharoplasty to remove excess upper eyelid tissue. In evaluating dermatochalasis of the upper eyelid, skin redundancy of the eyelid cannot be considered alone but must be considered as part of a single eyelid-brow-forehead esthetic and functional unit. To obtain the best cosmetic and functional improvement, the brow must be placed in the normal position prior to an upper eyelid blepharoplasty. It will, at least, reduce the amount of eyelid skin resection. Blepharoplasty alone may result in an undercorrection and may promote further brow descent. It is paramount that surgeons recognize and diagnose forehead/brow ptosis. If the primary problem is forehead/brow ptosis and an upper eyelid procedure is performed alone, the results may be less than ideal both esthetically and functionally.[17] A brow procedure may not be able to be performed secondarily if aggressive upper eyelid tissue removal has been performed (Fig 3-4). If upper eyelid dermatochalasis is mild, brow lift surgery alone may alleviate all excess upper eyelid tissue.

Compared with the female brow, the esthetic male brow is heavier in hair content, occupies a more inferior position, arches less laterally, and usually lies on the orbital rim (Fig 3-5). There are many variations to an esthetic female brow, but consistent generalities include the following:

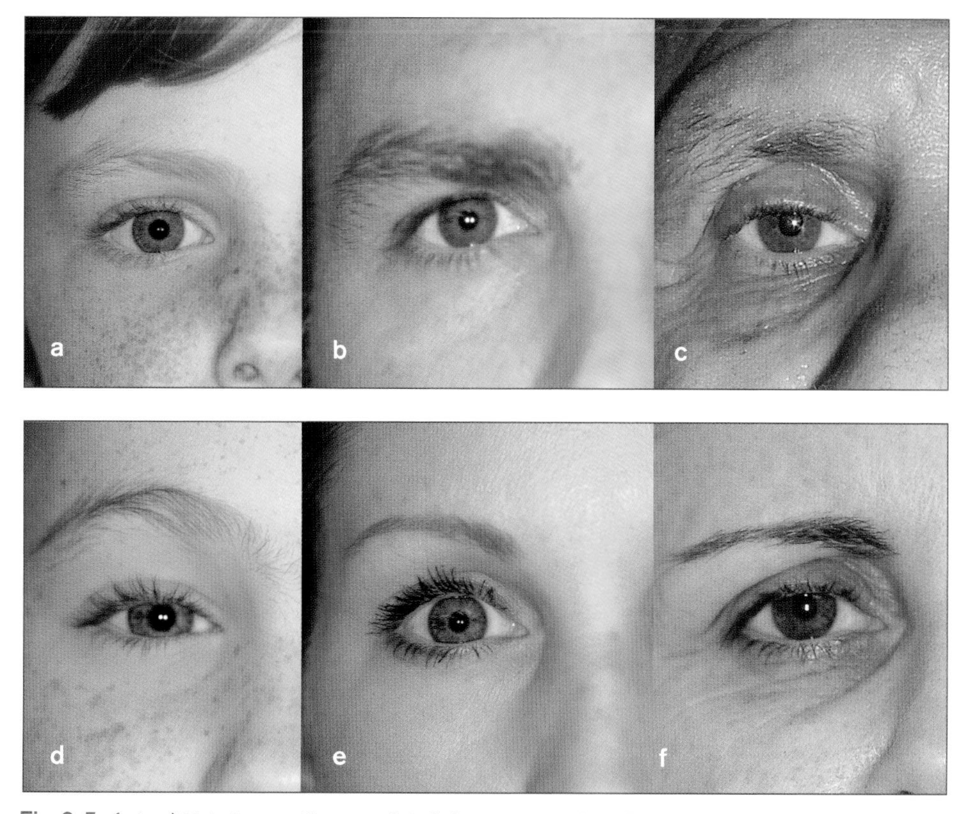

Fig 3-5 *(a to c)* **Male brow with age-related changes over time. The male brow remains horizontal, but over time, it descends and loses brow fat fullness as dermatochalasis develops.** *(d to f)* **Female brow with age-related changes over time. The female brow becomes ptotic and loses brow fat fullness as dermatochalasis develops.**

- The brow arches higher laterally than medially.
- The highest point is around the junction of the middle and outer third of the brow.
- The brow thins laterally.
- The medial aspect of the brow starts on a line superior to the medial canthus, and the lateral brow ends along a line from the lateral ala through the lateral canthus (Fig 3-6).
- The medial head and the lateral tail of the brow should be at the same horizontal level.

Numeric brow position has been evaluated by many and can aid in the evaluation. McKinney et al[18] found that the average distance from midpupil to the top of the brow was 2.5 cm. Booth's review summarized brow ptosis as less than 2.5 cm from the midpupil to the upper edge of the brow, less than 5 cm from the top of the brow to the hairline, and less than 1.5 cm of upper eyelid crease to brow.[4] With the evaluation of the patient, a complete series of standardized presurgical photographs should be taken. This series should consist of at least frontal, right and left oblique, and right and left lateral photographs, and close-up photographs of the hairline and the forehead-orbital unit. These photographs can be invaluable intraoperatively or for postoperative discussions.

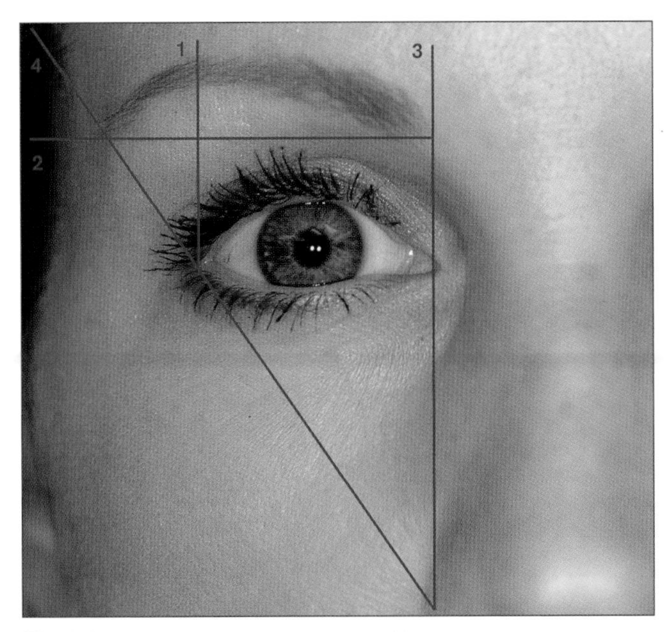

Fig 3-6 Ideal female brow esthetics. (1) The brow arches laterally with the highest point usually at the lateral third. (2) The medial and lateral brow lay on the same horizontal line. (3) The medial brow usually starts on a line perpendicular with the ala of the nose through the medial canthus. (4) The lateral extent is on a line from the ala through the lateral canthus.

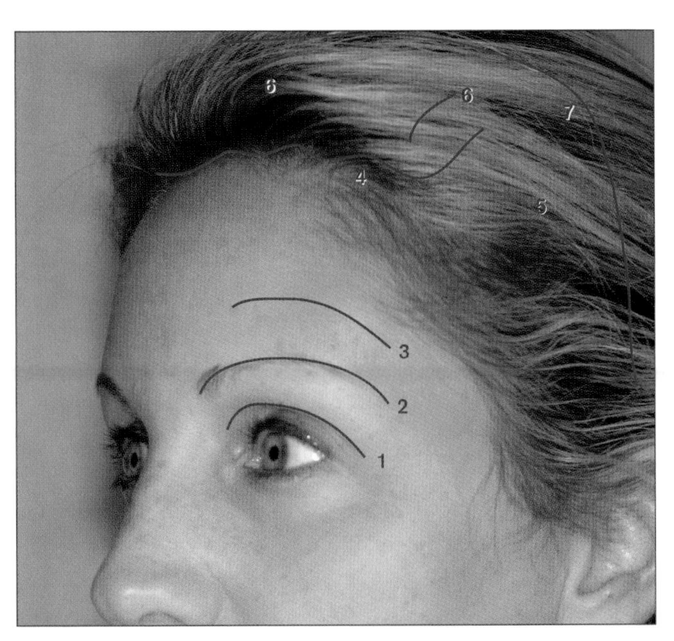

Fig 3-7 Different surgical options for brow and forehead lifting: (1) transblepharoplasty, (2) direct, (3) midforehead, (4) hairline, (5) temporal or endoscopic, (6) endoscopic, (7) coronal.

Surgical Procedures

Current surgical options for forehead and brow lifting are transblepharoplasty, direct, midforehead, temporal, hairline, coronal, and endoscopic (Fig 3-7). A comparison of each surgical option for indications and associated advantages and disadvantages are shown in Table 3-1. Nonsurgical treatments may include total and fractional ablative resurfacing, chemical peels, radiofrequency, fillers, and neurotoxin (ie, botulinum toxin) (see chapters 8 and 9).

All brow surgeries, regardless of the approach, share the following four steps:

1. Gaining access through the preferred incision design
2. Undermining and releasing tissue
3. Advancing and securing the elevated flap
4. Closing without tension

As with many surgeries, there does not appear to be one forehead or brow lifting procedure that is universally accepted as the "gold standard." The large body of published articles on forehead and brow lifting provides consensus on indications and techniques, but in many instances, the surgical approach seems to be the surgeon's personal preference.

This issue is probably best seen in open rather than endoscopic techniques. If the endoscopic approach is chosen, the surgeon may consider having the patient also consent to an open approach, in case it is required. One major difference between open and endoscopic techniques is that open procedures rely on skin excision to provide for brow fixation and elevation, whereas the endoscopic technique relies

Table 3-1 Comparison of surgical options for forehead and brow lifting

Technique	Advantages	Disadvantages
Transblepharoplasty	Simplicity Limited wound size Incision placement lends to esthetic scar Can treat two sites with one incision Can be applied with male-pattern baldness, previous hair transplants, and excessively high forehead	Brow elevation restricted to the lateral and middle segments Limited amount of brow lift Medial brow not addressed
Direct brow lift	Accurate brow elevation Preserves forehead and scalp sensation Corrects brow asymmetry	Visible scar Treats only the brow
Midforehead lift	Could be ideal for patient with prominent horizontal forehead creases Preserves the hairline Improved "fine-tuning" of the brow position More ideal in males	Possible visible scar Best to avoid in patients with thick, oily skin Not acceptable in patients prone to scar Potential for sensory deficit if performed below the frontalis
Temporal lift	Scar camouflage Improves brow position and temporal laxity Avoids raising the central hairline	Not useful for midforehead and glabellar creases No effect on medial aspect of the brow
Hairline lift	Ideal for high hairline No vertical forehead lengthening Preserves the hairline Treats all aspects of an aging forehead and brow Immediate scar camouflage (with hair)	Possible visible scar Possible prolonged sensory deficit Not indicated with male-pattern baldness or thin hairline
Coronal lift	Immediate scar camouflage Usually results in esthetic scar Treats all aspects of aging forehead and brow Ideal with low forehead hairlines Easily incorporated into facelift procedure Allows orbital and frontal bone reduction and reshaping	Some limitations with male-pattern baldness Elevates the hairline Vertically lengthens the upper third of the face Has an elongated scar Possible prolonged sensory deficit of the scalp Can induce alopecia Less "fine-tuning" of the brow position Facial nerve vulnerable to injury
Endoscopic lift	Small incisions No scalp resection Minimal motor and sensory nerve dysfunction Reduced possibility of inducing alopecia Reduced possibility of bleeding Possible faster recovery Possible higher patient acceptance Can be applied to bald patients	Cost Technique sensitive Possibly raises the hairline

on skin retraction to maintain the brow position following wound healing.[19] Postoperative light compression dressings can be applied for the first 24 to 48 hours. After this, a headband can be used for 1 to 2 weeks at night to help support the brow.

As with any surgery, appropriate surgical technique is paramount to having a successful outcome. The type of anesthesia may be local, oral sedation, intravenous sedation, or general, depending on the amount of surgery and the surgeon's comfort level. Presurgical antibruising medications, antibacterial hair washing, and antibiotics are the surgeon's choice. Incision design should be as cosmetic as possible, sparing the hair follicles. Local anesthesia is helpful for hemostasis and postoperative comfort. Tumescent anesthesia is also beneficial for many procedures to help facilitate tissue separation and make dissections easier, aid in surgical anesthesia, and decrease the amount of intravenous or general anesthesia for the case. There are many different modifications of tumescent mixtures. A common formulation is 500 mL of normal saline, 400 mg of lidocaine, and 1 mg of epinephrine.

Appropriate preoperative marking with the patient sitting in an upright position increases the accuracy and reliability of incision design and the amount of desired brow elevation. Many methods are advocated for addressing the depressor musculature: It may be released, divided, partially excised, or totally excised, though total excision may lead to a depression and an unacceptable esthetic result. Another option is to use chemical denervation (botulinum toxin) to maintain short- and long-term muscle relaxation. Two weeks before surgery, botulinum toxin can be injected into the depressor muscles alone, so elevation is less opposed, or into both the depressor muscles and forehead for brow and forehead relaxation.

When elevating the brow, less medial tissue excision is indicated to avoid a surprised look. As the incision becomes further from the brow, more tissue elevation and excision is required to gain the desired brow lift.

Transblepharoplasty

Transblepharoplasty may be the surgeon's choice if limited brow elevation is indicated and no medial brow elevation is desired. It can be incorporated through the traditional upper lid blepharoplasty incision. Presurgery, the brow is held in the desired position, and excess upper eyelid skin is marked. The traditional skin or skin-muscle excision is performed. At this time, dissection is carried just deep to the orbicularis oculi muscle along the orbital septum. The orbicularis oculi muscle interdigitates with the frontalis muscle at the level of the brows. If the brow fat pad (retro-orbicularis oculi fat pad) needs to be reduced, this also can be accomplished easily at this point. The superior orbital rim is palpated and, with care for the supraorbital neurovascular bundle, the arcus marginalis (periosteum) is incised from the midorbital rim to the lateral extent. Subperiosteal dissection is continued superiorly along the frontal bone for at least 2 cm. At this point, the brow is fixated, the orbital preseptal fat is addressed (if indicated), and the routine blepharoplasty closure is completed. Brow fixation can be performed with nonresorbable sutures to the periosteum or with a a resorbable tacking device (Endotine Brow, Coapt Systems).

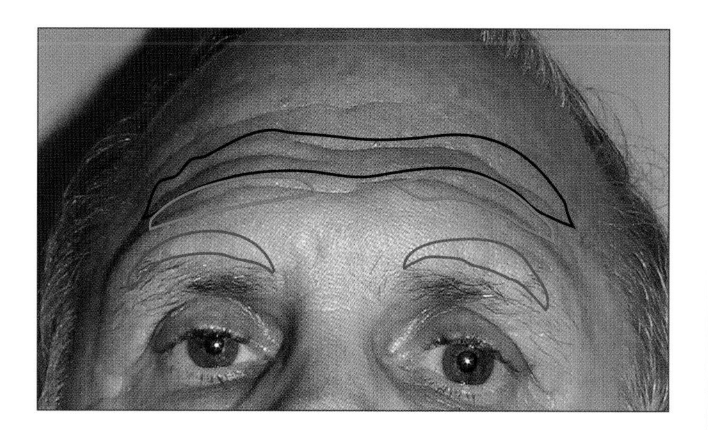

Fig 3-8 Different potential incision designs for direct *(pink)* and midforehead *(green and black)* brow lifts.

Direct brow lift

The direct brow lift is the oldest and simplest surgical approach for brow lifting.[20] It is the only brow lifting technique for which the ratio of elevation to excision is 1:1. With this technique, the patient has to be accepting of a scar, and the patient must understand that forehead rhytids and ptosis will not be addressed. Many times, this technique is reserved for those who medically cannot tolerate one of the other techniques or who desire the surgery for the purely functional reason of aiding vision.[4] The patient should have enough brow hair to aid in scar camouflage. If a horizontal rhytid exists, this should be used in the incision design (Fig 3-8). The patient should be closely evaluated for thick skin and tendencies for scar formation, which do not lend themselves well to this technique. The outline design can be variable, depending on the extent of brow elevation desired. The inferior incision line along the brow is marked first. Then, with the brow held in the desired position, a surgical marker is held next to the skin, the brow is released, and the skin is marked at the proposed site. This is done at the medial, central, and lateral brow, and then the lines are connected for the superior incision line. The dissection is to the subcutaneous plane; then, excision of the overlying skin is performed. The orbicularis muscle can be suspended to the periosteum,[13] and closure is then completed in two layers. Though this approach has limitations, it does preserve the sensory nerves and can give a predictable outcome with a less invasive procedure.

Midforehead lift

If a high hairline and deep forehead rhytids are present and the patient is accepting of a scar, then a midforehead lift may be performed in a relatively straightforward fashion. This approach should be avoided in patients with thick skin and those prone to scarring.[4] There are multiple incision designs depending on the forehead rhytids and desired area of brow elevation (see Fig 3-8). The dissection is performed in a subcutaneous plane and preserves the sensory nerves. One can perform a subgaleal or periosteal flap in the middle of the forehead to approach the depressor muscles from their undersurface in order to maintain the neurosensory supply. Forehead skin

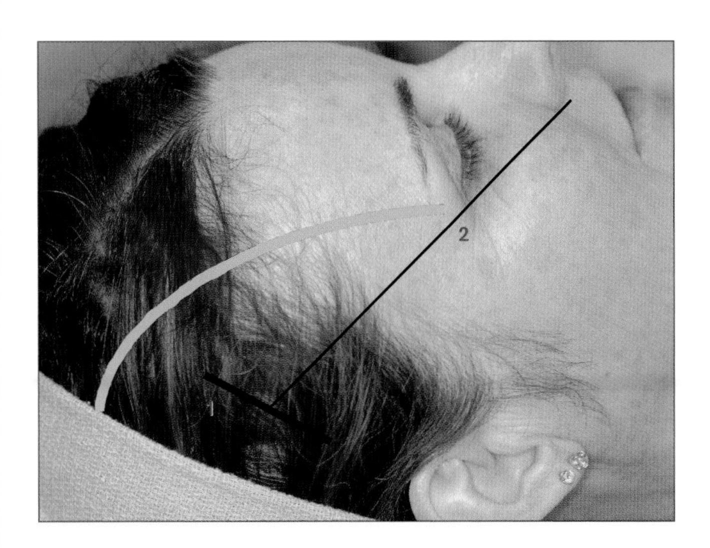

Fig 3-9 Access for temporal lift or the temporal portal of an endoscopic approach. The proposed access for temporal incision (1) lies at the hairline or up to 3 cm within the hairline and is identified by a line through the ala and lateral canthus (2). This incision line can be modified to correlate with the desired vector of lift. Gray line—temporal line of fusion.

excision is outlined, and the dissection is carried to just below the orbital rim level. The orbicularis may be suspended superiorly to nonmobile tissue.[5,20] Excision of redundant elevated skin is performed, and closure is in layers. Steri-Strips (3M) may be used. Some advocate 6 to 8 weeks of postoperative Steri-Strips for best scar maturation.[4] Patients should be educated preoperatively and told to expect a scar(s). They also need to understand that the scar will be variable in appearance until mature.

Temporal lift

If no midbrow and medial brow elevation is desired, the surgeon may choose access in the temporal region along the hairline or, more traditionally, around 2 to 3 cm within the hairline (Fig 3-9). The incision for temporal access is 3 to 4 cm in length and correlates to the desired vector of elevation and amount of proposed tissue to be excised. The surgeon needs to pay close attention to the position of the temporal tuft of hair as this may rise significantly if the incision is within the hairline. The dissection can be in the subcutaneous plane or along the superficial layer of the temporalis fascia. If the dissection is along the deep plane, some advocate releasing the arcus marginalis, conjoint tendon, and temporal line under direct visualization so the lateral brow is completely mobilized.[5] Regardless of the plane of dissection, undermining the temporal flap to the lateral extent of the eyebrow is performed with caution to avoid facial nerve injury. The flap is advanced along the desired vector, excess tissue is excised, and closure is in two layers.

Hairline lift

The hairline lift is described as *pretrichophytic* or *trichophytic*. *Pretrichial* is at or just anterior to the hairline; *trichial* is inside the hairline.[5] A hairline lift incision design is a good choice if the forehead is long, the hair is worn down, and a possible visible scar is accepted (Fig 3-10a). The pretrichial approach may be less esthetic as the hairline-skin margin can be more abrupt. The trichial approach, or modified pretrichial,[4] may help

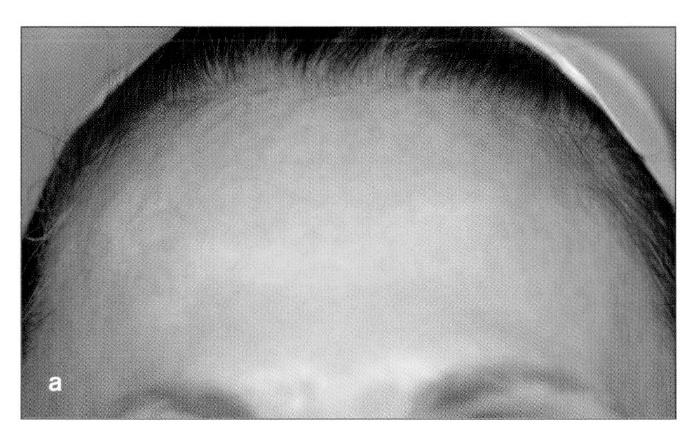

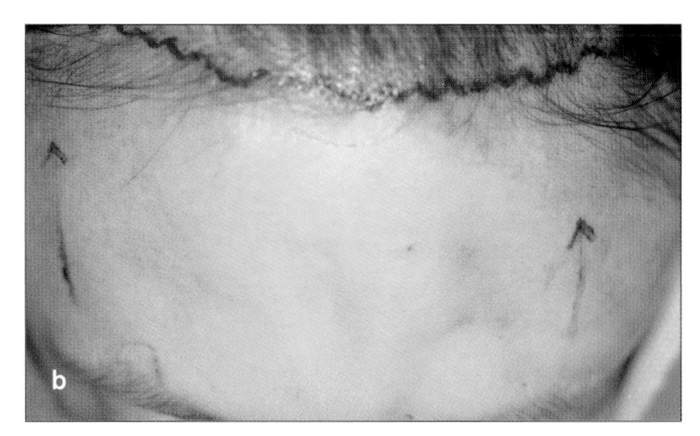

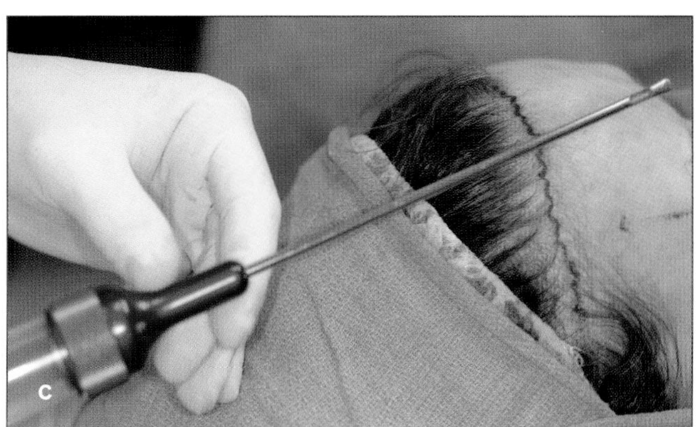

Figs 3-10a to 3-10c *(a)* Preoperative hairline. *(b)* Incision design for trichophytic approach. *(c)* A liposuction cannula can be used for initial undermining of tissues.

eliminate this esthetic concern by allowing hair to grow through the scar over time. The natural-appearing hairline is irregular and does not end abruptly; rather, it transitions through a 4- to 5-mm zone of decreasing follicle density to fine hair.[15] Many describe the incision as "irregular" for best cosmetic results (Fig 3-10b).

After appropriate markings are made, local anesthesia is used along the incision line and supraorbital nerve blocks. Tumescent anesthesia is infiltrated in the subcutaneous plane along the entire proposed forehead undermining unit. After an appropriate wait time of 10 to 15 minutes, the dissection can proceed. Undermining with liposuction spatulas (Fig 3-10c) without suction can be performed through two small, parasagittal stab incisions in the proposed incision line. Undermining should leave an even plane of subcutaneous tissue on the underside of the skin. This maneuver makes the flap elevation quick and uneventful.

If the incision is pretrichial, it is placed 3 to 4 mm into the hairline and on an exaggerated posterior to anterior bevel to transect through the hair follicle. The incision is made with a no. 11 blade and can taper posteriorly as the temporal region is approached. The dissection can be in the subcutaneous or the subgaleal/periosteal level. The subcutaneous dissection allows for preservation of sensation but does not lend itself well to addressing the corrugator muscles. The flap must be kept appropriately thick to reduce the risk for flap necrosis, especially if the patient smokes.

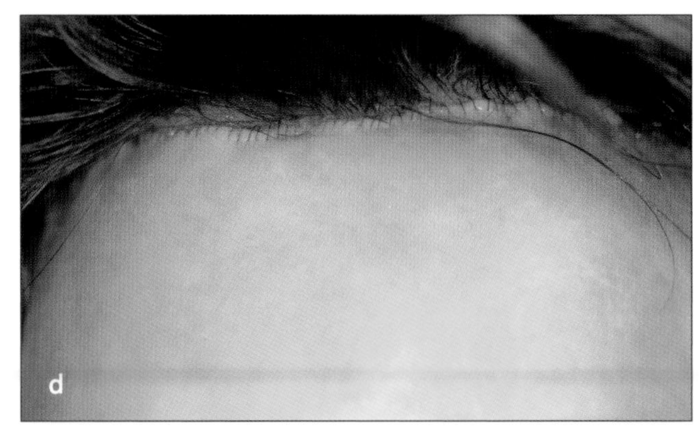

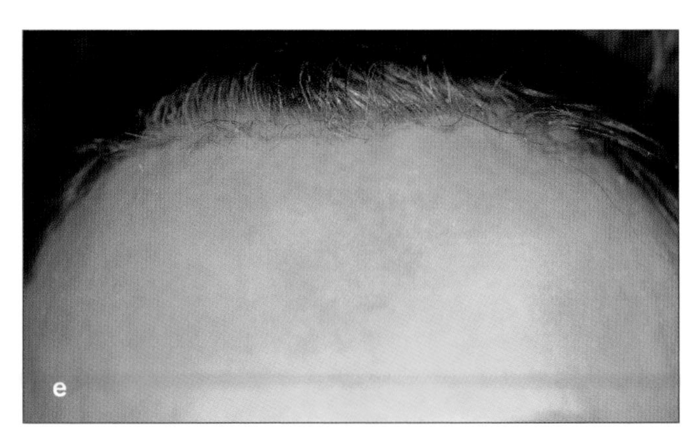

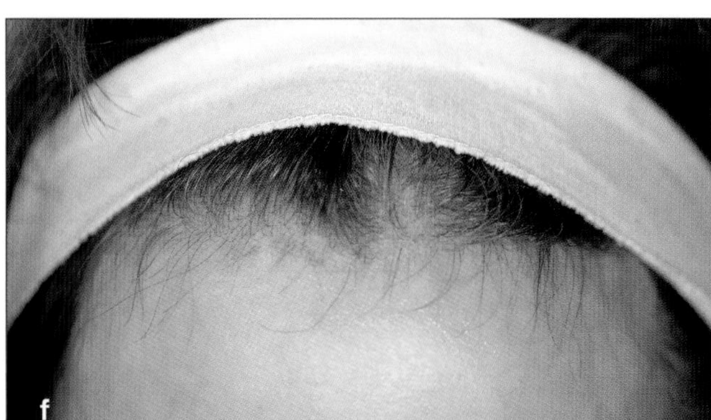

Figs 3-10d to 3-10f *(d)* Hairline at 1 week postoperative. *(e)* Hairline at 3 weeks postoperative. *(f)* Hairline at 3 months postoperative.

The flap is advanced, and multiple tacking sutures are placed. The excess skin should then be excised with the same bevel and closed in layers. The closure is critical if the initial incision was on a bevel (Figs 3-10d to 3-10f). An endoscope also may be used and the technique is described in the endoscopic lift section.

Coronal lift

The coronal lift is considered by many to be the workhorse[4] and gold standard of forehead and brow lifting. It was first described in 1926.[4] If the desired effect is to elongate the forehead, contour the underlying bone, or conceal an incision line, the coronal lift is an excellent choice.

Many incision designs can be used, depending on the hairline and the type of brow lift desired. It may be performed completely in either the subgaleal or subperiosteal plane, or the two techniques can be combined. If the subgaleal plane is started, the subperiosteal plane is usually entered about 2 cm above the orbital rim.[21] In either case, the incision is usually 4 to 5 cm posterior to the hairline.[4] The incision should try to spare hair follicles and should be beveled, if indicated.

At the subgaleal or subperiosteal level, the dissection is continued to the level of the bridge of the nose, just over the supraorbital rims, and may extend laterally to the zygomatic arches if the need for lateral elevation is significant or the desired vector requires. This allows complete visualization of the forehead and accompanying anatomy. The depressor muscles may be addressed as desired. The frontalis muscle can be scored, or partial resection may be performed. As the forehead tissue is advanced, the appropriate amount of excess tissue is excised accordingly. The ratio of desired elevation to amount of scalp excision is debatable, but a common rule is that for each 1 cm of elevation, 2 to 2.5 cm of scalp excision is indicated.[4] Closure of the incision is in layers. A dressing may be applied for 24 to 48 hours for tissue support and to reduce postoperative edema.

Endoscopic lift

With the advent of the endoscope, the endoscopic lift has become popular with many surgeons and has its widest application to date for forehead lifts.[22] This technique should be seen as one tool in the armamentarium that now has a proven long-term record. The endoscopic technique may be contraindicated for patients with a high brow, pattern baldness, or frontal bone irregularities, or if the surgeon is not trained in endoscopic techniques or does not possess the appropriate equipment and instrumentation. Some of the major advantages of the endoscopic lift include scalp excision, decreased bleeding, decreased risk of inducing alopecia, minimal risk of sensory or motor dysfunction, faster recovery[2,4] and, possibly, better patient acceptance. One commonly held but false idea about this approach is that it uses a smaller incision and results in less scarring; if the extent of the multiple access incisions is included in the measurement, then the overall incision length is usually comparable to that of other techniques. The basic required instrumentation includes the following: endoscopic unit composed of a camera; video monitor(s); xenon light; video recorder and printer; 4- to 5-mm, 30-degree rigid scope; and special elevators.[23]

Multiple endoscopic techniques have been advocated, including total subperiosteal, total subgaleal, subgaleal/subperiosteal without skin excision, and open biplanar techniques.[21] Some proposed advantages of the subperiosteal technique include a better optical cavity and bony landmarks that allow easier orientation, safety, and excellent vascularity. In addition, the periosteum may give a more rigid lift for long-term stability.[23] Some proposed advantages of the subgaleal dissections include less postoperative muscle movement, easier identification of and direct resection of muscles, improved forehead skin support resulting from the pericranium's adherence to the cut edges of the galea, and the ability to elevate the medial brow separately rather than having to elevate the entire brow as a unit.[24] Nassif et al[24] compared eyebrow and forehead elevation and tension among *(1)* subperiosteal dissection to the orbital rim, *(2)* subperiosteal dissection with release of the periosteum at the supraorbital rim, and *(3)* subgaleal dissection to the supraorbital rim. Their findings concluded that all three methods of dissection significantly elevated the brow at rest and both the brow and forehead when traction was applied. Brow and forehead elevation at rest and with 2.2 kg of traction did not significantly differ among the dissections. The subgaleal dissection was associated with less flap tension compared with the subperiosteal dissection, both with and without release. These data support the use of all three methods of forehead dissection for brow elevation.[24]

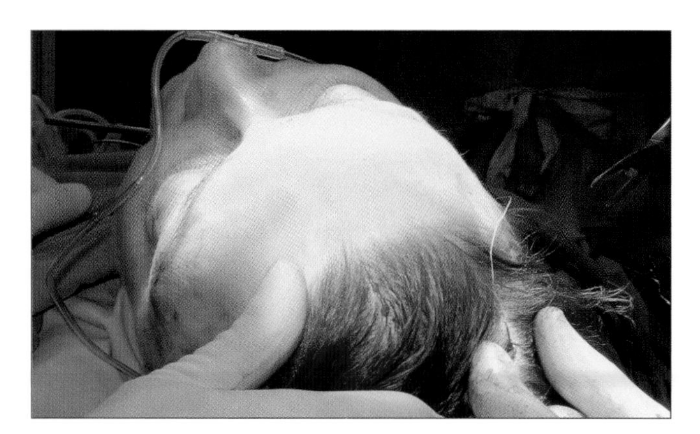

Fig 3-11a Midline and parasagittal access ports for the endoscope. (Courtesy of Dr King Kim, Melbourne, Florida.)

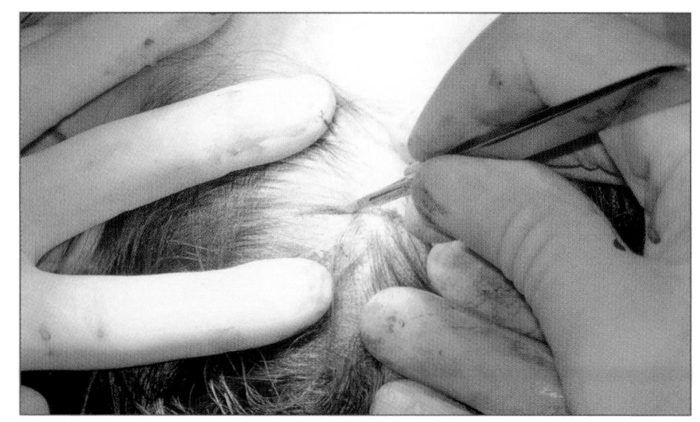

Fig 3-11b Lateral incision of the temporal access portal. (Courtesy of Dr King Kim, Melbourne, Florida.)

The endoscopic lift is started by marking the sites of the entry (portal) incisions (see Fig 3-9). The number of access incisions is variable. It can be as few as two, but more often, three or four are made. The shape of the skull, hairline position, underlying bony architecture, soft tissue thickness, and desired medial and lateral brow elevation help determine the number of access points. These are placed 1 to 3 cm into the hairline and are vertical in nature; they are usually about 1 cm long. If three access incision points are used, one is usually midsagittal and two are parasagittal (Fig 3-11a). If two temporal access incision points are used, they typically are placed over the temporalis muscle, measure about 3 cm in length, and are perpendicularly bisected by a line from the ala of the nose through the lateral canthus (Fig 3-11b). These access sites can also be used for an ellipse excision of tissue for assisting in elevating the lateral brow. The posterior branch of the superficial temporal artery may be encountered, and appropriate hemostasis is important to prevent a hematoma.

Once the forehead incision lines are accessed with sharp incisions, the dissection can be made in the subgaleal or subperiosteal plane (Fig 3-11c). For this example, the chosen plane will be in the subperiosteal. This dissection can be "blind" posterior to the occiput, lateral to the temporal fusion lines, and inferior to 2 to 3 cm above the orbital rim to protect the neurovascular anatomy (Fig 3-11d). The temporal access is to the superficial layer of the deep temporalis fascia (Fig 3-11e). If one is uncertain of this fascia, a small incision can be made through the fascia to visualize the temporalis muscle. This fascial layer is glistening white and does not move as a unit with the overlying scalp.

Once these two planes are completed, the endoscope is used in the forehead to complete the subperiosteal elevation inferiorly over the superior orbital rims and to the root of the nasal bones (Figs 3-11f to 3-11h). The supraorbital and supratrochlear nerves are noted and protected at all times. It is important to carry the dissection laterally to at least the zygomaticofrontal suture to allow appropriate release. At this time, the endoscope is introduced through the temporal access incision sites

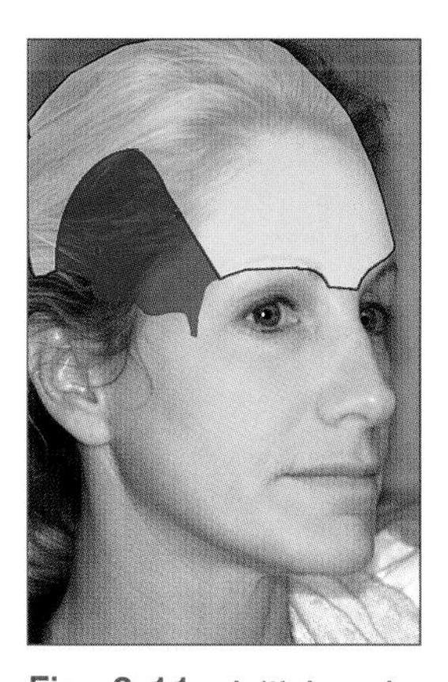

Fig 3-11c Initial endoscopic dissection is in the subperiosteal plane *(yellow)*. The temporal dissection follows just superficial to the temporalis fascia *(blue)*. The two planes are connected for completed undermining in the endoscopic approach.

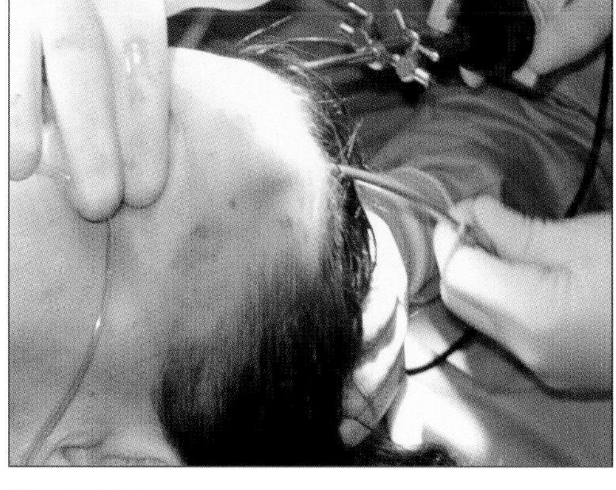

Fig 3-11d Initial access through the parasagittal access port allows for endoscopic dissection of the subperiosteal plane with an elevator. (Courtesy of Dr King Kim, Melbourne, Florida.)

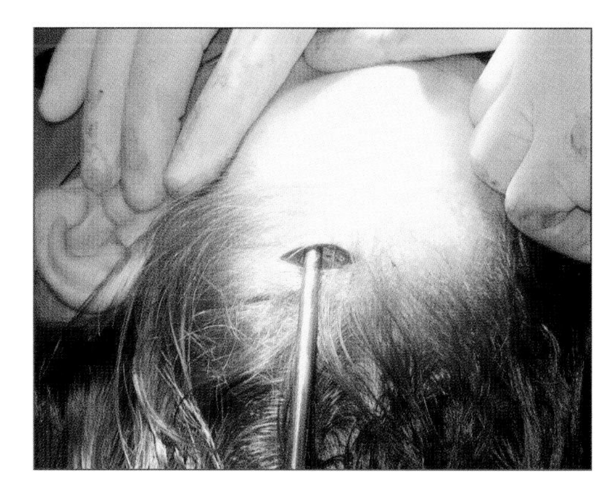

Fig 3-11e Endoscopic dissection superficial to the deep temporalis fascia. (Courtesy of Dr King Kim, Melbourne, Florida.)

Figs 3-11f to 3-11h Endoscopic view of the extent of the dissection. Dissection with endoscope to the nasal root *(f)*, around the supraorbital neurovascular unit *(g)*, and to the lateral orbital rim *(h)*.

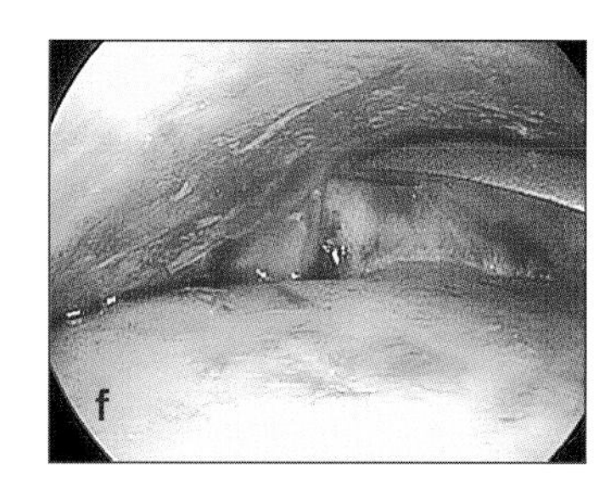

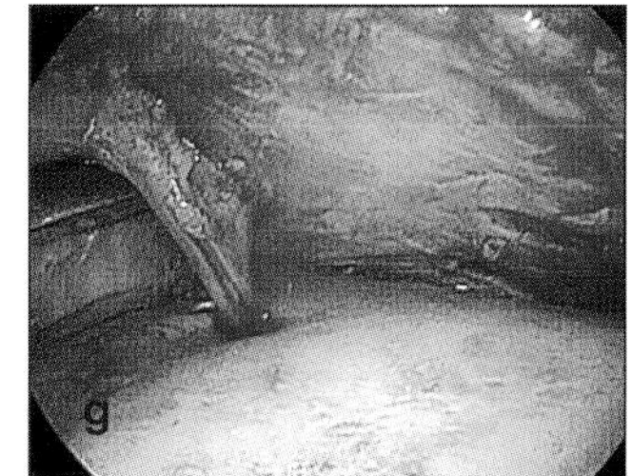

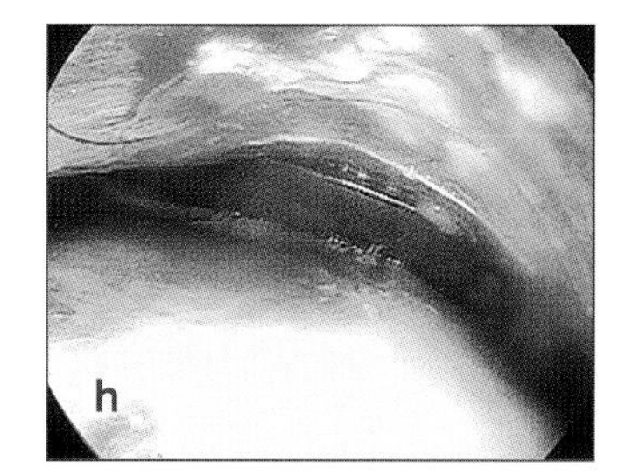

Figs 3-11i Temporal access with the endoscope. (Courtesy of Dr King Kim, Melbourne, Florida.)

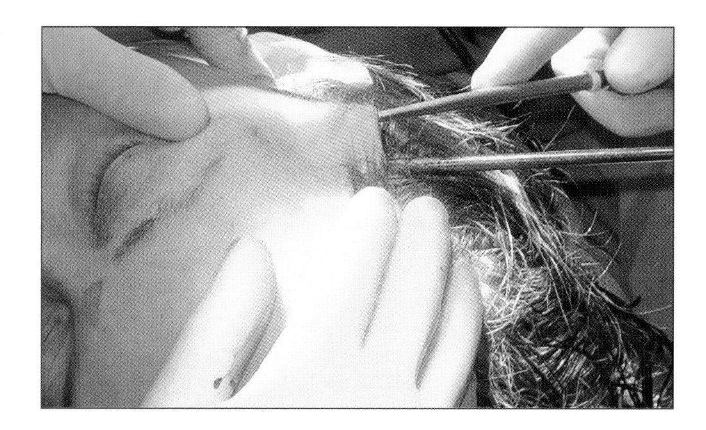

(Fig 3-11i). The instrumentation is kept intimately along the temporalis fascia as one nears the lateral orbit. The sentinel vein (medial zygomaticotemporal) is commonly visualized. The surgeon should attempt to keep this vein intact. If injury occurs and bleeding ensues, digital pressure usually alleviates this bleeding. If cautery is needed, one must be cognizant that the facial nerve is just superficial in the flap. Postoperative lateral orbital ecchymosis should be expected if bleeding occurs from this vein.

Establishing communication between the two planes is the next step. Communication through the temporal fusion line should be performed from the temporal plane under direct endoscopic visualization. If an attempt is made from the frontal plane, inadvertent communication to a more superficial plane can occur laterally. The temporal line of fusion should be released from the lateral orbit to as high as one can access through the lateral incision. Once this is complete, releasing of the periosteum with endoscopic hand instruments, radiofrequency, carbon dioxide laser, or another instrument of choice can be performed under endoscopic visualization through the forehead portals. The periosteal release is from the lateral orbit to the contralateral orbit at the level of the arcus marginalis. Care must be taken in the supraorbital and supratrochlear sites. The depressor corrugator and procerus muscles can be addressed at this time, if indicated.

Once these maneuvers are completed, the brow should be able to be freely advanced superiorly. Fixation of the brow with two Endotine resorbable plates (Coapt Systems) through the parasagittal incisions can be performed. The forehead incisions are closed in layers, and the two lateral temporal incisions can be closed in layers as well. The anterior incision line at the level of the SMAS can be secured to the posterior incision located in the deep temporalis fascia. The skin is then closed. The excess/redundant scalp skin posterior to the fixation points will subside over a short period of time.

Biplanar technique

With the biplanar technique, the open subcutaneous and endoscopic techniques are combined to take advantage of each procedure. This technique is indicated for patients who have high foreheads (7 cm or greater),[22,23] severe brow ptosis and hooding, and significant horizontal forehead rhytids.[9,21,23] The hairline incision is done as described previously. Lateral extension into the temporal region can vary, depending on the direction of elevation desired and the distance from the temporal hairline to the brow. If this distance is greater than 5 cm, the extension should be at the hairline so as to not increase this distance with the elevation.[25] The subcutaneous dissection can be from one-fourth to two-thirds of the vertical brow height, depending on the amount of horizontal rhytids and the amount of lateral extension needed. The dissection in the temporal scalp may be solely subcutaneous or along the temporalis fascia. Access incisions are made, usually one in the midline and one in each temporal region. The endoscope is then used to gain access into the subperiosteal plane. The procedure is much the same as the endoscopic approach described previously to undermine/elevate the desired periosteum, release the arcus marginalis, and address the depressor muscles as desired. Vertical anchoring sutures may be placed through the frontalis to decrease tension on the skin closure, with care to avoid the supraorbital nerves.[25] Excision of redundant skin and closure is as previously described.

Fixation Options

The surgeon can choose from many options for brow and forehead fixation. The goals of any fixation method include patient safety, simplicity, serviceability for the appropriate amount of time, and reproducibility. It is important to remember that whatever technique is used, the principal goal of fixation is to hold the brow in position and not to pull or release the brow. Every technique has its own risks and possible complications. These can include partial or total alopecia, loss of brow elevation, implant palpability, scalp pruritus, paresthesia, and potential dural injury.[26] The length of time required for healing to produce enough resistance to oppose the depressor muscles is unknown, but it is cited to be from as short as several days to as long as 6 weeks.[19]

Fixation devices can be endogenous or exogenous. Common endogenous methods are bolster, galea-frontalis-occipital release, lateral spanning suspension sutures, frontal periosteum and galea to occipital periosteum and galea suturing (galea-frontalis advancement), cortical tunnels, V-Y suture techniques, tissue adhesive, or no fixation. Common exogenous methods include internal screws and plates, pins, Mitek anchors, external screw fixation, Kirscher-wire fixation,[19,26,27] and resorbable fixation devices.

Complications

As with any surgery, complications are usually easy to manage if the proper diagnosis, planning, and patient counseling have been performed preoperatively. It is essential that every patient be informed and included in the treatment planning process. Patients will experience complications from surgery even when in the best of hands. Careful thought and planning done preoperatively, intraoperatively, and postoperatively will help lower the chance of complications, but a good result is not always guaranteed. Honesty and diligence is the rule. Listening to patients and giving immediate attention to their concerns is essential. In most cases, complications subside with time. Experienced surgeons know when to institute "watchful waiting" versus intervention and surgical management of a complication. Providing reassurance is a skill every cosmetic surgeon must develop.

The most common complications include temporary and permanent hair loss, bruising, prolonged edema, hematoma, scar widening, tissue necrosis, facial nerve injury, temporary and permanent scar pruritus, and neurosensory changes.[6,7] Skin flap necrosis is rare secondary to the abundant vascular supply. In patients who smoke, the subcutaneous dissection may be contraindicated. A light postoperative dressing also decreases the possibility of skin flap necrosis (Fig 3-12). If partial-thickness necrosis occurs, local tissue debridement and dressing will allow secondary healing. If full-thickness necrosis occurs in a flap that is too large for local wound care and secondary healing, a local flap may be indicated for primary closure. Hemorrhage under the flap can lead to infection and overlying skin flap necrosis. Good surgical technique and attention to bleeding is usually the best prevention. When identified—usually early—in the postoperative phase,[7] needle aspiration may be sufficient. Evacuation may be indicated for an expanding hematoma or liquefied clot. Management includes controlling the source of bleeding, removing the clot, and applying a new pressure dressing.

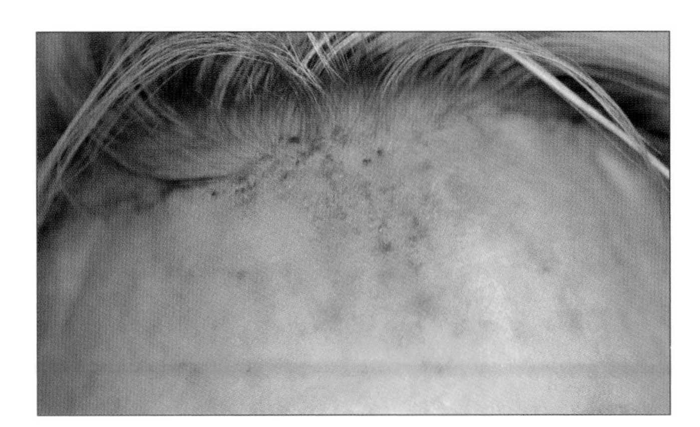

Fig 3-12 Superficial tissue necrosis secondary to pressure for postoperative dressing.

Infections are uncommon secondary to the excellent blood supply and short duration of brow surgery. If an infection does occur, it can lead to unsightly scar formation and hair loss. It must be treated diligently secondary to the direct communication with orbital anatomy. The inferior portion of the forehead drains into the ophthalmic vein, which continues into the cavernous sinus.[4,7] Possible sources of infection include underlying medical conditions or other habits that diminish wound healing (diabetes, immunosuppresion, smoking[4]), inadequate patient preoperative preparation, the presence of hair within the incision, and poor postoperative wound care. Alopecia can be induced by indiscriminant incision design, aggressive tissue handling, excessive use of electrocautery, closure of the incision under tension, poor postoperative wound care, and infection. With initial postoperative hair loss, hair may regrow over time. The uncommon condition of *telogen effluvium*, or spontaneous hair loss, occurs in a small percentage of patients. This rare condition is associated with physical or emotional trauma and usually resolves over time.[7] If appropriate time passes and no hair growth occurs, topical minoxidil, a local flap, or hair grafts may be indicated.

As evidenced by preoperative photographs, a certain percentage of patients have preoperative asymmetries. If no plan is made to alter the asymmetry with surgery, the same asymmetry should be expected to be present postoperatively. If the asymmetry is to be corrected, appropriate differential correction should be planned. An asymmetry may be caused by injury to the temporofrontal branch of the facial nerve. If this occurs, it is usually temporary. Depending on the extent, the patient may need to be educated regarding appropriate eye care. Daily eye drops, a lubricant, and taping of the eyelid at night may be required to prevent corneal insult. Contralateral forehead neurotoxin injections may be administered to mask the asymmetry and give time for the injured nerve to return to function. In rare cases, if function does not return, a gold eyelid weight may be indicated.

Sensory disturbances are not uncommon but usually resolve within a short amount of time. Patients should be educated that postoperative paresthesia or anesthesia posterior to the incision is likely to occur when the coronal or trichial approaches are used if the dissection plane is below the frontalis muscle, but sensation usually improves over time. Regardless of the approach, delicate dissection and tissue manipulation around the exit points of the supraorbital and supratrochlear nerves should be adhered to at all times. If a postoperative dysesthesia occurs, some surgeons advocate nerve blocks with 0.5% bupivacaine 1:200,000, which can last for hours, followed by potential days of pain relief.[4]

Pruritus at the incision line or in areas of sensory deficit has been described[4,28] but usually subsides over the first few months. Postoperative lagophthalmos should be anticipated (2 to 3 mm is desired) early in the healing process. If unexpected lagophthalmos arises from a facial nerve injury, it is managed as described previously, with ointments and eye taping. If the lid incompetence is secondary to aggressive upper lid skin excision or brow elevation, constant eye care may be needed as well as ophthalmic consultation.

Summary

With the popularity of facial cosmetic surgery, the facial surgeon must be cognizant of the upper face and the early effects of the aging process. When the diagnosis of forehead and brow rhytids and/or ptosis is made, appropriate preoperative planning and competent surgery produce results that can satisfy both surgeon and patient. Currently, there are multiple brow elevation procedures to choose from. It is clear that no single technique is universally applicable to all patients. As with all surgeries, complications can arise, but these are usually infrequent and temporary.

Endoscopic Brow/Forehead Lift Tray

- Mandibular awl (KLS-Martin)
- Zygomatic awl (KLS-Martin)
- Scalpel handle, two (KLS-Martin)
- Adson-Brown forceps, two (KLS-Martin)
- Dean scissors (KLS-Martin)
- Towel forceps, four (KLS-Martin)
- No. 9 periosteal elevator (KLS-Martin)
- Iodine bowl (Biomet)
- Ramirez EndoFacelift dissector (Snowden-Pencer)
- Crile-Wood needle holder (Snowden-Pencer)
- Ramirez EndoForehead "T" dissector (Snowden-Pencer)
- Daniel quarter-curved EndoForehead elevator (Snowden-Pencer)
- Daniel full-curved EndoForehead elevator (Snowden-Pencer)
- Daniel half-curved EndoForehead dissector (Snowden-Pencer)
- Daniel half-curved EndoForehead elevator (Snowden-Pencer)
- Ramirez EndoForehead parietal elevator (Snowden-Pencer)
- Ramirez EndoForehead spreader (Snowden-Pencer)
- Emory endoplastic dissector (Snowden-Pencer)
- Daniel EndoForehead suction (Snowden-Pencer)
- Ramirez EndoForehead grasper (Snowden-Pencer)
- Ramirez EndoForehead scissors (Snowden-Pencer)
- Aspirating syringe, two (KLS-Martin)
- Mosquito hemostat, four (Snowden-Pencer)

References

1. Arteaga DM, Taylor CO. Esthetic evaluation and treatment of the upper one third of the face. J Oral Maxillofac Surg 1991;49:27–32.
2. Taylor CO, Green JG, Wise DP. Endoscopic forehead lift: Technique and case presentations. J Oral Maxillofac Surg 1996;54:569–577.
3. Griffin JE, Frey BS, Max DP, Epker BN. Laser-assisted endoscopic forehead lift. J Oral Maxillofac Surg 1998;56:1040–1048.
4. Taylor CO, Lewis JS. Cosmetic surgery of the forehead and brow. In: Fonseca RJ, Baker SB, Wolford LM (eds). Oral and Maxillofacial Surgery. Vol 6: Cleft/Craniofacial/Cosmetic Surgery. Philadelphia: Saunders, 2000:382–394.
5. Henderson J, Larrabee W. Analysis of the upper face and selection of rejuvenation techniques. Facial Plast Surg North Am 2006;14:153–158.
6. Adamson PA, Johnson CM Jr, Anderson JR, Dupin CL. The forehead lift: A review. Arch Otolaryngol 1985;111:325–329.
7. Beeson WH, McCollough EG. Complications of the forehead lift. Ear Nose Throat J 1985;64:575–583.
8. Ozerdem OR, Vasconez LO, de la Torre J. Upper face-lifting. Facial Plast Surg North Am 2006;14:159–165.
9. Isse NG. Endoscopic facial rejuvenation: Endoforehead, the functional lift. Case reports. Aesthetic Plast Surg 1994;18:21–29.
10. Vinas JC, Caviglia C, Cortinas JL. Forehead rhytidectomy and brow lifting. Plast Reconstr Surg 1976;57:445–454.
11. Liebman EP, Webster RC, Berger AS, DellaVecchia M. The frontalis nerve in the temporal brow lift. Arch Otolaryngol 1982;108:232–235.
12. Cuzalina AL, Holmes JD. A simple and reliable landmark for identification of the supraorbital nerve in surgery of the forehead: An in vivo anatomic study. J Oral Maxillofac Surg 2005;63:25–27.
13. Morgan J, Farrior E. Rejuvenation of the aging forehead. Facial Plast Surg North Am 2006;14:167–173.
14. Michelow BJ, Guyuron B. Rejuvenation of the upper face: A logical gamut of surgical options. Clin Plast Surg 1997;24:199–212.
15. Owsley TG. Subcutaneous trichophytic forehead browlift: The case for an "open" approach. J Oral Maxillofac Surg 2006;64:1133–1136.
16. Ramirez OM. Why I prefer the endoscopic forehead lift. Plast Reconstr Surg 1997;100:1033–1039.
17. Flowers RS, Caputy GG, Flowers SS. The biomechanics of brow and frontalis function and its effect on blepharoplasty. Clin Plast Surg 1993;20:255–268.
18. McKinney P, Mossie RD, Zukowski ML. Criteria for the forehead lift. Aesthetic Plast Surg 1991;15:141–147.
19. Rohrich RJ, Beran SJ. Evolving fixation methods in endoscopically assisted forehead rejuvenation: Controversies and rationale. Plast Reconstr Surg 1997;100:1575–1582.
20. Cook TA, Brownrigg PJ, Wang TD, Quatela VC. The versatile midforehead browlift. Arch Otolaryngol Head Neck Surg 1989;115:163–168.
21. Ramirez OM. Classification of facial rejuvenation techniques based on the subperiosteal approach and ancillary procedures. Plast Reconstr Surg 1996;97:45–55.
22. Oslin B, Core GB, Vasconez LO. The biplanar endoscopically assisted forehead lift. Clin Plast Surg 1995;22:633–638.
23. Ramirez OM. Endoscopic subperiosteal browlift and facelift. Clin Plast Surg 1995;22:639–660.
24. Nassif PS, Kokoska MS, Homan S, Cooper MH, Thomas JR. Comparison of subperiosteal vs subgaleal elevation techniques used in forehead lift. Arch Otolaryngol Head Neck Surg 1998;124:1209–1215.
25. Ramirez OM. Endoscopically assisted biplanar forehead lift. Plast Reconstr Surg 1995;92:323–333.
26. Walden JL, Orseck MJ, Aston SJ. Current methods for brow fixation: Are they safe? Aesthetic Plast Surg 2006;30:541–548.
27. Paul MD. The evolution of the brow lift in aesthetic plastic surgery. Plast Reconstr Surg 2001;108:1409–1424.
28. Wolfe SA, Baird WL. The subcutaneous forehead lift. Plast Reconstr Surg 1998;83:251–256.

4

Rhytidectomy (Facelift)

MANOLIS G. MANOLAKAKIS, DMD

The goal of rhytidectomy, or facelift surgery, is to restore and rejuvenate the youthful appearance of the face and neck that has been lost to the normal aging process (Fig 4-1). For those patients who have unrealistic goals, it is the job of the surgeon to educate them and to present them with realistic outcomes of a rhytidectomy procedure. Once a procedure for the "rich and famous," facelifts have crossed all lines of socioeconomic and ethnic groups, partly due to mass media coverage and widespread Internet exposure, which have catapulted facial cosmetic surgery into the mainstream. This surge in popularity has also produced much misinformation and confusion for patients, which in turn have made the initial consultation with interested patients more challenging. To further complicate matters, marketing campaigns such as "lunchtime facelift" and "mini-facelift" have patients asking for minimal to no downtime.

The most common misconception encountered is the belief that a rhytidectomy will erase all lines and signs of aging. Surgeons are well aware that cervicofacial rhytidectomies correct only a defined and limited set of problems of the lower third of the face: neck laxity, jowling, melolabial folds, and, with more limited success, nasolabial folds. The severity of the aging process determines what type of rhytidectomy and adjunctive procedures are used (see Fig 5-2). To address aging of the upper and middle thirds of the face, endoscopic forehead (see chapter 3) and midface lifting procedures typically are performed in conjunction with cervicofacial rhytidectomy. Oral and maxillofacial surgeons possess the precise knowledge and surgical skills required to perform facial rejuvenating procedures in the complex anatomy of the upper, middle, and lower thirds of the face. Training in orthognathic, reconstructive, and traumatic facial surgery provides the necessary expertise to evaluate, diagnose, and treat underlying skeletal deficiencies to enhance esthetic results of traditional cervicofacial rhytidectomies. In some patients, a facelift is the answer to all of their facial aging concerns, but the majority require simultaneous facial rejuvenation procedures such as forehead lifts, midface lifts, fillers, facial implants, malarplasty, genioplasty, and/or laser resurfacing to provide them with the balanced, esthetic appearance they seek.

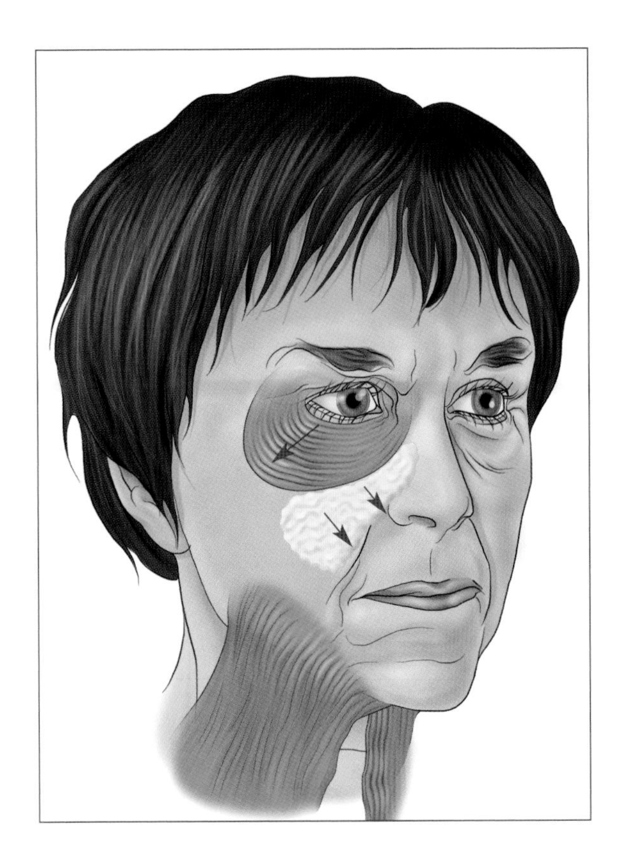

Fig 4-1 Structural effects of middle and lower face aging include weakening of the underlying muscles, inferior descent of suborbicularis and molar fat pads *(arrows)*, deepening of nasolabial folds, and platysmal banding. (Redrawn from Friedman[1] with permission.)

Preoperative Evaluation

A thorough medical history and physical examination of potential patients are absolutely necessary prior to any elective facial cosmetic surgical procedure. It is important to have at least three to four patient interactions prior to performing a rhytidectomy, including the initial consultation with preoperative photographs, the case presentation, the history and physical examination, and the consent-signing appointment with a final review of pre- and postoperative instructions. These patient interactions help the practitioner get a complete understanding of patients' desires, motivations, and dedication toward their facial cosmetic surgeries. It also makes the postoperative course easier not only for the patient but also for the doctor. Patients who smoke are instructed that smoking cessation is required 8 weeks prior to the procedure for better blood supply to facial skin flaps as well as less potential for anesthesia complications.[2] It also is imperative to educate facelift patients on what medications, herbs, and vitamins to avoid prior to surgery. Likewise, it is important to counsel them on what supplements promote healing and recovery. Three weeks prior to surgery, it is recommended that facelift patients start a regimen of supplements that promote cellular activity, healing, and boosting of the immune system. They are placed on multivitamins, vitamin C with glutathione and L-cysteine, free-form amino acids, arnica/bromelain, and the complete vitamin B complex.

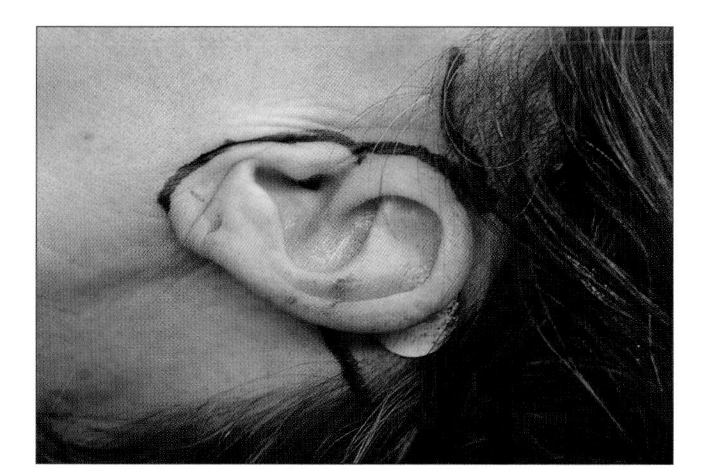

Fig 4-2a Planned incision design.

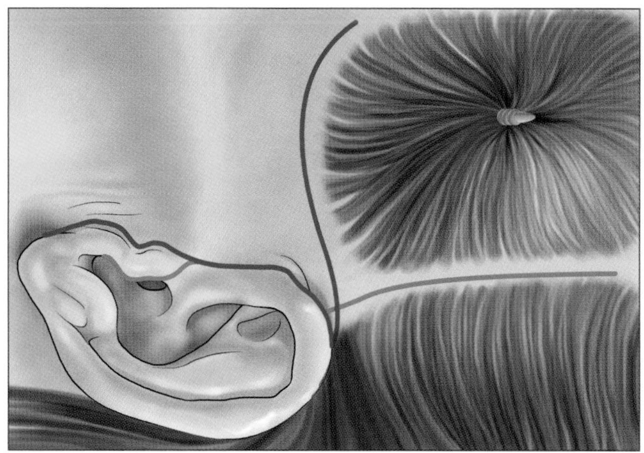

Fig 4-2b A pretrichial incision preserves the temporal tuft, and a preauricular incision *(blue line)* is planned in the natural skin crease. A retrotragal incision *(red line)* is performed if requested.

Surgical Procedures

Patient preparation

After the patient arrives at the surgical center, he or she is asked to change into the patient robe and to wash the face and hair with Phisohex (Bayer) to reduce the amount of skin bacteria. The patient is then brought to the preoperative holding area. Here, the signed consent forms are verified, preoperative baseline vital signs are obtained, last-minute questions are answered, and the patient is reassured that everything will go as planned. At this point, a scopolamine patch is placed behind the patient's ear. An 18-gauge angiocatheter is used to gain intravenous access in the antecubital fossa, and 60 mL of venous blood is drawn and prepared to make platelet-rich plasma to be used under the facial skin flaps prior to closure. The superconcentrated platelets aid in hemostasis and accelerate healing of the soft tissue flaps. The patient is marked in a an upright position and then brought into the operating room, where he or she is induced under general anesthesia with a combination of inhalational and intravenous anesthetics, then intubated with a cuffed oral endotracheal tube (Figs 4-2a to 4-2c). As the patient is prepared and draped in the standard sterile surgical fashion for this type of procedure, the anesthesiologist administers preoperative medications: Unasyn (Pfizer) 3 g intravenous piggyback (IVPB) (clindamycin 600 mg IVPB, if the patient is allergic to penicillin) to reduce the chance of surgical infection, dexamethasone 12 mg to reduce swelling, and ondansetron hydrochloride 4 mg to reduce the risk of postoperative nausea and vomiting. The entire length of the planned incisions is injected with 2% lidocaine with 1:100,000 epinephrine. Next, a modified Klein tumescent anesthesia solution of 500 mL of 0.9% normal saline, 20 mL of 2% plain lidocaine, 1 mL of triamcinolone 10 mg, and 1 mL of 1:1,000 epinephrine is injected into the subcutaneous layer of the face, cervical area, neck, and postauricular regions.[3] Approximately 100 mL of tumescent anesthesia is injected into each side of the face, and another 50 to 75 mL is injected into the submental region (Fig 4-2d). Exactly 10 minutes is allowed to elapse prior to incision, which allows vasoconstriction of the superficial vessels in the subcutaneous layer to take effect and provides a drier surgical field.

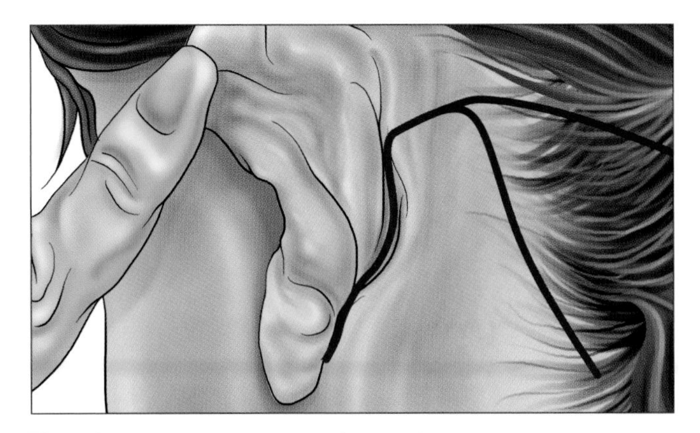

Fig 4-2c Postauricular incision *(blue line)* is placed on conchal cartilage and turns into the hairline at the level of the external auditory canal.

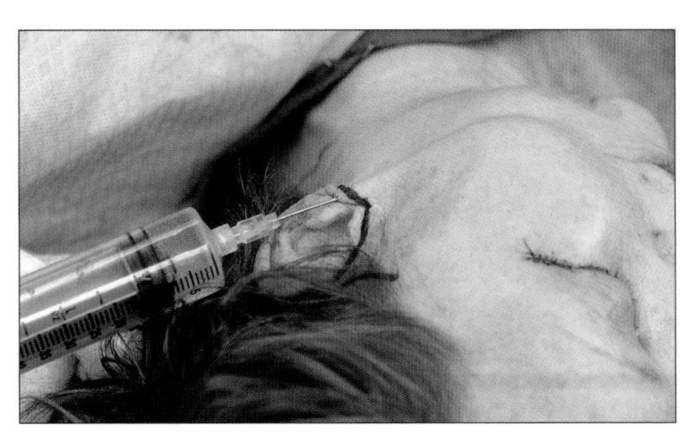

Fig 4-2d Tumescent anesthesia is used to provide local anesthesia and for hemostasis during the case. A 60-mL syringe with an 18-gauge spinal needle is used to inject the solution. The incision line itself is injected with 2% lidocaine with 1:100,000 epinephrine.

Dissection

Attention is first directed to the cervical portion of the procedure. A 2-cm transverse curvilinear incision is made in the midline in a submental crease (see Fig 5-5a). The dominant submental crease should not be used; rather, a crease that is slightly inferior (posterior) should be used. Use of the dominant submental crease can potentially accentuate the crease in the healing phase. The dissection is started by grasping the inferior edge of the incision with a lightweight straight skin hook, and gentle traction of the skin is applied in a direction away from the subcutaneous fat. Kaye facelift scissors are used to carry out a subcutaneous dissection of the submental region (see Fig 5-5b). Once the dissection is carried to the level of the inferior border of the thyroid cartilage, the skin hook is replaced with a small right-angled facelift retractor. At this point, the cervical dissection proceeds laterally within the subcutaneous layer, inferior to the mandibular border and lateral to the anterior border of the sternocleidomastoid muscle (SCM). With Cushing tissue forceps and Kaye facelift scissors, a direct lipectomy of the midline subcutaneous fat is performed. This helps to identify the medial borders of the platysma muscle.

If required, an open suction–assisted lipectomy with a 6-mm spatula liposuction cannula is performed (see Fig 5-7). The spatula is connected to gentle wall suction that provides adequate negative pressure to perform cervicofacial liposuction. When performing submental liposuction, it is wise not to be overly aggressive, because this could lead to scarring of the skin down to the deeper tissues or "cobra neck" deformity. In addition, when performing submental and cervicofacial liposuction, the skin and underlying fat layer should be inspected using a "pinch-and-roll" technique; when the surgeon can feel a thin layer of adipose tissue remaining between two opposing skin layers, an adequate amount of fat has been removed.[4]

Fig 4-2e Endoscopic-assisted subperiosteal midface lift with Endotine Midface ST (Coapt Systems). Temporal dissection is performed through the same incision used for the endoscopic brow lift. A 1.5-cm intraoral vestibular incision is made 4 to 5 mm above the mucogingival line.

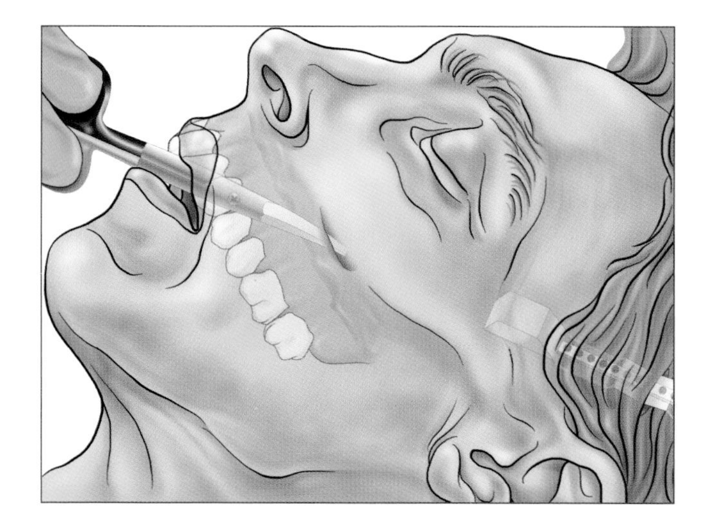

The platysma is addressed next. A 3-0 clear nylon suture is used for platysma suspension. The suture is placed at the edge of the platysma at the level of the new cervicomental angle, which is later suspended to the contralateral mastoid fascia[5] (see Fig 5-6). Some surgeons advocate a horizontal back-cut of the platysma muscle at the level of the hyoid bone, paralleling the inferior border of the mandible for approximately 5 to 7 cm to re-create a more defined cervicomental angle.[6] The author of this chapter has seen patients from other surgeons at 6 months to 1 year postrhytidectomy without submentoplasty or platysmaplasty and believes that submentoplasty is almost always necessary when performing a facelift to provide a longer-lasting, rejuvenated cervicomental angle. Now that both medial edges of the platysma muscle have been identified and isolated, a 3-0 Vicryl (Johnson & Johnson) suture is used in an interrupted fashion, starting at the submental incision and proceeding inferiorly to the level of the thyroid cartilage. This creates a nice muscular sling and tightens the platysmal banding. Hemostasis is evaluated, and open, moist gauze is placed under the submental skin flap.

Attention is now directed toward the facial dissection of the procedure. The objective of the incision design is to prevent temporal hair loss, postauricular step-off, tragal distortion, and pixie ear deformity.[7] At this point, the author typically has already performed an endoscopic forehead lift and addressed the midface lift through the temporal incision and a 1.5-cm intraoral vestibular incision approximately 4 to 5 mm above the mucogingival line (Fig 4-2e). A subperiosteal dissection is carried out over the maxilla and body of the zygoma onto the zygomatic arch. The two planes of dissection are joined through a small incision of bridging fascia at the junction of the zygomatic arch and body. The subperiosteal plane and the previously dissected temporal portion from the endoscopic brow lift (between the temporoparietal and the temporal fascia) are elevated and fixed with the Endotine Midface ST (Coapt Sys-

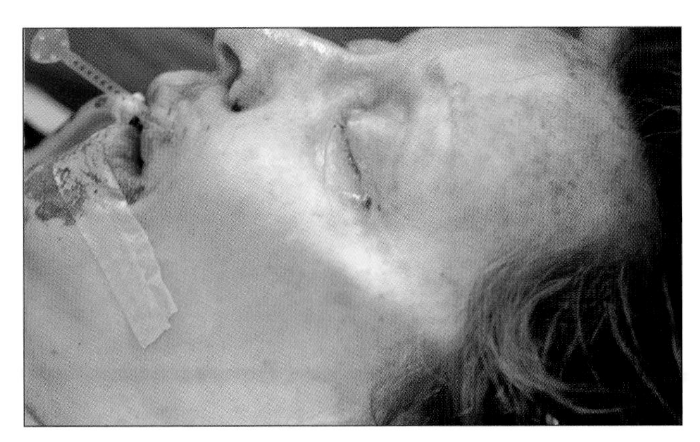

Fig 4-2f A subperiosteal dissection is performed, exposing the entire zygoma and anterior half of the zygomatic arch. The endoscope is introduced into the temporal pocket, directed toward the inferolateral orbital rim. With blunt scissor dissection via an intraoral approach, a 1-cm pocket is created to connect the two dissection pockets. The Endotine Midface ST is introduced via an intraoral approach, pulled through the temporal incision, and secured to the temporal fascia.

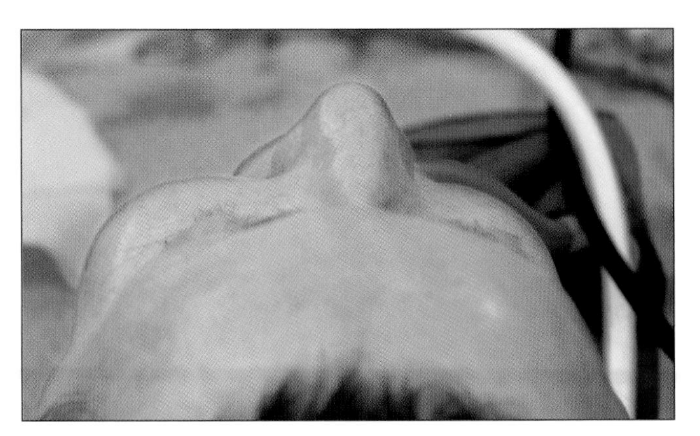

Fig 4-2g Subperiosteal midface lift. The left side is lifted with Endotine Midface ST. A significant difference is appreciated between the left and right sides. Midface lifting restores malar volume, corrects malar ptosis, and decreases lower eyelid length.

tems; Figs 4-2f and 4-2g). Because an endoscopic forehead lift and midface lift are usually performed simultaneously with a facelift, the temporal incision design used is a pretrichial incision with a severe bevel directed superiorly. It is then continued inferiorly into a pretragal incision around the ear lobule attachment, with special care not to incise on the cheek side and not to place the incision on the posterior lobule. Next, the incision travels in the postauricular sulcus for a short distance and then rises on the posterior surface of the conchal cartilage to the level of the external auditory canal. At this level, the incision turns posteriorly into and through the hairline with a very slight inferior downturn (see Fig 4-2a). This incision design prevents poor scar formation, hairline step defects, and pixie ear deformity. Once the incision is complete, the skin flap is elevated.

The subcutaneous dissection is carried to approximately 2 to 3 cm away from the oral commissure and over the malar eminence (Figs 4-2h to 4-2j). Inferiorly, the dissection is carried to the level of the inferior border of the mandible and is connected with the previous cervical dissection. Postauricular dissection is also carried out in a subcutaneous level, and care is taken to protect the great auricular nerve that crosses the SCM at about 6.5 cm inferior to the bony edge of the external auditory canal.[8] The posterior border of this dissection is the anterior border of the trapezius muscle.

There are many variations with regard to superficial musculoaponeurotic system (SMAS) management.[9,10]The author of this chapter uses a sub-SMAS flap with imbrication of the SMAS, unless performing a modified S-lift. The horizontal component originates at the root of the zygoma about 0.5 cm below the zygomatic arch (Fig 4-2k). It continues posteriorly to approximately 1 cm anterior to the tragus. At this point, the incision turns inferiorly and parallels the skin incision line, approximately 1 cm ant-erior to the skin incision. At the level of the ear lobule, the SMAS incision

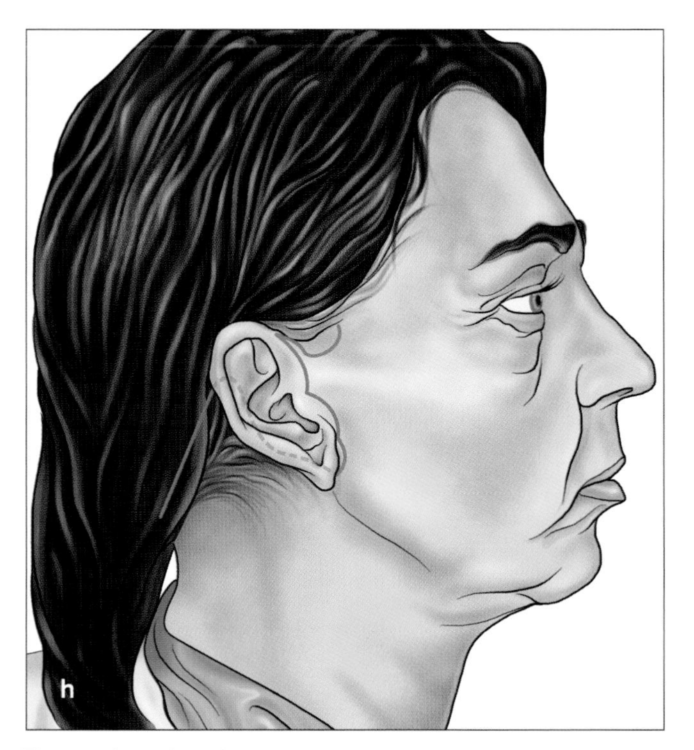

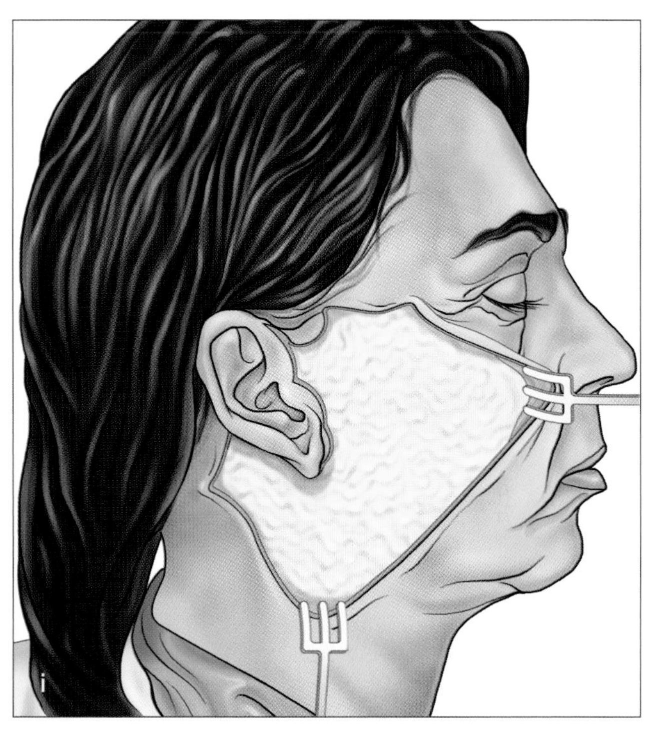

Figs 4-2h and 4-2i *(h)* Facelift incision *(red line)*. Note the pretrichial design to maintain the temporal tuft of hair. The upper face is lifted via an endoscopic approach. *(i)* Subcutaneous dissection.

Fig 4-2j Subcutaneous dissection. Under the skin flap, the dark blue markings indicate the planned incisions of SMAS.

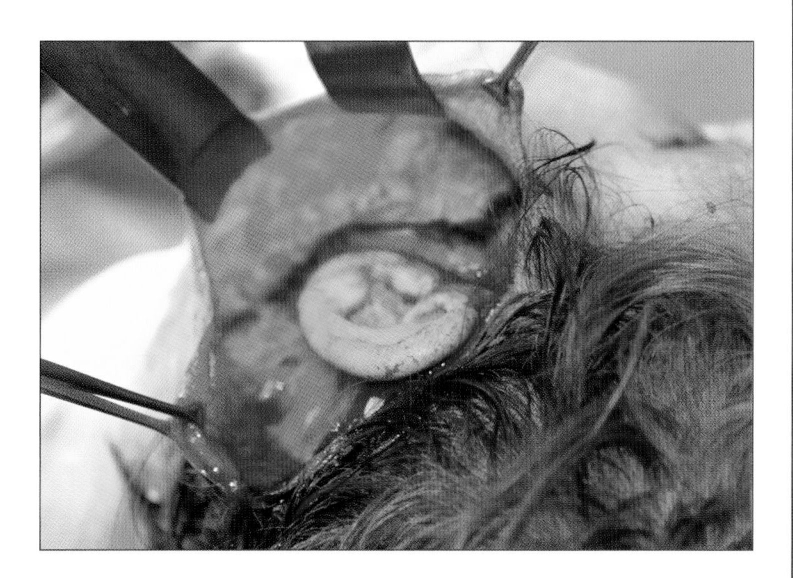

turns slightly posteriorly and continues into the posterior edge of the platysma muscle. The sub-SMAS and subplatysma dissections are carried for approximately 2 to 3 cm (Fig 4-2l). Moderate superoposterior traction is placed on the mobile SMAS flap (Fig 4-2m). A back-cut is made at the most superior and posterior point and is fixed to nonmobilized SMAS with 2-0 Vicryl suture. The remainder of the SMAS flap is

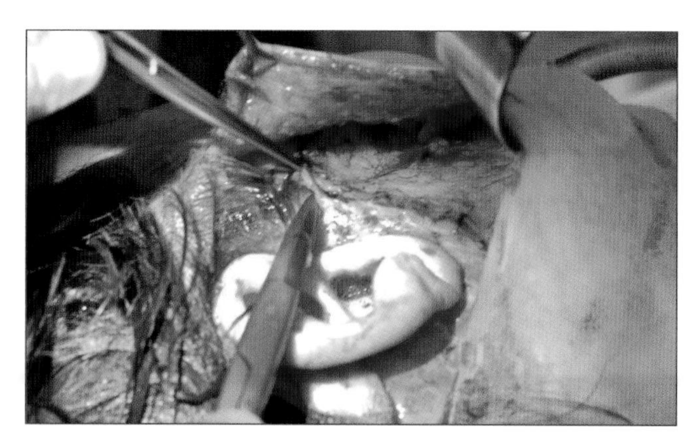

Fig 4-2k Following the planned incision, the SMAS flap is developed to the level of the parotidomasseteric fascia.

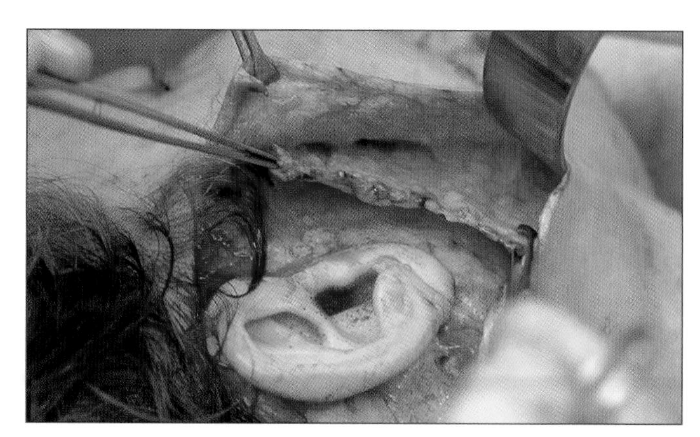

Fig 4-2l Elevated SMAS flap.

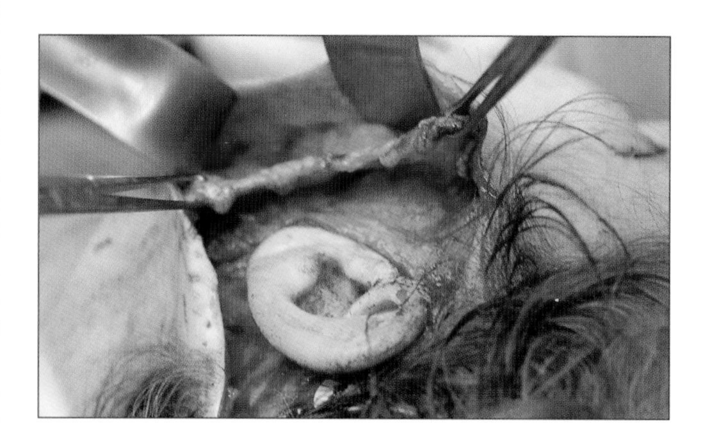

Fig 4-2m Superoposterior vector of pull of elevated SMAS flap.

then positioned, back-cut, and sutured into a more posterosuperior position. It is the positioning of the SMAS and platysma flaps that provides the long-term stability as well as the improvement in the neck and jowl contour. The posterior edge of the platysma is gently grasped, and traction is placed in a posterosuperior direction and sutured with 2-0 Vicryl suture to the mastoid fascia. The excess SMAS and platysma are excised.

The previously marked platysma suspension sutures are now passed under the cervical flap to the contralateral side. The head is slightly turned away while the suture is fixed to the fascia overlying the mastoid process. The suture should be tightened until slight indentation of the underlying soft tissue is appreciated. This is then repeated on the other side. At this time, meticulous control of bleeding is achieved with Bovie cautery. Prior to skin closure, platelet-rich plasma is sprayed under the facial flaps, and pressure is gently applied to the flap while any excess platelet-rich plasma is expressed from under the flap.

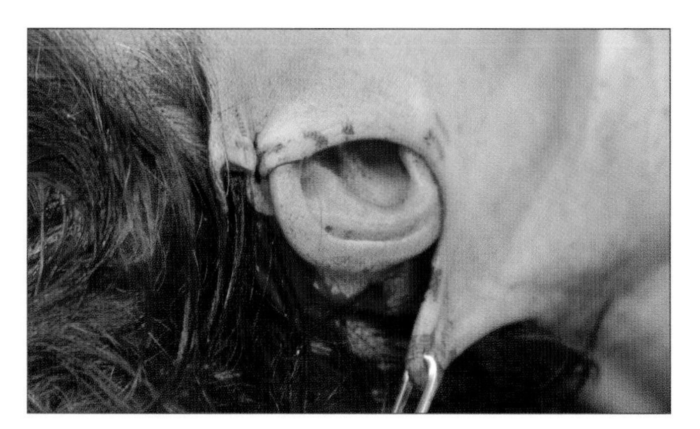

Fig 4-2n Skin flap closure. The initial holding suture is placed at the temporal area just above the ear. A 3-0 silk suture is used. The second suture is placed in the postauricular area, with care to line up the hairline. Slight anterior rotation of the flap is crucial in this part of the flap closure.

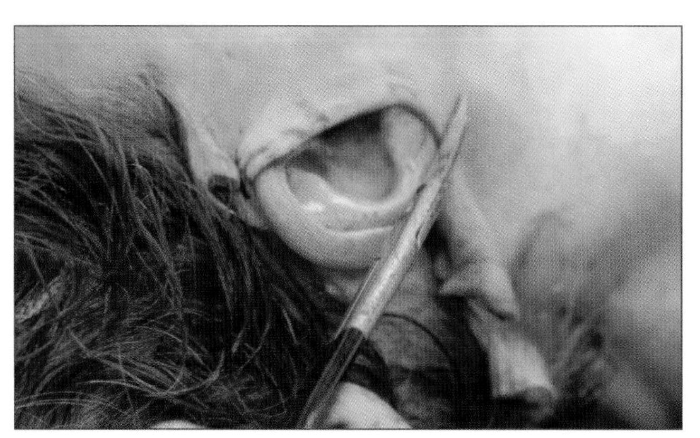

Fig 4-2o Re-create the natural earlobe. Scissors are used to incise the skin flap to the level of the superior lobule. The direction of skin incision should follow the helical cartilage. When the earlobe is brought out from underneath the skin flap, there should be slight bunching of the earlobe, which prevents pixie ear defect.

Skin flap closure

Skin closure is now undertaken. It is vital that the skin be closed under minimal tension, which reduces the chances of scar widening, lessens the risk of flap necrosis, and minimizes the lifted appearance. It is also important that the head be placed in a neutral position. Extension and flexion of the head influence how much tissue is excised and can adversely affect the results.[11] The skin flap should primarily be pulled in a superior position with a posterior component. The initial stitch is placed near the temporal area, just above the ear (Fig 4-2n). The second stitch is placed in the postauricular region, where the incision turns into the hairline. It is very important to have the hairline and incision lined up to prevent a step deformity in the hairline. Once both of these sutures are in place, the lobule rests under the flaps. Scissors are used to part the flap and expose the lobule. The direction of the cut outlines the helical rim and stops at a level approximating the level of the superior portion of the lobule (Fig 4-2o). The incision does not extend to the inferior aspect of the lobule; doing so would create unnecessary tension and risk a pixie ear deformity.[7]

The excess skin is precisely excised with facelift scissors, and 5-0 polydioxanone suture (PDS, Ethicon) is placed in the subdermis layer. In the mastoid process and hair-bearing area, 3-0 silk is used. The postconchal portion is closed with 5-0 PDS in the subdermal layer and 6-0 nylon on the skin. The temporal portion of the flap is closed with 3-0 silk. The submental incision is then closed with 5-0 PDS in the subdermal layer and then with 6-0 nylon on the skin. The incisions are dressed with nonadherent bandages and antibiotic ointment. The ears are padded on the anterior and posterior surfaces to prevent pressure damage. A Kerlix bandage (Covidien) is wrapped first around the head and submental area in a coronal fashion, and then it is wrapped from the forehead around the occiput. Coban (3M) is then wrapped around the head and neck to provide a light pressure. Care must be taken to avoid applying too much pressure to the facial flaps, because this may cause flap necrosis.

Postoperative Care

Postoperative care starts immediately after the facial wrap is applied and prior to extubation. It is very important that the anesthesiologist be aware that a nice, calm extubation is required, because anything else may cause coughing, choking, and straining. This type of wake-up may lead to hematoma formation. The patient is observed in the recovery room for 2 to 3 hours while vital signs are monitored and clear liquids are allowed. Postoperative nausea and vomiting are evaluated, and appropriate medications are administered. Prior to discharge, the facial wrap is removed, and the incision lines and flaps are evaluated. The facial dressing is then reapplied. The postoperative course for rhytidectomy typically is anxiety ridden but not painful. Valium and postoperative analgesics are prescribed. The author suggests that valium be taken rather than analgesics, unless they are absolutely necessary. The benzodiazepines help with postoperative nausea as well as anxiety. Almost all patients report that valium is very beneficial during the postoperative course. The patient is provided a neckroll pillow and instructed to sleep with the head elevated with three pillows. If the patient has a recliner at home, he or she is instructed to sleep in it. The patient is evaluated at 24 hours postoperatively in the office to evaluate skin flap perfusion, edema, bleeding, and the need for evacuation of hematomas and/or the placement of a pressure dressing. The patient is then reevaluated after 48 hours and provided with a facioplasty garment to be worn at night for 3 weeks. Sutures should be kept clean of eschar with a 1:1 mixture of hydrogen peroxide and water. This provides the best healing environment. The patient can resume hair washing at 5 days. Skin sutures and hair sutures are removed at 5 and 10 days postoperatively, respectively. The patient is advised to limit head turning for 2 to 3 weeks to decrease the potential of widening of postauricular scars. Ultraviolet protection and limiting sun exposure help facial scars heal without hyperpigmentation.

Adjunctive Procedures

It is quite common to perform other simultaneous facial cosmetic surgical procedures with a facelift. As mentioned before, a rhytidectomy procedure mainly addresses the lower third of the face. To achieve a well-balanced, rejuvenated, esthetic result, it is important that the upper and middle portions of the face resemble the lower third. It is equally important that the patient's skin condition be addressed prior to surgery. Typically, some form of prescription skin care with 0.05% tretinoic acid and 4% hydroquinone is started at the time of initial consultation. This prepares the skin for future treatments such as chemical peels or laser resurfacing, depending on its condition. By improving the appearance of the skin with topical prescriptions and resurfacing procedures, the facelift is greatly enhanced. Chemical peels and laser resurfacing can be performed before, after, or concomitantly with the facelift. Some surgeons perform laser resurfacing at the same time the facelift is performed. Extreme care must be taken with laser treatment of the facial skin near the incision line.

Changes seen with midfacial aging are not adequately addressed with traditional rhytidectomy alone.[12] The descent of the malar fat pads is in an inferomedial direction and results in midfacial aging signs that include lengthening of the lower eyelid, skeletonization of the infraorbital rim, pseudoherniation of the orbital fat, and a more pronounced nasolabial fold.[13] It also creates a double convexity midface deformity (Fig 4-3) with loss of cheek projection, which is observed in the senescent

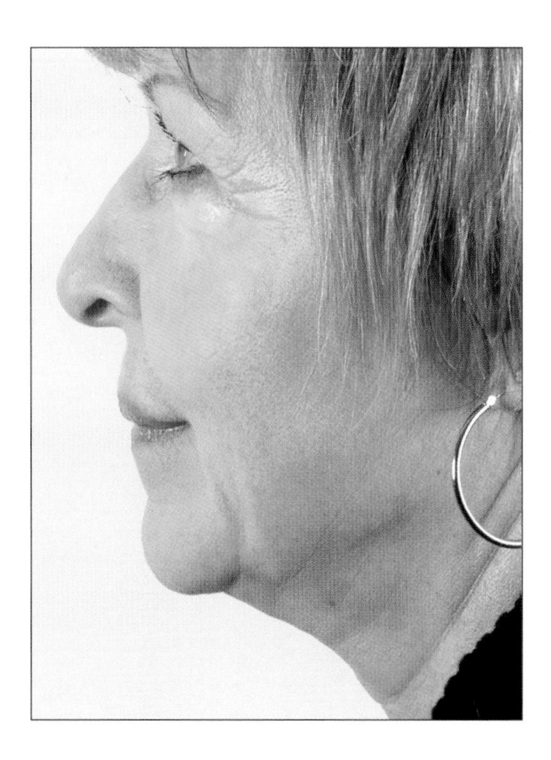

Fig 4-3 Midfacial aging signs: Lengthening of the lower eyelid, pseudoherniation of the orbital fat pads, ptotic midface, and skeletonization of the infraorbital rim. Descent of malar fat pads causes a double convexity midface deormity.

population.[14] This part of the face has been addressed via multiple approaches and multiple surgical planes. When there are many different ways to address certain aging processes, there are usually some limitations to each of the procedures. As the malar fat pads descend in the aging face, the resultant loss of volume can be restored with midface lifting procedures, fat augmentation, fillers, or malar/submalar silicone implants.[15–17] The author's preferred method of addressing the midface is through a subperiosteal midface lift or malar/submalar silicone implants.

The surgical method for the midface lift is an endoscopic approach via the same temporal incision that is used for the endoscopic forehead lift. An incision that is approximately 2.5 cm in curvilinear fashion is made approximately 2.5 cm behind the hairline. The middle of the incision is bisected by a line from the lateral aspect of the ala of the nose through the lateral canthus of the eye into the hair. The incision is made with a severe bevel that allows for hair growth through the scar. This incision is carried down to the level of the temporal fascia, just inferior to the temporoparietal fascia. This is the same plane of dissection for the endoscopic brow lift. After the endoscopic brow dissection is completed, the midface dissection is addressed. Dissection is carried inferiorly to the level of the zygomatic arch. At this point, attention is directed intraorally. A 1.5-cm incision 4 to 5 mm above the mucogingival line is made with a Bovie cautery or radiofrequency. This incision is carried down to bone. A subperiosteal dissection is performed with a periosteal elevator to the inferior orbital rim, above the zygoma and onto the zygomatic arch. Visualization of the infraorbital nerve is accomplished. At this point, the assistant inserts the endoscope into the temporal pocket that was dissected. Through the intraoral approach, long facelift scissors are used to dissect through the remaining bridge of tissue that separates the temporal pocket from the subperiosteal pocket.

The Endotine Midface ST is used to lift the midface tissues into a more superolateral position. The tail of the endotine is inserted in a retrograde fashion through the vestibular incision. Through the temporal incision, a large tonsillar clamp is used to grasp the endotine and pull it superiorly through the temporal incision. The tines are then engaged to the malar soft tissue at the level of the nasolabial fold. Once the malar fat pads are lifted to the desired level, the endotines are then fastened to the temporal fascia with a 2-0 Vicryl suture. Midface lifting may create bunching of the lower eyelid. If no fat is to be removed from the lower eyes, then lower skin excision blepharoplasty is to be performed after the midface lift (see chapter 7). If needed, fat is removed via a transconjunctival approach, and then lower eyelid skin is removed. This technique does not violate the muscle layer of the lower eyelid, and it significantly reduces the chance of ectropion or scleral show.

Complications

Complications after surgery can be stressful for both the patient and the surgeon. The best mechanism a surgeon has for avoiding complications is to be as meticulous as possible in all aspects of the rhytidectomy. Preoperatively, the surgeon must sit down with the patient and educate him or her about the upcoming procedure. Most importantly, the patient must be aware of the common, expected, and temporary complications, including decreased sensation, tightness, and bruising.

Hematoma

Hematoma is the most common complication of the rhytidectomy procedures. It occurs with a reported frequency of 1% to 15%.[18–21] Hematomas can range from small collections of blood to large expanding clots. The need for surgical intervention ranges from 1.9% to 3.6%.[20,21] The majority of large expanding hematomas that occur within the first 24 hours after surgery are associated with acute pain, swelling, and ecchymosis. Other signs include hardness of overlying skin, tightness, trismus, anxiety, and dyspnea. Late signs include more swelling and discoloration of the lips and buccal mucosa.[22] Management of hematomas ranges from placing sterile suction through the postauricular incision to releasing some sutures to expressing the blood through the incision line. Expanding hematomas require immediate surgical intervention, including wound exploration, clot evacuation, and hemostasis of any bleeding vessels. Failure to treat these emergencies could lead to flap necrosis.

Postrhytidectomy hematomas can be associated with multiple events, including coughing, vomiting, and straining. Perioperative hypertension has been shown to be closely linked to postrhytidectomy hematomas. A preoperative systolic pressure greater than 150 mm Hg has been shown to be associated with increased hematoma formation, 9.2% compared with an overall incidence of 1.6%.[23] Postoperative hypertension has also been shown to increase hematoma formation. Berner et al[24] studied 202 facelift patients. They observed that patients' postoperative blood pressures during the first 2 hours of recovery were similar to their preoperative blood pressures. During the subsequent 3 hours, most patients' blood pressures were in excess of their preoperative systolic blood pressures. This reactive hypertension increases with pain and anxiety and can be properly controlled with

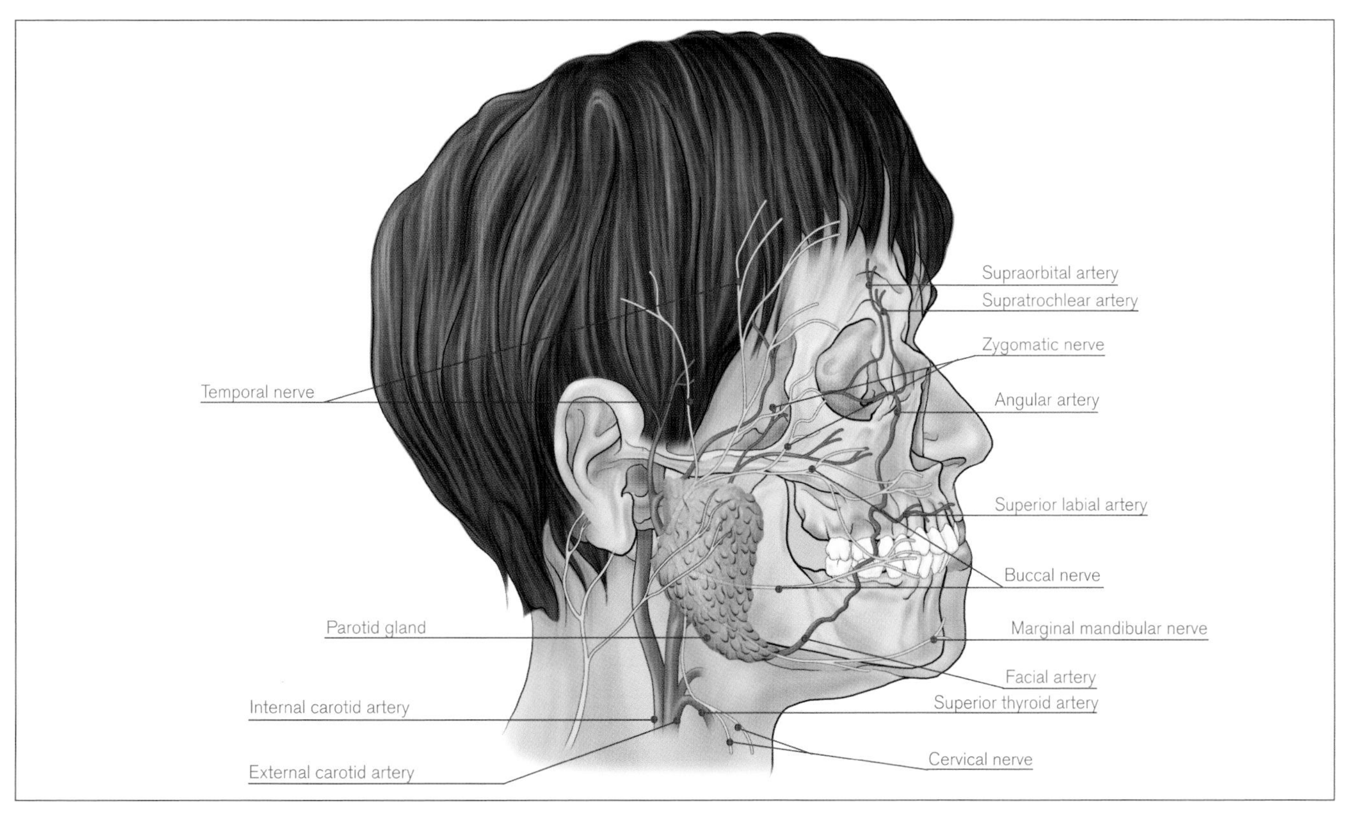

Fig 4-4 Facial nerve anatomy and arterial supply.

analgesics and benzodiazepines. Furthermore, Kamer and Kushnick[25] found a twofold increase in expanding hematoma when propofol was used for anesthesia (2% in the nonpropofol group versus 4.2% in the propofol group). Treatment with propofol caused a 26% drop in systolic blood pressure, compared with a 16% drop in the nonpropofol group. This finding indicates that antihypertensive medications should be continued throughout the perioperative period. Adjunctive methods for hemostasis, such as fibrin glue, desmopressin acetate, and platelet-rich plasma, have been used and reported on with conflicting results.[18,26–28] Meticulous hemostasis prior to closure is the most important aspect of preventing large expanding hematomas.

Nerve injury

The most common nerve injury is to the great auricular nerve (Fig 4-4). This nerve consistently crosses the SCM at 6.5 cm below the caudal edge of the bony external auditory canal (Erb point). It travels under the SMAS and the platysma to reach the anterior border of the SCM.[8] A superficial dissection of the skin over the SCM helps prevent injury to the great auricular nerve. Less common are injuries to the facial nerve. The majority of these injuries are neurapraxia from excessive retraction, the heat of cautery, or needles. Baker[20] reviewed over 7,000 facelifts reported in the literature and found only 55 cases of paralysis, 7 of which were permanent. The most common branch injured was the marginal mandibular, followed by the temporal nerve, followed by the buccal branch. The marginal mandibular nerve lies below the platysma muscle in the superficial layer of the deep cervical fascia.[29] When a subplatysma flap is developed, care must be taken to avoid injuring the marginal mandibular nerve. The temporal branch is at risk when a forehead or brow lift is combined with a facelift. Pitanguy and Ramos[30] noted that the temporal branch has a consistent course extending from 0.5 cm below the tragus to 1.5 cm above the lateral brow. In the area superior to the arch, the nerve travels within the temporoparietal fascia. Safe dissection to avoid the temporal nerve during the forehead lift is in a surgical plane immediately superior to the temporalis fascia. Although permanent motor nerve injuries are rare, sound surgical skill and expert knowledge of facial anatomy are of the utmost importance in preventing them.

Necrosis

Skin flap necrosis is associated with either vascular congestion or arterial compromise, which is frequently related to unrecognized hematoma, tobacco use, diabetes, or excessive wound closure tension. The most susceptible areas of skin sloughing are the postauricular and mastoid regions because of the thinness of the skin and its distance from the vascular supply. Reese et al[2] determined that the risk of flap necrosis increases by a factor of 12 in patients who use tobacco products. The author of this chapter requires patients to stop smoking for 8 weeks prior to facelift procedures, which helps reduce both the risk of skin necrosis and anesthesia complications.

Scarring

Unsightly rhytidectomy scars are mainly caused by increased wound tension and poor suture technique. After the SMAS/platysma flap is elevated and imbricated, excess skin should be trimmed in such a fashion that the skin flap rests passively in the preauricular region. Placing buried sutures relieves some of the tension on the skin and provides a better chance of thin scar formation. Widened scars occur mostly in the postauricular area. Even modest wound closure tension may result in a widened scar. Poorly placed incisions and excessive skin removal result in subsequent scar contracture, which can lead to pixie ear deformity or obliteration of the sulcus between the earlobe and cheek (Fig 4-5). Tragal retraction is a common complication with a retrotragal incision (Fig 4-6).

Hair loss

Hair loss is most likely to occur in the preauricular region. Distortion of the temporal tuft may occur by elevating the tuft to an unnatural level (Fig 4-7). This can easily be avoided by placing a pretrichial, severely beveled incision at the temporal tuft area. Posterior hairline distortion occurs when the postauricular flap is not pivoted in the anterior direction and alignment of the hairline is neglected.

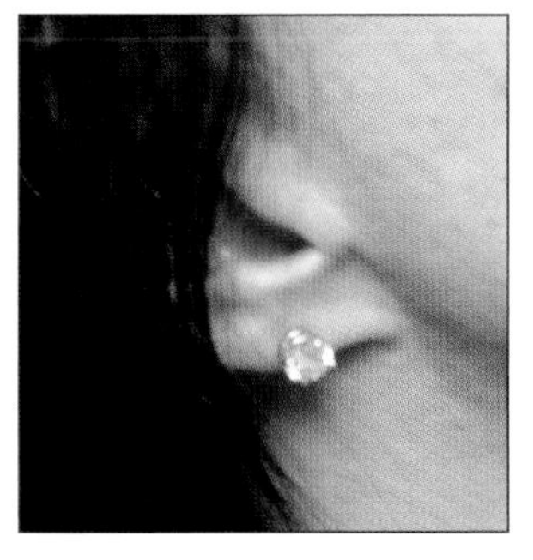

Fig 4-5 Pixie ear deformity.

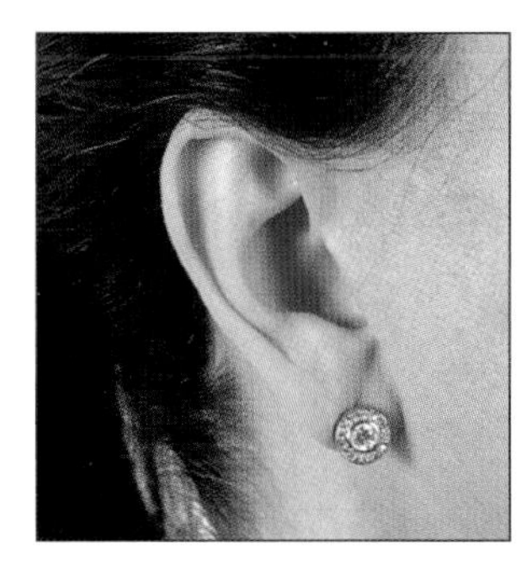

Fig 4-6 Tragal retraction.

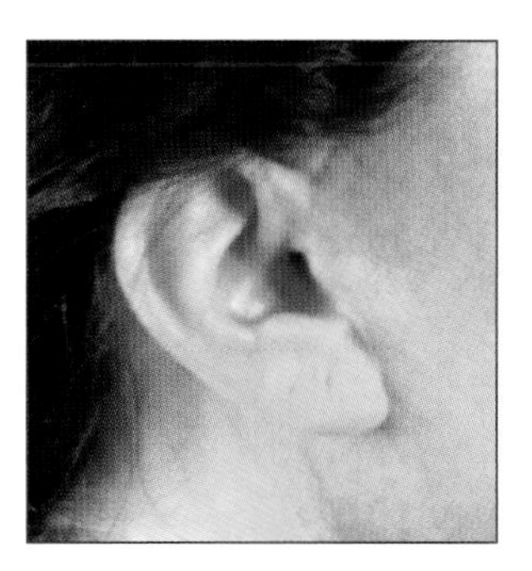

Fig 4-7 Loss of temporal tuft.

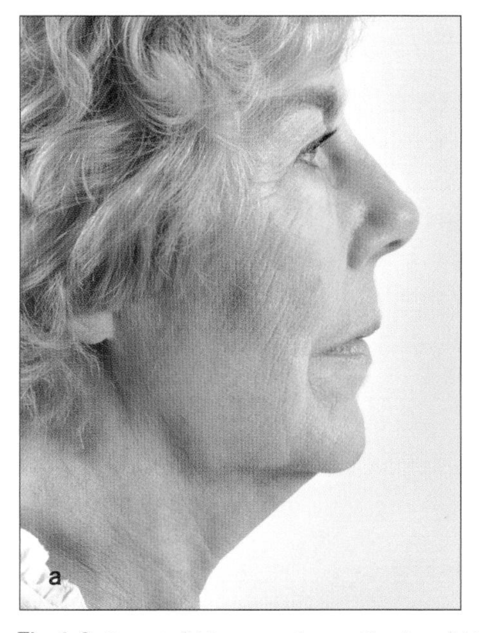

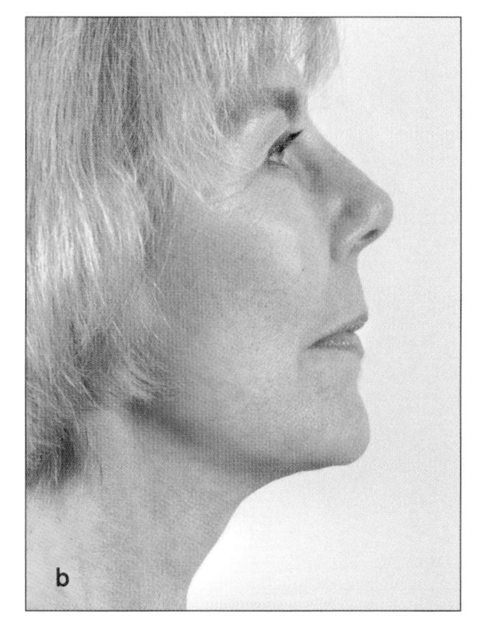

Fig 4-8 Case 1. *(a)* Preoperative profile view. *(b)* Postoperative subperiosteal midface lift, sub-SMAS rhytidectomy, and platysmaplasty with necklift.

Depression

Depression occurs in about 30% of women undergoing rhytidectomy and is usually related to facial edema, bruising, and distortion.[31] Generally, all that is needed is emotional support and reassurance.

Case Reports

Case 1

A 66-year-old woman with advanced facial aging presented with submental lipomatosis, deep nasolabial folds, malar ptosis, and jowling (Fig 4-8a). She underwent rhytidectomy with sub-SMAS dissection and imbrication, platysmaplasty with neck suspension, and subperiosteal midface lift with Endotine Midface ST (Fig 4-8b).

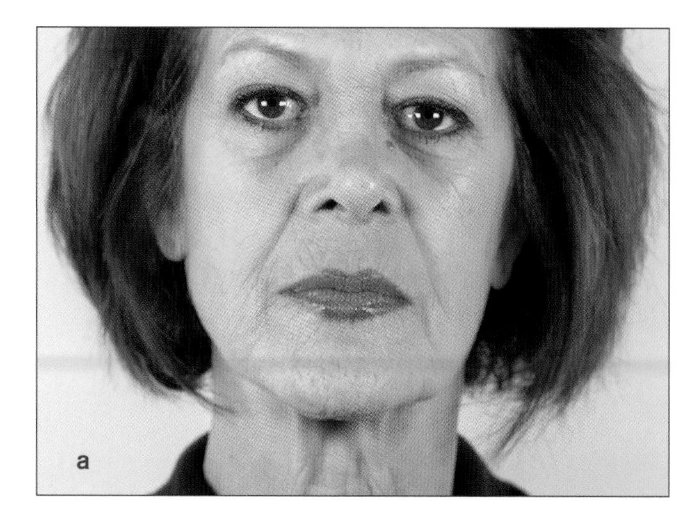

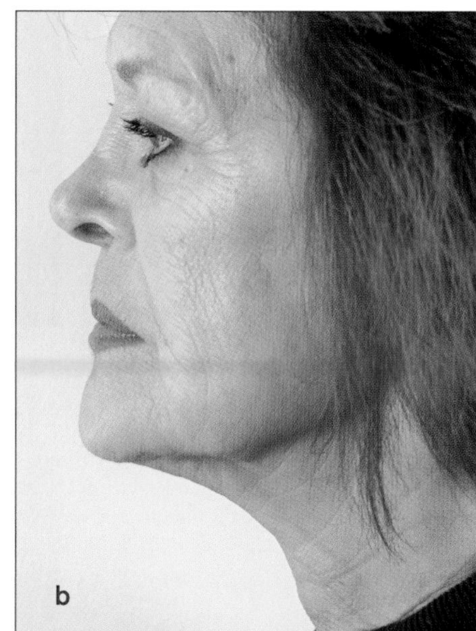

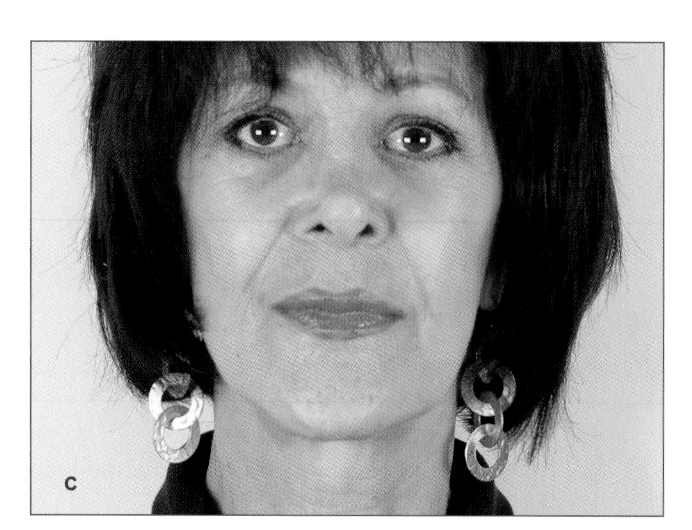

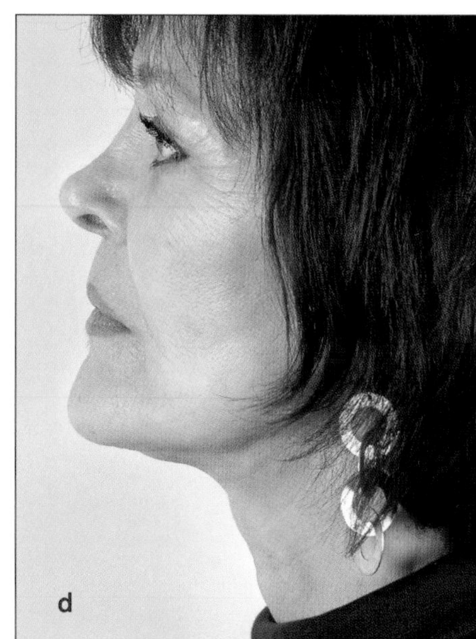

Fig 4-9 Case 2. *(a and b)* Preoperative views. *(c and d)* Postoperative views.

Case 2

A 62-year-old woman with advanced facial aging presented with photodamaged skin, brow ptosis, upper and lower eyelid dermatochalasis with pseudoherniation of fat pads, malar ptosis, deep nasolabial folds, jowling, platysmal banding, and submental lipomatosis (Figs 4-9a and 4-9b). She underwent endoscopic brow lift, subperiosteal midface lift with Endotine Midface ST, lower blepharoplasty, sub-SMAS dissection and elevation rhytidectomy, platysmaplasty with neck suspension, and fractionated CO_2 laser resurfacing. After 6 months, she returned for upper blepharoplasty (Figs 4-9c and 4-9d).

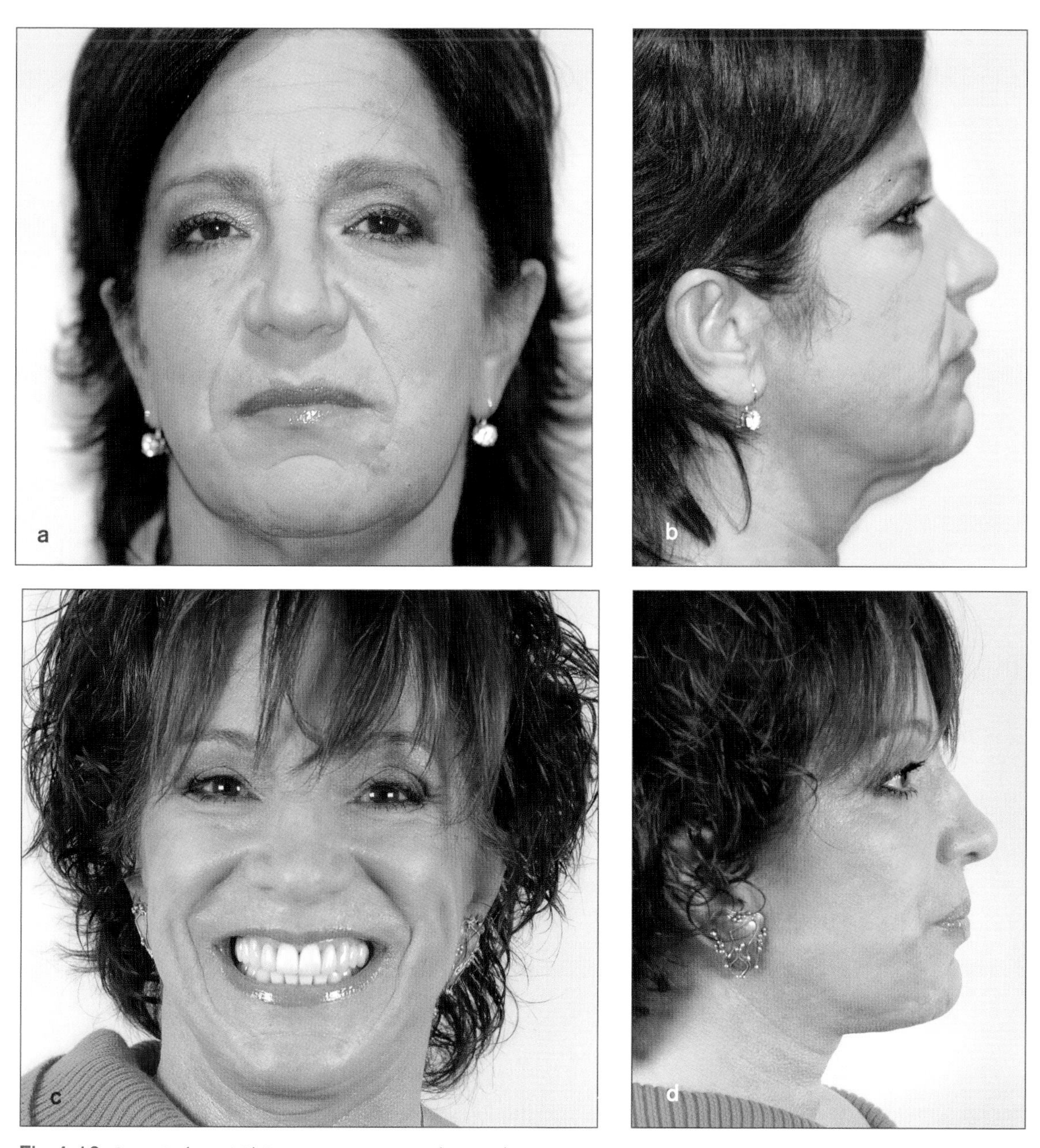

Fig 4-10 Case 3. *(a and b)* Preoperative views. *(c and d)* Postoperative views.

Case 3

A 51-year-old woman with advanced facial aging presented with severely photodamaged skin and dynamic and static rhytids of the forehead, glabella, and periocular areas. She exhibited brow ptosis, upper and lower eyelid dermatochalasis with pseudoherniation of fat pads, deep nasojugal folds, malar ptosis, deep nasolabial folds, melolabial folds, jowling, platysmal banding, and submental lipomatosis with skin laxity (Figs 4-10a and 4-10b). She underwent endoscopic brow lift, upper and lower blepharoplasty, subperiosteal midface lift with Endotine Midface ST, sub-SMAS dissection and imbrication rhytidectomy, submental open liposuction/lipectomy, platysmaplasty with neck suspension, and erbium laser resurfacing (Figs 4-10c and 4-10d).

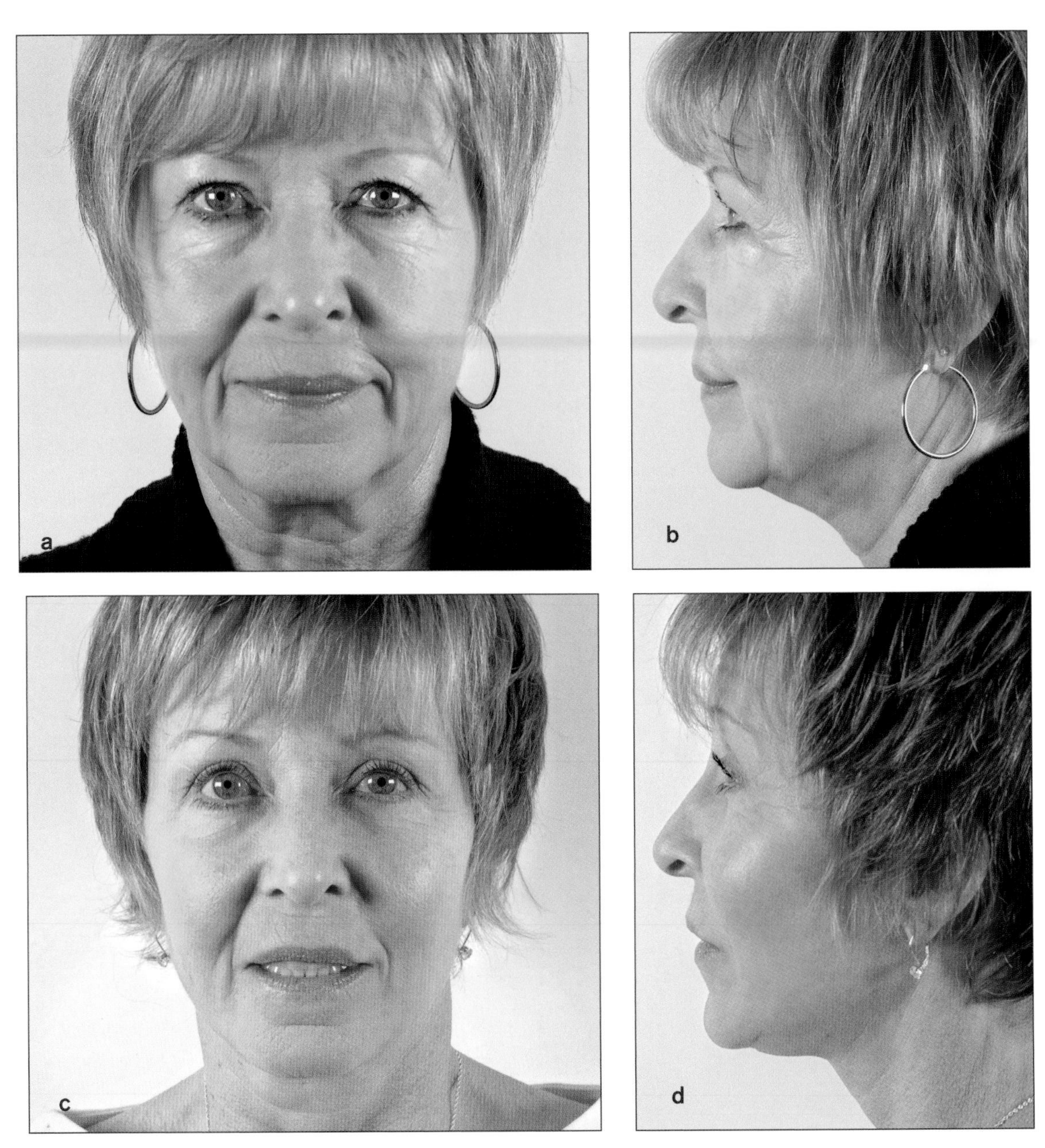

Fig 4-11 Case 4. *(a and b)* Preoperative views. *(c and d)* Postoperative views.

Case 4

A 53-year-old woman presented with advanced facial aging, photodamage, brow ptosis, upper and lower dermatochalasis, malar ptosis, deep nasolabial folds, melolabial folds, jowling, perioral rhytids, submental lipomatosis, and platysma banding (Figs 4-11a and 4-11b). She underwent endoscopic brow lift, subperiosteal midface lift with Endotine Midface ST, lower eyelid blepharoplasty, sub-SMAS dissection and imbrication rhytidectomy, submental open liposuction/lipectomy, platysmaplasty, and neck suspension. Three months later she underwent upper eyelid blepharoplasty and laser resurfacing (Figs 4-11c and 4-11d).

Summary

Cervicofacial rhytidectomy is arguably the most image-altering cosmetic procedure performed. Many different types of rhytidectomy procedures exist. Constant evolution of the technique with regard to incision design, SMAS manipulation, suturing, and adjunct procedures has improved rhytidectomy results and provided a more natural, well-rested appearance. Several factors that optimize facelift results include working with healthy skin, addressing the midface, and performing adjunctive procedures.

Rhytidectomy Tray

- Scalpel handle no. 3, two (Biomet)
- Scalpel handle no. 15, two (Biomet)
- Kaye lightweight knife handle, two (Snowden-Pencer)
- Webster diamond-lite titanium needle holder (Snowden-Pencer)
- Adson-Brown forceps (tungsten carbide), two (Biomet)
- Kaye facelift 7-inch diamond SerEdge scissors (Snowden-Pencer)
- Cushing 7-inch tissue forceps (tungsten carbide), two (Snowden-Pencer)
- Cottle retractor (Snowden-Pencer)
- Lightweight straight skin hook (Snowden-Pencer)
- Kelly forceps, two (Snowden-Pencer)
- Backhaus towel forceps, two (Snowden-Pencer)
- Small facelift retractor (Snowden-Pencer)
- Large facelift retractor, baby deaver (Biomet)
- Allis atraumatic tissue clamps (Biomet)
- Mayo scissors (Snowden-Pencer)
- Iodine cup (Biomet)
- Strabismus scissors (Snowden-Pencer)
- Blepharoplasty scissors (KLS-Martin)
- Frazier-tip suction (KLS-Martin)
- Aspirating syringe, two (KLS-Martin)
- Mosquito hemostat, four (Snowden-Pencer)

References

1. Friedman O. Changes associated with the aging face. Facial Plast Surg Clin North Am 2005;13: 371–380.
2. Reese TD, Liverett DM, Guy CL. The effect of cigarette smoking on skin-flap survival in the facelift patient. Plast Reconstr Surg 1984;73:911–913.
3. Schoen SA, Taylor CO, Owsley TG. Tumescent technique in cervicofacial rhytidectomy. J Oral Maxillofac Surg 1994;52:344–347.
4. Watson D. Submentoplasty. Facial Plast Surg Clin North Am 2005;13:459–467.
5. Giampapa VC, Di Bernardo BE. Neck recontouring with suture suspension and liposuction: An alternative for the early rhytidectomy candidate. Aesthetic Plast Surg 1995;19:217–223.
6. Cuzalina LA, Koehler J. Submentoplasty and facial liposuction. Oral Maxillofac Surg Clin North Am 2005;17:85–98.
7. Miller TR, Eisbach KJ. SMAS facelift techniques to minimize stigmata of surgery. Facial Plast Surg North Am 2005;13:421–431.
8. McKinney P, Katrana DJ. Prevention of injury to the greater auricular nerve during rhytidectomy. Plast Reconstr Surg 1980;66:675–679.
9. Baker DC. Minimal incision rhytidectomy (short scar face lift) with lateral SMASectomy. Aesthet Surg J 2001;21:68–79.
10. Hamra ST. Composite rhytidectomy. Plast Reconstr Surg 1992;90:1–13.
11. Ghali GE, Milton D. Rhytidectomy. In: Fonseca RJ, Turvey TA, Marciani RD (eds). Oral Maxillofacial Surgery. Vol III: Orthognathic Surgery, Esthetic Surgery, Cleft and Craniofacial Surgery, ed 2. Philadelphia: Saunders, 2009:497–512.
12. Pontius AT, Williams EF 3rd. The extended minimal incision approach to midface rejuvenation. Facial Plast Surg Clin North Am 2005:13:411–419.
13. Williams EF 3rd, Lam SM. Upper and midfacial rejuvenation. In: Williams EF 3rd, Lam SM (eds). Comprehensive Facial Rejuvenation: A Practical and Systemic Guide to Surgical Management of the Aging Face. Philadelphia: Lippincott, Williams & Wilkins, 2004:54–104.

14. Owsley JQ Jr, Zweifler M. Midface lift of the malar fat pad: Technical advances. Plast Reconstr Surg 2002;110:674–685.
15. Quatela VC, Marotta JC. Pitfalls of midface surgery. Facial Plast Surg Clin North Am 2005:13: 401–409.
16. Coleman SR. Facial contouring with lipostructure. Clin Plast Surg 1997;24:347–367.
17. Niamtu J 3rd. Accurate and anatomic midface filler injection by using cheek implants as an injection template. Dermatol Surg 2008;34:93–95.
18. Jones BM, Grover R. Avoiding hematoma in cervicofacial rhytidectomy: A personal 8-year quest. Reviewing 910 patients. Plast Reconstr Surg 2004; 113:381–387.
19. Grover R, Jones M, Waterhouse N. The prevention of haematoma following rhytidectomy: A review of 1078 consecutive facelifts. Br J Plastic Surg 2001;54:481–486.
20. Baker DC. Complications of cervicofacial rhytidectomy. Clin Plast Surg 1983;10:543–562.
21. Rees TD, Barone CM, Valauri FA, Ginsberg GD, Nolan WB 3rd. Hematomas requiring surgical evacuation following face lift surgery. Plast Reconstr Surg 1994;93:1185–1190.
22. Moyer JS, Baker SR. Complications of rhytidectomy. Facial Plast Surg Clin North Am 2005;13: 469–478.
23. Straith RE, Raju DR, Hipps CJ. The study of hematoma in 500 consecutive facelifts. Plast Reconstr Surg 1977;59:694–698.
24. Berner RE, Morain WD, Noe JM. Postoperative hypertension as etiological factor in hematoma after rhytidectomy: Prevention with chlorpromazine. Plast Reconstr Surg 1976;57:314–319.
25. Kamer FM, Kushnick SD. The effect of propofol on hematoma formation in rhytidectomy. Arch Otolaryngol Head Neck Surg 1995;121:658–661.
26. Man D, Plosker H, Wildland-Brown JE. The use of autologous platelet-rich plasma (platelet gel) and autologous platelet-poor plasma (fibrin glue) in cosmetic surgery. Plast Reconstr Surg 2001;107: 229–237.
27. Marchac D, Sándor G. Facelifts and sprayed fibrin glue: An outcome analysis of 200 patients. Br J Plast Surg 1994;47:306–309.
28. Oliver D W, Hamilton SA, Figle AA, wood SH, Lamberty BG. A prospective, randomized, double-blinded trial of the use of fibrin sealant for face lifts. Plast Reconstr Surg 2001;108:2102–2105.
29. Ziarah HA, Atkinson ME. The surgical anatomy of the cervical distribution of the facial nerve. Br J Oral Maxillofac Surg 1981;19:171–179.
30. Pitanguy I, Ramos AS. The frontal branch of the facial nerve: The importance of its variations in face lifting. Plast Reconstr Surg 1966;38:352–356.
31. Goin MK, Burgoyne RW, Goin JM, Staples FR. A prospective psychological study of 50 female face-lift patients. Plast Reconstr Surg 1980;65: 436–442.

5

Cosmetic Management of the Neck

CORTLAND S. CALDEMEYER, DDS
ELIE M. FERNEINI, DMD, MD, MHS

Most people are concerned with the cosmetic appearance of their neck and are aware of changes that occur in this area as they age. As a result, facial cosmetic surgery continues to increase.[1] Those patients who seek treatment for these changes frequently desire a more defined jawline, removal of excess fat under the chin, and tightened skin in the neck. The success of a cosmetic surgery practice is driven by patient satisfaction and predictable surgical outcomes. Like all areas of facial cosmetic surgery, a thorough understanding of anatomy and adequate patient assessment are critical to setting realistic expectations and obtaining successful surgical outcomes in the neck region.[2]

Applied Anatomy

The main muscles to identify in the neck are the platysma and the sternocleidomastoid (SCM) (Fig 5-1). The platysma is a superficial muscle that overlaps the SCM muscle. It is a broad-based, flat, thin muscular sheet that extends across the neck. Inferiorly, the platysma is attached to the subclavicular and acromial soft tissues and runs obliquely and medially to the mandible. It functions in facial expression by lowering the inferior lip. The superficial layer of the deep cervical fascia extends between the trapezius and SCM in the posterior triangle and between the SCM in the anterior triangle. The marginal mandibular branch of the facial nerve may be located close by, within, or just deep to the superficial layer of the deep cervical fascia. Superiorly, the platysma is continuous with the superficial musculoaponeurotic system (SMAS). Posteriorly, the platysma and SMAS are continuous with the fascia surrounding the SCM. The sternal head of the SCM originates at the anterior surface of the manubrium and its clavicular head at the medial third of the clavicle. It inserts at the mastoid process. The SCM turns the chin toward the opposite side. The carotid sheath lies deep to the SCM. Overlying the platysma is a fat layer that is variable in volume, especially at the anterior third of the mandible and at the suprahyoid region. Fat in the submental regions can be either supraplatysmal or in the subplatysmal space. This subplatysmal space is bounded laterally by the digastrics, superficially by the platysma muscle, and deeply by the mylohyoid muscle. On average, 30% of the submental fat is located at the subplatysmal level, but the amount can be as much as 57%.[3] Also located in this space are the submental artery[4] and the anterior jugular veins in the midline, as well as the facial artery and vein, the marginal mandibular nerve, and the submandibular gland laterally. Finally, the medial fibers of the platysma muscle typically interlace at the midline, forming an inverted V shape. The platysma has three types of fibers distributed in the suprahyoid region (Box 5-1).

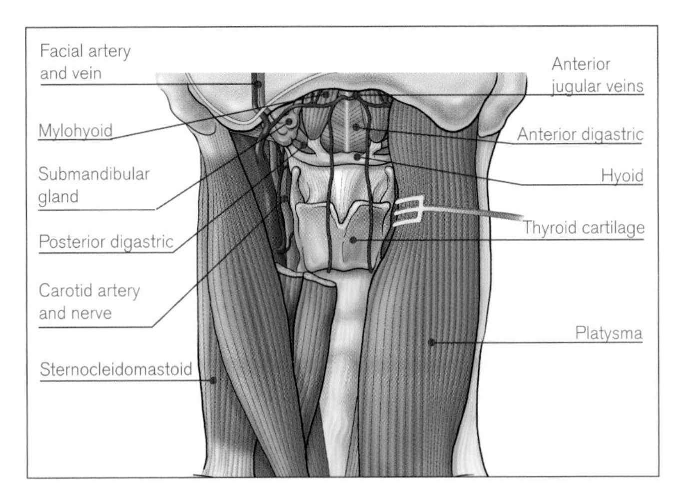

Fig 5-1a **Anterior anatomical view of the neck region.**

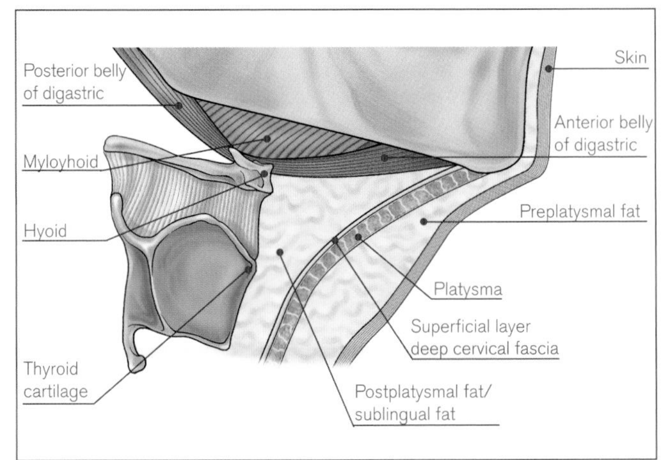

Fig 5-1b **Sagittal anatomical view of the neck.**

Box 5-1	Types of platysmal muscle fiber distribution in the suprahyoid region of the neck[4,5]
Type I	Medial muscle fibers that decussate 1 to 2 cm below the chin but are separate in the suprahyoid region. Occurs in 75% of patients.
Type II	Medial muscle fibers that decussate all the way down to the thyroid cartilage, covering the submentum like a sling. Occurs in 15% of patients.
Type III	Medial muscle fibers that are separate and do not decussate at all in the submental region. The fibers insert directly at the chin. Occurs in 10% of patients.

Preoperative Evaluation

During any cosmetic surgical consultation, it is necessary to review the patient's general health status, past medical history, medications (including vitamins and supplements), allergies, and previous surgeries. Tobacco history must be elicited and documented. The effects of nicotine are important to wound healing and critical to planning any elective facial cosmetic surgical procedure. Discontinuing tobacco use before and after a cosmetic neck surgery may be recommended, depending on the invasiveness of the planned procedure. In addition, any history of anticoagulation must be elicited from the patients. Patients are usually advised to avoid aspirin, vitamin E, and nonsteroidal anti-inflammatory drugs for 2 to 3 weeks prior to surgery. It is important to remember that many nutritional supplements taken by patients today should be investigated thoroughly for anticoagulation properties and managed appropriately. A patient's Fitzpatrick skin type should be assessed. Patients with a higher Fitzpatrick skin type are more prone to hypertrophic scar and keloid formation as well as pigmentation changes in the surgical area. Pathologic conditions such as salivary gland or thyroid disease should also be ruled out.[2] After the baseline preliminary history, attention can be turned to the cosmetic aspects of the case. Features of a youthful neck include a distinct inferior mandibular border, a subthyroid depression, a visible thyroid cartilage, and a visible anterior SCM border[6,7] (Fig 5-2a). A cosmetic evaluation of the submental area should begin with the patient's hyoid position. An ideal neckline or cervicomental angle ranges from 105 to 120 degrees. In general, the more posterior and superior the hyoid bone positioning, the more youthful and esthetic the neckline. This angle becomes more obtuse with the aging process. It is critical that the position of the hyoid bone be identified because it determines where the cervicomental angle will likely measure after surgery.[9] The patient's skin laxity, neck asymmetry, consistency and content of adipose tissue, and platysmal integrity should be assessed. Submental skin laxity, also termed *submental cutis laxis*,[1] increases with age because of the breakdown of collagen and elastin. As a result, wrinkles develop due to the pull of the facial musculature and gravitational effects (Fig 5-2b). This laxity causes skin sag at the mandibular line and accentuates the jowls. In addition, prejowl sulci and submandibular gland prolapse can occur.[10] Fat and soft tissue descent along the mandibular line obscures the fine bony definition of the mandible. Fat accumulation in the neck and ptosis of the skin result in jowling (Fig 5-2c). With the aging process, fat deposits in the neck occur. This fat usually localizes in the submental and submandibular areas. The platysma muscle becomes flaccid. However, the medial portion becomes fibrous and contracted, resulting in platysmal bands (Fig 5-2d).[11] Sometimes a chin implant is recommended to address retrognathia or microgenia or to camouflage an anteriorly positioned hyoid bone (Figs 5-2e and 5-2f).

Patients should be allowed to express their concerns about the face and neck. Following this initial work-up, a cosmetic assessment can be performed. During a consultation, it should be communicated that younger patients with more elasticity of the skin are usually good candidates for less invasive procedures such as liposuction and isolated open lipectomy without platysmaplasty. Older patients with decreased skin elasticity have lower predictable outcomes with these procedures and can be better treated by more invasive open procedures such as submentoplasty and isolated necklift procedures. A reasonable understanding of these aspects of patient assessment is critical to setting realistic patient expectations.[9]

With an understanding of the anatomy of the area, acceptable patient assessment, and an informed patient consent that includes drawings indicating the proposed facial incision lines, cosmetic surgery of the neck can be considered. The remainder of this chapter focuses on five surgical techniques in order from least invasive (most predictable) to most invasive (least predictable): *(1)* serial release of platysmal bands, *(2)* submental liposuction, *(3)* submental lipectomy with or without platysmal plication, *(4)* submentoplasty, and *(5)* posterior necklift with platysmal suspension.

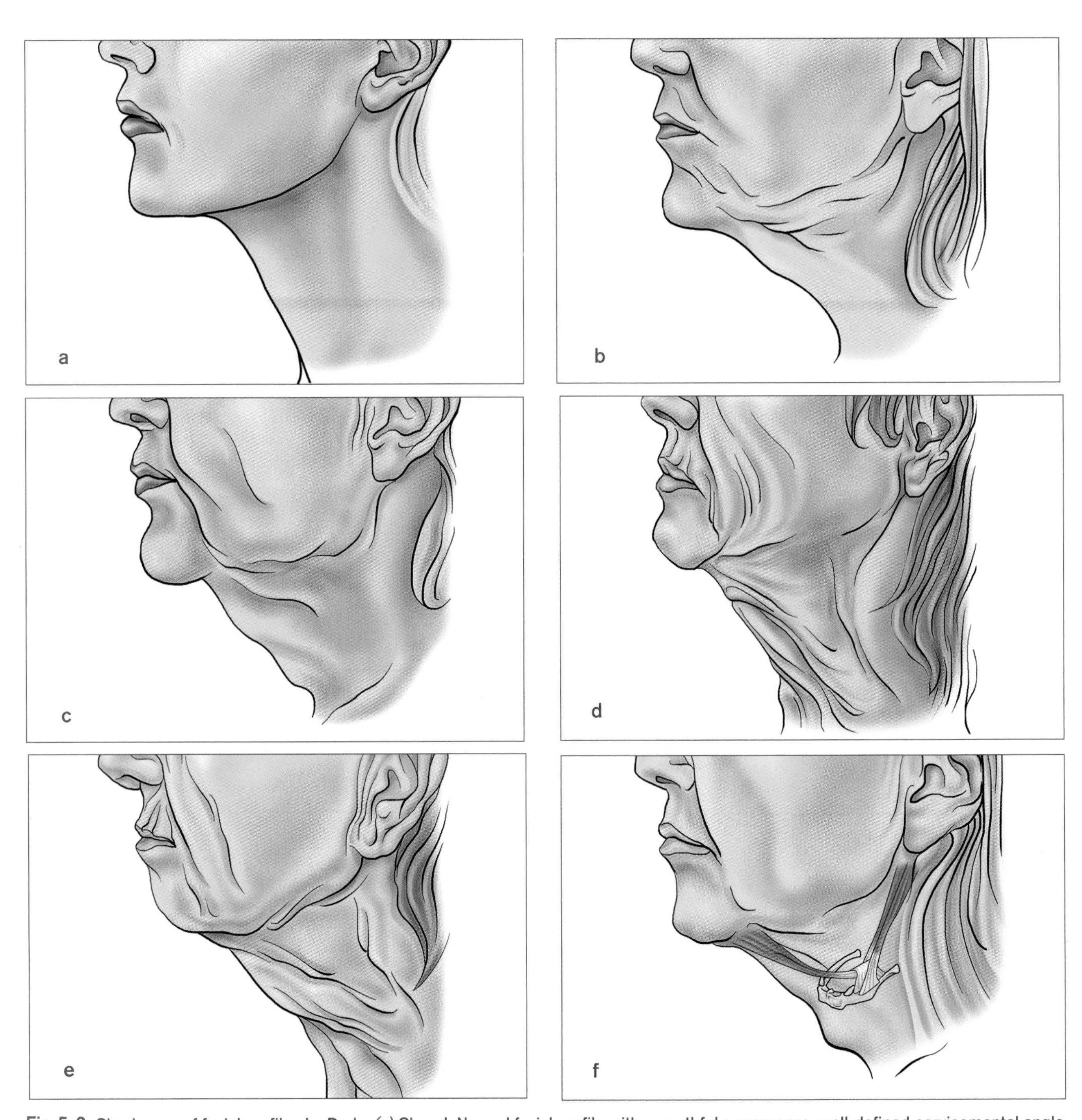

Fig 5-2 Six classes of facial profiles by Dedo. *(a)* Class I: Normal facial profile with a youthful appearance, well-defined cervicomental angle, good muscle tone, and no submental fat. *(b)* Class II: Skin laxity creates an obtuse cervicomental angle. *(c)* Class III: Submental fat accumulation results in an obtuse cervicomental angle. *(d)* Class IV: Platysma muscle banding. *(e)* Class V: Retrognathia and/or microgenia diminish the cervicomental angle. *(f)* Class VI: Inferior hyoid bone placement reduces the cervicomental angle. (Modified from Ghali and Evans[8] with permission.)

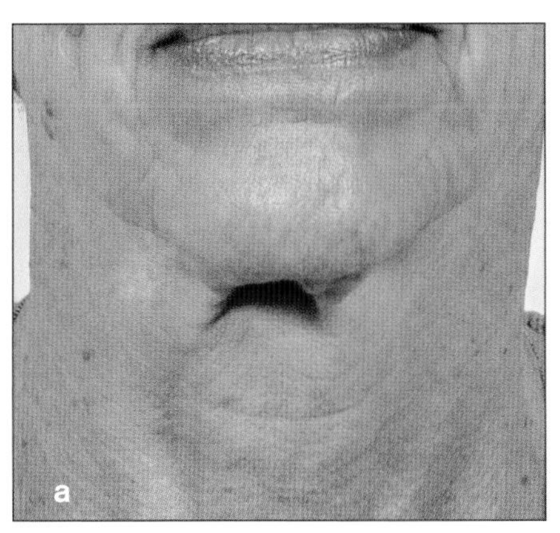

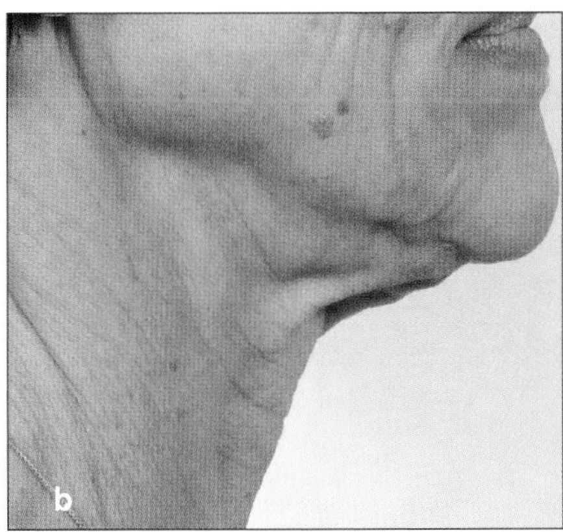

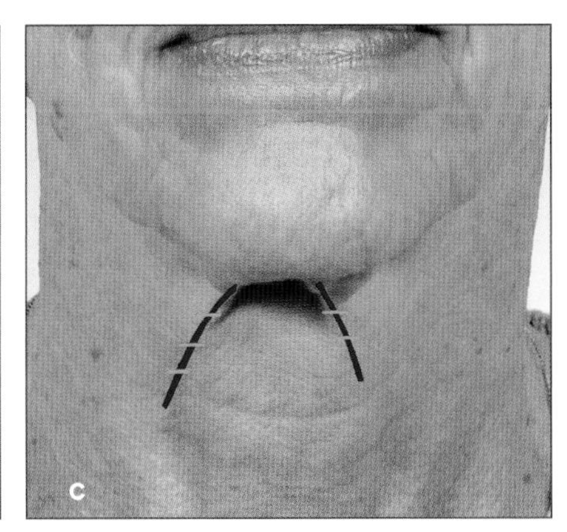

Fig 5-3 *(a and b)* **Frontal and profile views of a patient with platysmal banding.** *(c)* **Serial platysmal notching.**

Surgical Procedures

Serial release of platysmal bands

With the more invasive open procedures described in the following sections of this chapter, a submental incision is used to gain access to the platysma muscle, which allows for traditional platysmaplasty. Sometimes, however, a patient's sole concern is isolated platysmal banding. The submental approach may seem overly invasive for those who require only minor platysmaplasty without simultaneous lipectomy or submentoplasty. These patients are usually those who have been satisfied with the results of botulinum toxin for the treatment of isolated platysmal banding but unhappy with its duration and the need for repeated treatment. These patients are good candidates and often will be receptive to the idea of serial notching of the platysma as described by Saylan.[12]

The procedure is carried out in the following way: The patient is placed in the upright position and prepared in a standard fashion (Figs 5-3a and 5-3b). The platysmal bands are marked with a vertical line. The band is divided into fourths or fifths, and the two middle fourths, or the three middle fifths, are marked with small 1- to 2-mm horizontal incisions (Fig 5-3c). It is recommended with all surgical markings that the proposed surgical area be cleaned with alcohol and allowed to dry before preparing the area with scrub solutions (Betadine, Purdue Pharma). This prevents the ink from the surgical marker from rubbing off with application of the surgical preparation.[4] Next, the patient is prepared, local anesthesia with epinephrine is administered, and 5 to 7 minutes is allowed for vasoconstriction to take effect. A no. 11 blade is then used to make a stab incision in the proposed site through the skin. The platysmal band is carefully dissected, delivered through the incision with a hemostat, and released with either the no. 11 blade or electrocautery. The incision is then closed with a 6-0 nylon suture, and the patient is scheduled for follow-up in 1 week.

Fig 5-4 Planned submental liposuction to address minimal fat accumulation in the submental area.

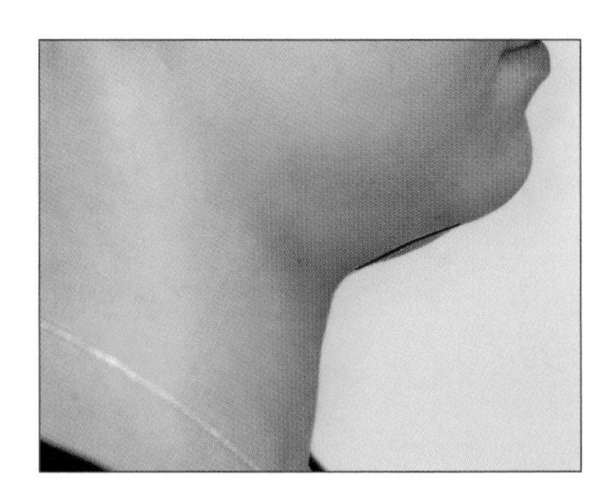

Box 5-2 Tumescent solution[14]

- 500 mL normal saline
- 20 mL 2% lidocaine (400 mg of lidocaine) (35 mg/kg maximum dosage in highly dilute form for tumesence[1])
- 1 mL epinephrine 1:1,000 (1 mg epinephrine)
- 1 to 2 mL triamcinolone (10 to 20 mg)

Optional: Bicarbonate can be added at 10 mEq/L to reduce the burning on injection if the procedure is being done under local anesthesia[1]

Submental liposuction

For patients with minimal platysmal banding, minimal submental fat deposits, and good skin elasticity, supraplatysmal submental liposuction is a good treatment option (Fig 5-4). It is important to keep in mind that the goal of submental liposuction is not complete removal of the fat in the supraplatysmal submental region[13] but rather a resculpting of the fat from this area to facilitate cosmetic future readaptation and shrinking of the overlying skin. This controlled process is facilitated by the use of smaller 1- to 2-mm cannulas rather than the large spatulated cannulas of the past.[9] Before starting this procedure, the surgeon must recognize that there are potential drug interactions with the tumescent solution recommended in liposuction (Box 5-2). Drugs that inhibit the hepatic enzyme cytochrome P-450 can increase lidocaine toxicity. These include selective serotonin reuptake inhibitors (eg, sertraline hydrochloride), benzodiazepenes, proton pump inhibitors, antifungal medicines, calcium channel blockers, and macrolide antibiotics. The maximum dose of lidocaine should be decreased by half in patients taking these drugs.[9] In addition, caution should be used in patients taking monoamine oxidase inhibitors or β-blockers and in patients with hyperthyroidism because of the epinephrine content in the tumescent solution.[9] Clonidine as a premedicant has been shown to greatly reduce the incidence of intraoperative and postoperative tachycardia with the use of tumescent solution.[9]

The procedure is carried out in the following manner: The skin is cleaned with alcohol. A 1- to 2-mm incision is marked in the midline just inferior to the submental crease, and the areas of greatest concern are outlined with a surgical marker[9] (see Fig 5-4). Next, the patient is prepared in a standard fashion, and a 22-gauge spinal needle is then used to inject 75 to 100 mL of tumescent solution (see Box 5-2) through the proposed incision site into the subcutaneous supraplatysmal plane to distend the subcutaneous submental plane.[2] Five to 7 minutes is allowed for vasoconstriction to take effect, after which a no. 11 blade is used to make a stab incision through the skin of the proposed incision site. A 1- to 2-mm liposuction cannula is inserted through the skin with the liposuction tip opening directed toward the platysma. Liposuction is safely performed between, but not crossing, the inferior borders of the mandible laterally (to prevent injury to the marginal mandibular nerve), the angles of the mandible posteriorly, and the superior border of the thyroid cartilage inferiorly. Each pass of the cannula should be directed with the dominant hand through new openings in the tissue, with the nondominant hand palpating the tip of the cannula and contour of the tissue.[9] When an adequate amount of fat has been removed and recontouring of the tissue is considered acceptable, the incision is closed with one or two 6-0 nylon sutures. A standard gentle pressure dressing is then applied with a 4-inch-wide rolled gauze, and fluffed standard 4 × 4–inch gauze pads are placed between the rolled gauze and the surgical area. The patient is seen for follow-up on the first postoperative day, and the dressing is removed. The patient is then given a facelift bra to be worn as much as possible for the first week and at night for the second postoperative week.

Submental lipectomy

For patients with platysmal banding, supraplatysmal fat deposits, and moderate skin laxity, submental lipectomy with platysmal plication, when indicated, is a sound but slightly more invasive treatment option. Submental lipectomy is carried out through a 2- to 3-cm submental incision[15] that allows adequate access for the direct removal of larger amounts of adipose tissue than can be removed with liposuction. The direct visual access also helps facilitate contouring of the area to better promote the expected future readaptation of the overlying skin. In addition, this open submental approach also allows for inspection of the platysma muscle. If a dehiscence is diagnosed and entrance into the subplatysmal space is not indicated, repair, or plication, of the platysma can then easily be performed.

The procedure is carried out in the following manner: The patient is prepared in a fashion similar to the liposuction patient, but the proposed incision is a 2- to 3-cm curvilinear site just inferior to, but not directly in, the submental crease (Fig 5-5a). Placing the incision directly in the submental crease can lead to accentuation or deeping of the crease with healing.[4] Next, a no. 15 blade is used to incise the skin along the proposed incision line. No liposuctioning is recommended at this point because a thick, healthy submental flap is desired.[9] Facelift scissors are used to undermine the subcutaneous tissue in the supraplatysmal plane, identical to the area of liposuction proposed, and create a healthy skin flap (Fig 5-5b). Next, supraplatysmal lipectomy with direct adipose tissue recontouring is performed with facelift scissors or electrocautery. When removal and contouring of the fat is considered adequate, the platysma is inspected for integrity. If a dehiscence is noticed, a platysmal plication is performed in a posterior to anterior direction, beginning at the level of the thyroid cartilage with 4-0 Vicryl sutures

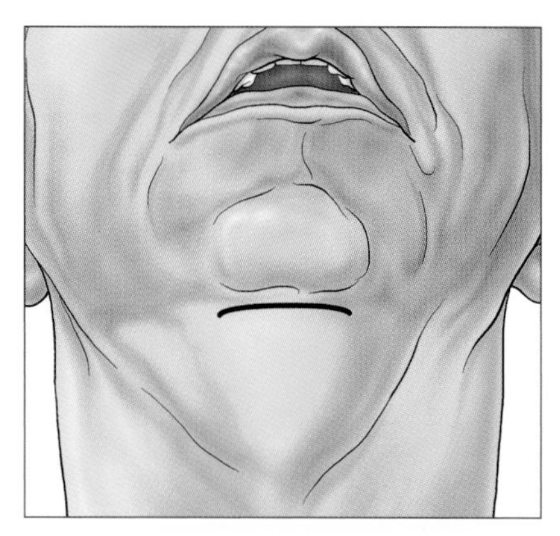

Fig 5-5a Planned submental incision design. An incision, approximately 2.5 cm wide with a slight posterior curve, is made just posterior (inferior) to the prominent submental crease.

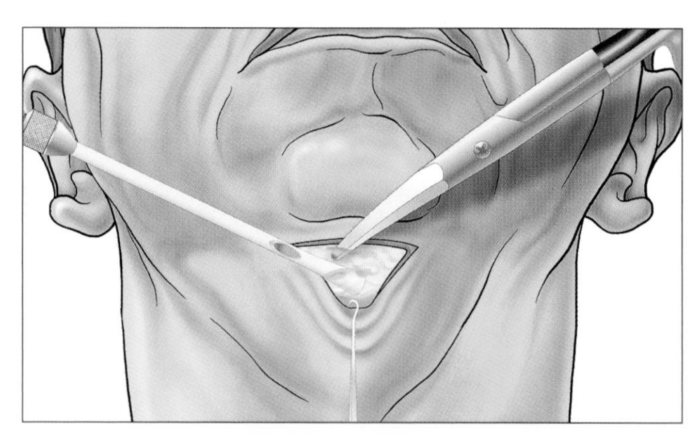

Fig 5-5b Dissection in the subcutaneous level using Kaye facelift scissors.

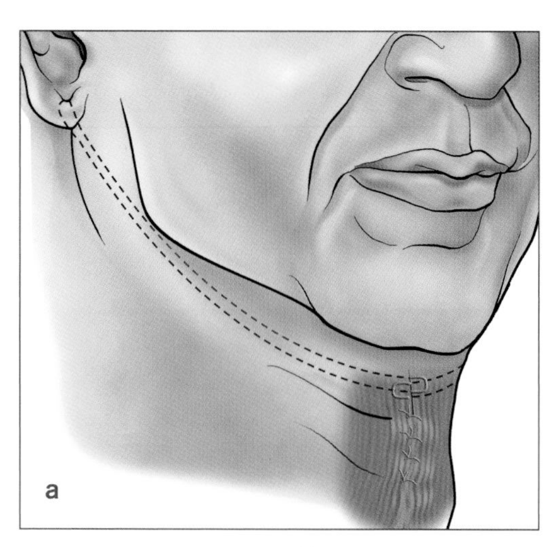

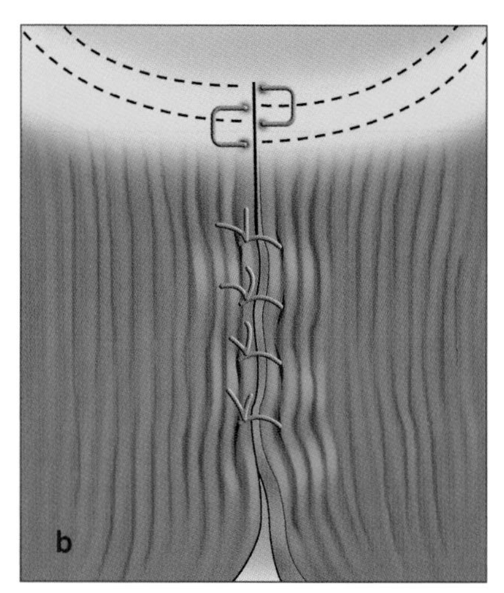

Fig 5-6 *(a)* Platysmal plication technique. *(b)* Detailed view showing the medial edge of the platysma muscle tagged with 3-0 clear nylon sutures at the level of the hyoid bone. The platysma decussation is then repaired with 4-0 Vicryl sutures. The clear nylon is later passed underneath the neck skin flap to the contralateral side and sutured to the mastoid fascia to re-create a more defined cervicomental neck angle.

(Johnson & Johnson) in an interrupted fashion (Fig 5-6). Finally, liposuction is performed with a 4-mm or 6-mm flat cannula introduced through the submental incision for final sculpting of the supraplatysmal fat (Fig 5-7). The submental incision is then closed with one or two midline subcutaneous 5-0 polydioxanone sutures (PDS, Ethicon) and a 6-0 running nylon suture for approximation of the skin. The postoperative dressing and care are identical to that of the liposuction patient.

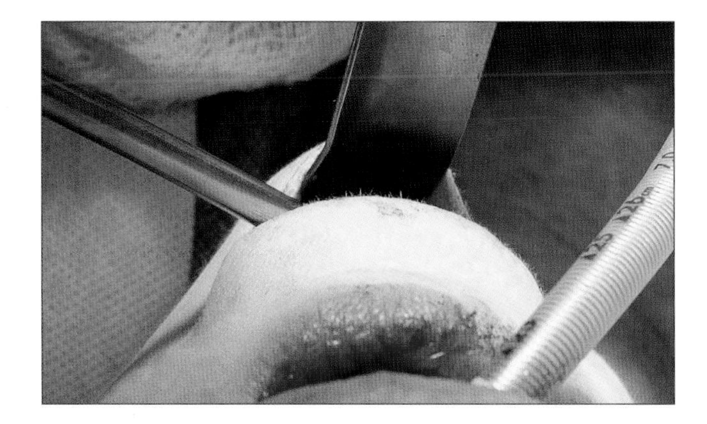

Fig 5-7 Open suction–assisted lipectomy with a 6-mm spatula liposuction cannula tissue pick-up is performed. The opening of the cannula is always directed away from the skin flap. (Courtesy of Dr Manolis Manolakakis, Shrewsbury, New Jersey.)

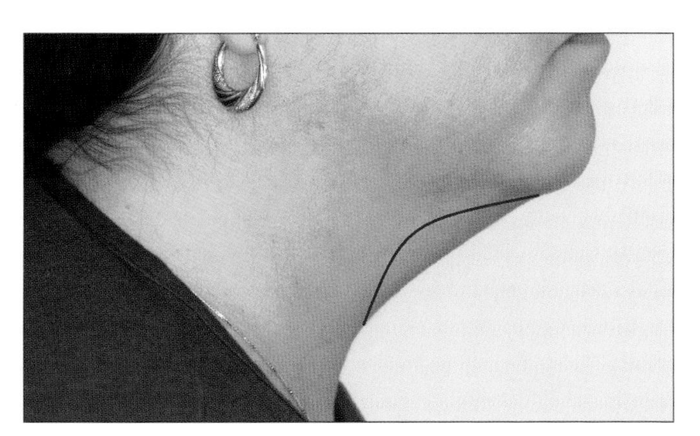

Fig 5-8a Candidate for submentoplasty with fat accumulation localizing in the submandibular area.

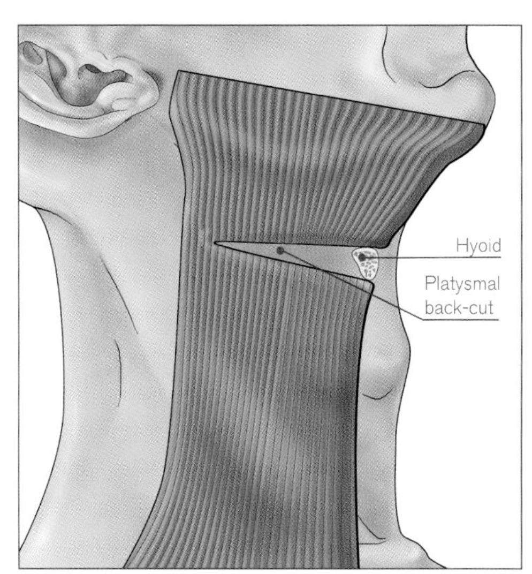

Fig 5-8b Platysmal back-cut technique.

Submentoplasty

Submentoplasty as described by Cuzalina and Koehler[9] is a slightly more invasive option in the cosmetic surgical management of the neck than those previously described. This procedure is indicated for those patients with a greater amount of suspect submental fat in the subplatysmal space (Fig 5-8a). The procedure is identical to that used for open lipectomy until the management of the platysma muscle. After completion of the supraplatysmal lipectomy, the dehisced platysma is entered—or the platysma is incised in the midline—and dissected to the inferior border of the mandible laterally and to the superior border of the thyroid cartilage inferiorly, with care to avoid the anterior jugular veins and submental artery. This allows access to the subplatysmal fat, which can then be carefully sculpted with facelift scissors and electrocautery. A 5- to 7-cm back-cut in the platysma muscle, inferior to the submandibular gland and lateral to the hyoid bone, is then considered (Fig 5-8b). If indicated, partial submandibular gland resection can be carefully completed, with great care to avoid injury to the marginal mandibular nerve and to manage bleeding of the facial artery and vein if encountered. The platysma is then cosmetically reapproximated with a partial midline resection and plicated with a 2-0 Vicryl suture as described in the previous section. Alternatively, if further submental debulking is desired in patients with a heavy neckline, an effective complete suprahyoid platysmaplasty is performed. This procedure is considered an aggressive submentoplasty, and if performed, it is very important to leave a thick submental skin flap. The submental incision is then closed, a dressing is placed, and postoperative instructions similar to those for the submental lipectomy with plication are given. This surgical procedure should be reserved for only those experienced facial cosmetic surgeons comfortable with submental anatomy and cosmetic surgery in this area.

Posterior necklift with platysmal suspension

In patients who are borderline candidates for an aggressive submentoplasty and are accepting of a postauricular incision, often a posterior necklift with platysmal suspension is the treatment of choice (Figs 5-9a and 5-9b).[16] Because of the additional access allowed by the postauricular modified rhytidectomy incision, this is considered a more invasive procedure.[1] This additional access allows for the removal of redundant neck skin and an actual mastoid suspension of the platysma, rather than relying on debulking of the submental area and skin shrinkage for treatment of the redundant neck skin. The procedure is carried out in a fashion similar to the direct lipectomy with platysmal plication, with the following additions: The posterior extent of a standard facelift incision is also marked beginning just posterior to the attachment of the earlobe, extending into the postauricular crease and 2 mm onto the conchal bowl before extending posteriorly at the level of the external auditory canal, then traveling inferiorly and posteriorly once in the occipital scalp area.[17,18] An extra 75 to 100 mL of tumescent solution is also injected, for a total of 150 to 200 mL, through the proposed postauricular incision area along the long access, superior to the SCM and inferior to the mandibular angle.

When lipectomy is completed and removal and contouring of the fat are considered adequate, the platysma is inspected for integrity, and a plication is performed, if necessary. Some surgeons advocate entering the subplatysmal space for removal of the subplatysmal fat or submandibular gland and partially or fully resecting the platysma in conjunction with this procedure.[9] The authors of this chapter do not routinely enter the subplatysmal space during this procedure but rather proceed directly to a platysmal imbrication as previously described, if necessary, and then to mastoid suspension of the platysma in the following fashion: The medial borders of platysma muscle are tagged at the depth of the cervicomental angle with 3-0 clear nylon sutures and clamped for later use. A no. 15 blade is then used to incise through the skin of the postauricular modified rhytidectomy incision. Facelift scissors are used to dissect the neck in a subcutaneous plane below the mandibular angle and anterior to the SCM, avoiding the greater auricular nerve. Communication between the posterior neck and submental flaps is then accomplished. The anterior platysmal tagging sutures are crossed through the midline and tunneled underneath the contralateral

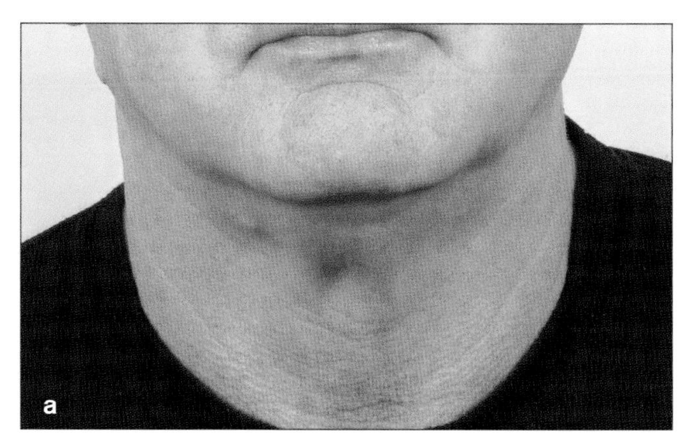

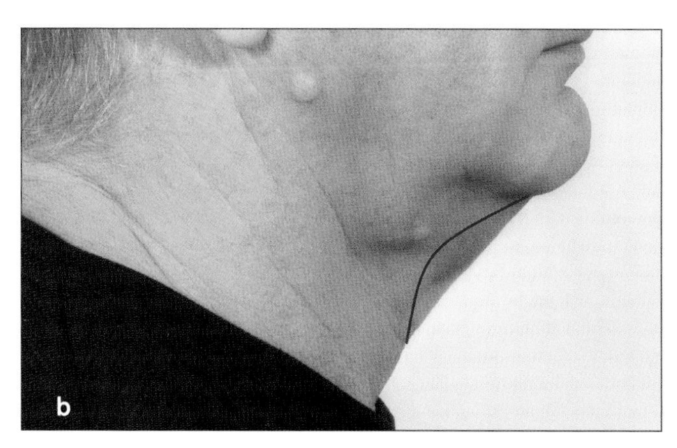

Figs 5-9a and 5-9b Typical features of the aging neck include skin laxity and accentuated jowls. A posterior necklift with platysmal suspension is planned.

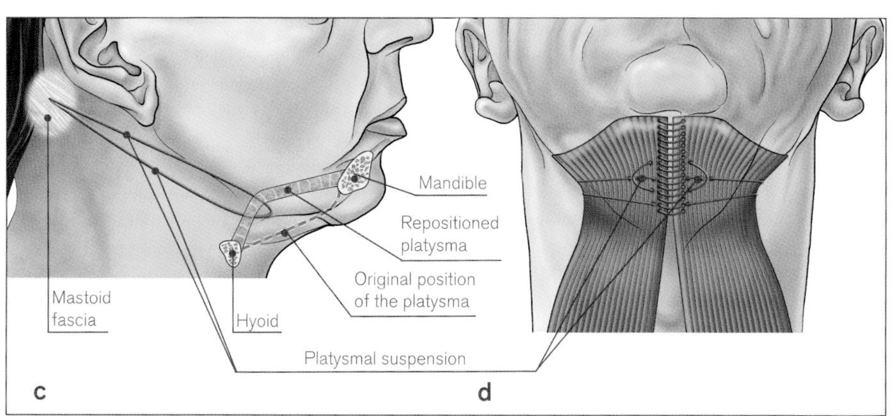

Figs 5-9c and 5-9d Platysmal suspension technique: *(c)* lateral view; *(d)* submental view.

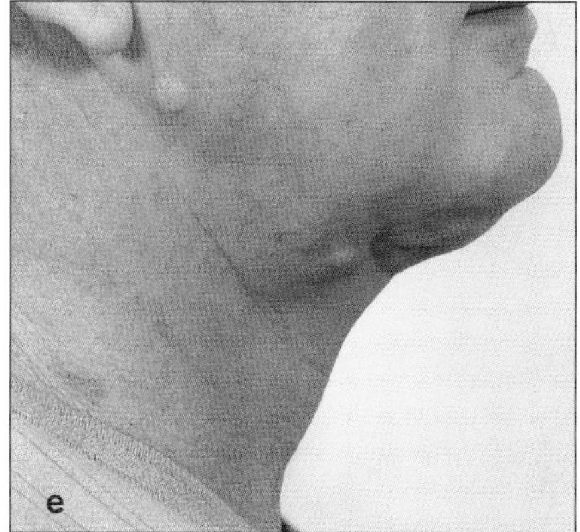

Fig 5-9e Postoperative view of posterior necklift.

posterior neck skin flap, exiting the postauricular incision. They are then tied to the contralateral mastoid fascia, while the head is turned to the ipsilateral side (Figs 5-9c and 5-9d). Finally, liposuction is performed through both incisions with a 4-mm flat cannula, which is also used for final sculpting of the platysmal/SMAS fat. The modified rhytidectomy skin flaps are then redraped with a superolateral vector in the neck. Because of this larger flap, the use of fibrin glue[14] or platelet-rich plasma can be considered prior to closure. Back-cuts are then made in the postauricular area of the modified rhytidectomy flap to gauge skin excess, and key 3-0 silk sutures are placed in a standard fashion. The skin flaps are then trimmed, and final closure is carried out. The scalp is closed with 3-0 silk sutures. Next, 5-0 PDS sutures are used to close the subcutaneous layer of the postauricular skin. The postauricular skin is closed with 6-0 nylon suture without tension. The submental incision is then closed, a compressive dressing is placed, and postoperative instructions similar to those for the submental lipectomy are given (Fig 5-9e).

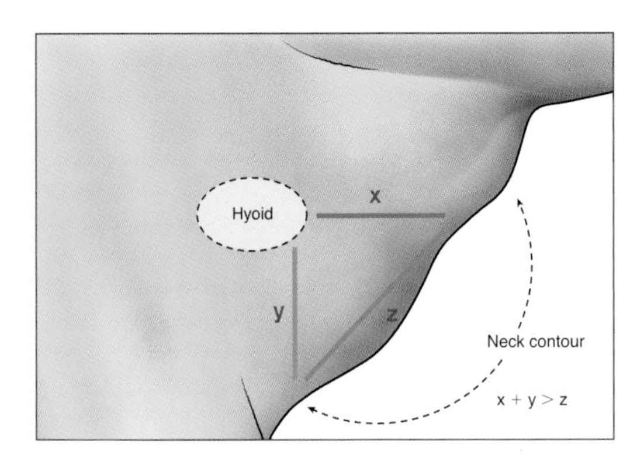

Fig 5-10 Mathematic depiction of submental cutis laxis: $x + y > z$. In conjunction with submental lipectomy, the submental cutis laxis is necessary to passively redrape the new, better-defined neck contour.

Techniques not recommended

The following techniques are described in the literature. However, the authors of this chapter do not recommend using these techniques to correct an aged neck.

Submental skin excision with advancement of the flap and Z-plasty

When a patient refuses a standard or modified rhytidectomy incision, it may be tempting to offer a less invasive option. There are descriptions in the literature of submental skin excision with or without a Z-plasty.[19,20] It is the authors' opinion that, although a limited elliptical skin excision with advancement of the skin flap and/or Z-plasty may have some relative indications, it does not seem to make mathematic sense in most cases and can result in unnecessary scarring (Fig 5-10). A few indications for this procedure include male patients wishing to avoid the stigma of male facelifts,[21] patients with extreme skin laxity in the neck, and patients in whom a posterior necklift is undesirable. The authors of this chapter believe that similar results can usually be obtained with one or a combination of the procedures described in this chapter. Because significant skin shrinkage and readaptation is expected to occur in most Z-plasty cases,[4] it has not been included among the treatment algorithms covered in this chapter.

Facial percutaneous suspension

Percutaneously placed regular or barbed sutures have been suggested and used in the neck region.[22,23] Although this procedure can have an immediate cosmetic benefit, long-term patient satisfaction is reported to be low.[24] It is the authors' experience that this procedure carries a high rate of relapse as well as a possible need for removal of the sutures due to their being painful, palpable, or visible. Because the authors do not recommend these procedures in the cosmetic management of the neck, they have been excluded from the treatment algorithms.

Complications

In general, complications stemming from the procedures discussed in this chapter are rare. However, they can include skin irregularities, prolonged swelling, seromas, hematomas, prolonged indurations, transient and permanent injury of the marginal mandibular nerve, postinflammatory hyperpigmentation, and sialoceles.[4,5,8,12,14,23]

Skin irregularities, a skeletonized appearance, or "cobra neck" are due to uneven surgical technique. They can be treated with massage or external ultrasound therapy and may require re-excision or fat grafting if conservative treatment is insufficient.

Seromas can result from inadequate pressure dressing or from the surgical technique. They are treated with aspiration and compression dressing. If further treatment is required, surgical exploration and antibiotics are indicated.

Hematomas usually occur within the first 24 hours and most often result because of an unknown anticoagulant that the patient was taking or because of the surgical technique. They are managed in a fashion similar to seromas. On rare occasions when the hematoma is large or small hematomas do not resolve following treatment, postoperative antibiotics and surgical drainage are indicated. If not managed in a timely fashion, hematoma can lead to hyperpigmentation as well as rippling and induration of the skin.

Indurations are usually secondary to dermal injury or hematoma and are treated with massage or external ultrasound therapy. If the indurations persist, injectable steroids can be considered (0.1 to 0.2 mL of triamcinolone).

Although permanent injury to the marginal mandibular nerve is very rare, transient nerve injury is more common and results from postoperative swelling and surgical technique. Observation is recommended, and if the injury lasts more than 2 weeks, botulinum toxin injection to the opposite side might be indicated.

Postinflammatory hyperpigmentation can result from patient variation in skin type, sun exposure, and delayed treatment of hematoma. It is usually managed with 4% hydroquinone or sunscreen. If it persists, camouflage makeup may be considered.

Sialoceles are rare (occur in less than 0.5% of cases) and result from damage to submandibular ducts and/or the sublingual gland. Management of sialoceles requires postoperative serial aspirations, pressure dressing, and an antisialogauge. They rarely require surgical management, unless the volume does not decrease after each aspiration.

Summary

Cosmetic management of the neck can involve many different procedures and techniques. The aim of this chapter is to mention a variety of reliable surgical options to address the concerns of the facial cosmetic patient. There are many nonsurgical modalities that should be discussed during treatment planning, either as treatment alternatives for those patients who are not good candidates for surgery or for those patients who are not yet ready to proceed with surgery. These nonsurgical modalities include skin care regimens, chemical peels, laser skin resurfacing, radiofrequency treatments, and botulinum toxin. These nonsurgical treatment techniques can also be incorporated into a surgical treatment plan to enhance or help maintain surgical outcomes.

When making the decision to surgically treat an isolated neck condition, it is critical to do a thorough physical examination not only to rule out pathologic conditions but also to make an accurate diagnosis and offer the patient a complete list of surgical options. Cosmetic surgery in the neck region can sometimes be performed solely with local anesthesia, but many times, intravenous sedation or general anesthesia is recommended. Often, less invasive procedures are more attractive to patients. However, though less invasive procedures are sometimes adequate for success, some patients may be disappointed by the results. Of utmost importance is the preoperative consultation, where previous cases can be presented to a prospective cosmetic surgery patient and the appropriate procedure can be selected that balances the patient's expectations with his or her tolerance for invasiveness. Whatever procedure is chosen, it should be understood that most patients expect the creation of a cosmetically pleasing neck. If a surgical procedure is chosen that is not likely to produce the results demonstrated in the figures, consideration should be given to an alternative, more invasive procedure or to the possibility of performing no surgical treatment. Also, it should always be mentioned to the patient that "touch-up" or additional procedures will possibly be necessary.

References

1. Adamson PA, Litner JA. Evolution of rhytidectomy techniques. Facial Plast Surg Clin North Am 2005;13:383–391.
2. Dayan SH, Bagal A, Tardy ME Jr. Targeted solutions in submentoplasty. Facial Plast Surg 2001; 17:141–149.
3. Lambros V. Fat contouring in the face and neck. Clin Plast Surg 1992;19:401–414.
4. Fattahi TT. Management of isolated neck deformity. Atlas Oral Maxillofac Surg Clin North Am 2004;12:261–270.
5. Grover R, Jones BM, Waterhouse N. The prevention of haematoma following rhytidectomy: A review of 1078 consecutive facelifts. Br J Plast Surg 2001;54:481–486.
6. Friedman O. Changes associated with the aging face. Facial Plast Surg Clin North Am 2005;13: 371–380.
7. Watson D. Submentoplasty. Facial Plast Surg Clin North Am 2005;13:459–467.
8. Ghali GE, Evans WT (eds). Peterson's Principals of Oral and Maxillofacial Surgery, vol 2. Part 9: Facial Esthetic Surgery. Shelton CT: People's Medical, 2005:1367.
9. Cuzalina LA, Koehler J. Submentoplasty and facial liposuction. Oral Maxillofac Surg Clin North Am 2005;17:85–98.
10. Brennan HG, Koch RJ. Management of aging neck. Facial Plast Surg 1996;12:241–255.
11. Guerroerosantos J. Surgical correction of the fatty fallen neck. Ann Plast Surg 1979;2:389–396.
12. Saylan Z. Serial notching of platysma bands. Aesthet Surg J 2001;21:412–417.
13. Schoen SA, Taylor CO, Owsley TG. Tumescent technique in cervicofacial rhytidectomy. J Oral Maxillofac Surg 1994;52:344–347.
14. Oliver DW, Hamilton SA, Figle AA, Wood SH, Lamberty BG. A prospective, randomized, double-blind trial of the use of fibrin sealant for face lifts. Plast Reconstr Surg 2001;108:2101–2105.
15. Wang T. Patient selection for aging face surgery. Facial Plast Surg Clin North Am 2005;13:381–382.
16. Kaminer MS, Bogart M, Choi C, Wee SA. Long-term efficacy of anchored barbed sutures in the face and neck. Dermatol Surg 2008;34:1041–1047.
17. Griffin JE Jr, Epker BN. Correction of cervicofacial deformities. Atlas Oral Maxillofac Surg Clin North Am 2004;12:179–197.
18. Miller TR, Eisbach KJ. SMAS facelift techniques to minimize stigmata of surgery. Facial Plast Clin North Am 2005;13:421–431.
19. Schaar C, Wolters M, Lampe H. Yes to a tight neck, no to a rhytidectomy: What can be obtained with a platysmaplasty? Eur J Plast Surg 2002;25:130–138.
20. Miller T. Excision of redundant neck tissue in men with platysma plication and Z-plasty closure. Plast Reconstr Surg 2005;115:304–313.
21. Brissett E, Hilger P. Male face-lift. Facial Plast Surg Clin North Am 2005;13:451–458.
22. Vasquez GD. Facial percutaneous suspension. Plast Reconstr Surg 2005;116:656–660.
23. Saylan Z. Posterior neck lift. Aesthet Surg J 2004; 24:155–158.
24. Moyer JS, Baker SR. Complications of rhytidectomy. Facial Plast Surg Clin North Am 2005;13: 469–478.

6

Minimal Incision Facelift

JOHN E. GRIFFIN, DMD
KING KIM, DMD

The minimal incision facelift is a very useful procedure for the cosmetic surgery practice. Often, patients present with only a minimal amount of jowling, ptosis, rhytids, and skin laxity. For these patients who desire a fresher appearance but only exhibit limited signs of facial aging, the minimal incision facelift is successful in producing optimal results.

Applied Anatomy

Anatomical considerations when performing this procedure are vital to achieving a favorable outcome. Recognition of the location of certain structural elements allows the surgeon to perform the procedure with increased confidence and skill.

From superficial to deep, the layers encountered during the minimal incision facelift dissection are skin, subcutaneous fat, dense fibrous septae, and the superficial musculoaponeurotic system (SMAS), which is the layer that is crucial when lifting and suspending the soft tissues of the face. Over time, the descent of the SMAS, due to the forces of gravity, contributes significantly to the signs of facial aging. Adequate lifting of this layer in key anatomical areas leads to significant, positive results.

From cadaveric dissections, 80% of subcutaneous fat in the face and neck superficial to the SMAS has been shown to be above the inferior border of the mandible, whereas 20% of subcutaneous fat is below the mandible in the neck. This superficial fat is densest in the regions of the cheek, nasolabial folds, jowls, chin, anterior neck, and glabella.[1]

The SMAS is a fibromuscular layer that rests in the cheek and midface areas. It is continuous with the galea and temporoparietal fascia superiorly and with the platysma inferiorly. It lies superficial to the parotidomasseteric fascia and buccal fat pad and is an intermediary between the skin and muscles during facial animation. The branches of the facial nerve all lie deep in the SMAS layer and will be discussed later. The SMAS is densest in the parotid area and thinnest in the anterior cheek, and it is a key component in amplifying movement of the facial musculature.[1]

Osseocutaneous retaining ligaments anchor the skin to the underlying periosteum (Fig 6-1). One bundle of such ligaments is the zygomatic retaining ligaments, also known as the *McGregor patch*. These ligaments are located at the junction of the zygoma and zygomatic arch. An artery and sensory nerve course within this bundle of ligaments, and the zygomatic branch of the facial nerve travels deep and inferior to the ligaments.[1] In addition, extending from the junction of the anterior and middle thirds of the mandibular body to the skin of the anterior jowl lies the mandibular retaining ligament. Adjacent to this ligament are an artery and vein that may be encountered during the dissection. The strong adherence of the ligaments between the skin and periosteum makes dissection more challenging in these areas.[1,2]

Beneath the SMAS reside the muscles of facial expression. These muscles include the buccinator, orbicularis oris, zygomaticus minor and major, levator labii superioris, levator labii superioris alaeque nasi, levator anguli oris, depressor anguli oris, depressor labii inferioris, mentalis, risorius, and platysma. The muscles that are enveloped by the SMAS on their superficial and deep surfaces are the risorius, zygomaticus major and minor, platysma, depressor anguli oris, and orbicularis oris. The muscular movements of the face work congruously in such a way that as one group contracts, the others oppose and pull in opposite directions.[1]

Innervation

It is important to understand the path in which the facial nerve (cranial nerve VII) travels, because this nerve supplies motor innervation to the muscles of facial expression. After leaving the stylomastoid foramen, the main trunk of the facial nerve enters the parotid gland, where it separates the gland into superficial and deep lobes. There, the nerve divides into superior and inferior divisions, and it then divides even further into the frontal, zygomatic, buccal, marginal mandibular, and cervical branches. These branches leave the parotid gland and travel superficial to the masseter muscle within or just deep to the parotidomasseteric fascia and further arborize to innervate the muscles of facial expression. It should be noted that the nerve supplies all of these muscles from their undersurfaces, with the exception of the levator anguli oris, buccinator, and mentalis. These three muscles are innervated on their superficial surfaces (Fig 6-2) for facial nerve distribution.

The marginal mandibular nerve courses deep to the platysma muscle inferiorly to loop below the inferior border of the mandible anywhere from 1 to 4 cm below the mandibular edge. It then travels anteriorly and superiorly toward the facial artery and vein, after which it crosses superficial to these vessels.[2] It has been shown that, posterior to the facial artery, this nerve is above the inferior border of the mandible in 81% of patients and up to 2 cm below the mandible in 19% of patients.[3] In 15% of patients, the nerve has direct connections with the buccal branch of the facial nerve, meaning that preservation of function can occur if the marginal mandibular branch were injured. It has also been shown that by extending the neck during the procedure, the nerve descends more inferiorly.[1] The frontal branch has been shown to have the highest risk of permanent muscle paralysis, with an overall risk of 0.53% to 2.60% after conventional rhytidectomy.[2,4–6] This risk is lessened with the minimal incision facelift procedure because of the limited dissection. The typical course of the anterior ramus of the frontal branch crosses the zygomatic arch approximately 2 cm posterior to the lateral canthus, just deep to the temporoparietal fascia, which is a continuation of the SMAS layer above the zygomatic arch (Fig 6-3). The posterior

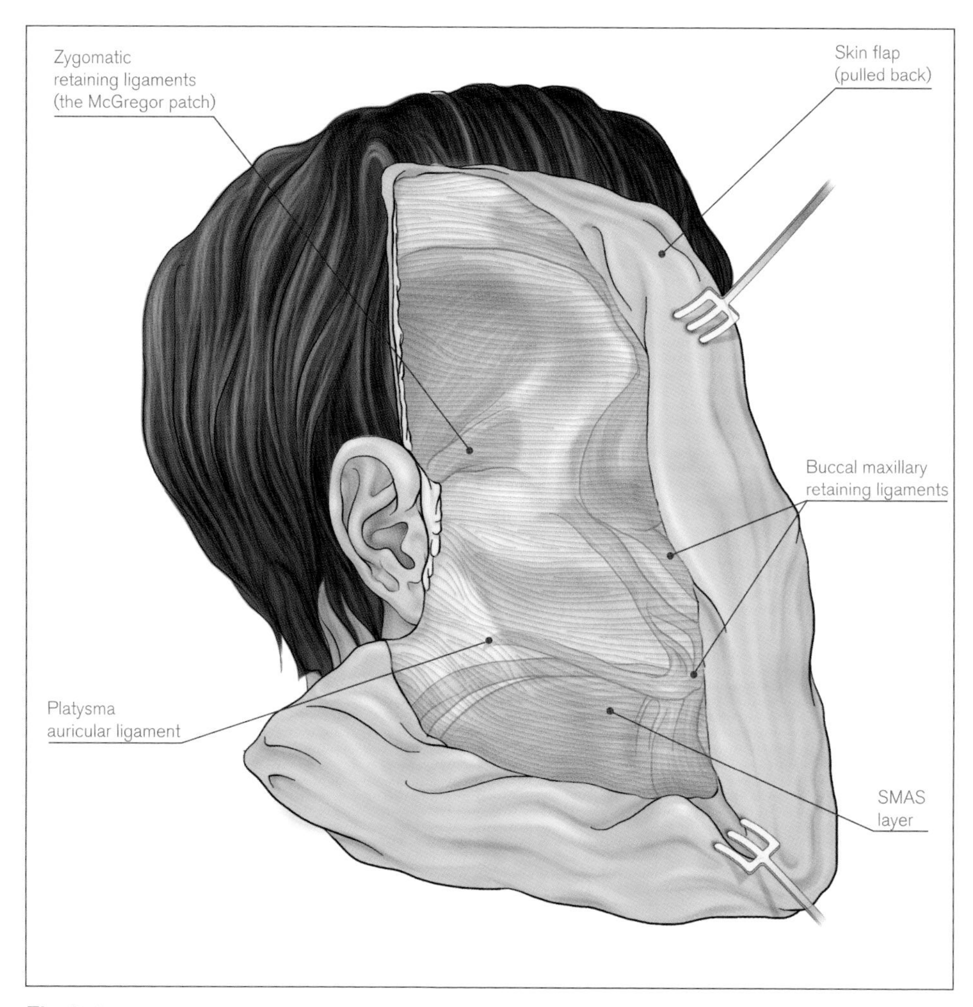

Fig 6-1 Osseocutaneous retaining ligaments that anchor the skin and the underlying periosteum.

ramus of the frontal branch courses about 1.8 cm anterior to the superoanterior helix of the ear.[2] The area encompassing the zygomatic arch should be handled with careful attention during the dissection (Fig 6-4). A zone of safety in regard to the facial nerve is typically at the inferior edge of the anterior zygomatic arch and body.[1]

Sensory innervation of the face is via the trigeminal nerve and cervical plexus. The infraorbital nerve (V2) innervates the skin from the orbital rim to the commissure. The buccal branch (V3) of the mandibular nerve innervates the area between the commissure and the mandible. The preauricular region is innervated by the auriculotemporal branch of the mandibular nerve (V3). The greater auricular nerve innervates the skin overlying the posterior ear and originates from the cervical branches from C2 and C3. It leaves the deep cervical fascia and crosses over the sternocleidomastoid fascia approximately 6.5 cm inferior to the ear lobule. This region where it crosses the muscle has been termed *Erb point*.

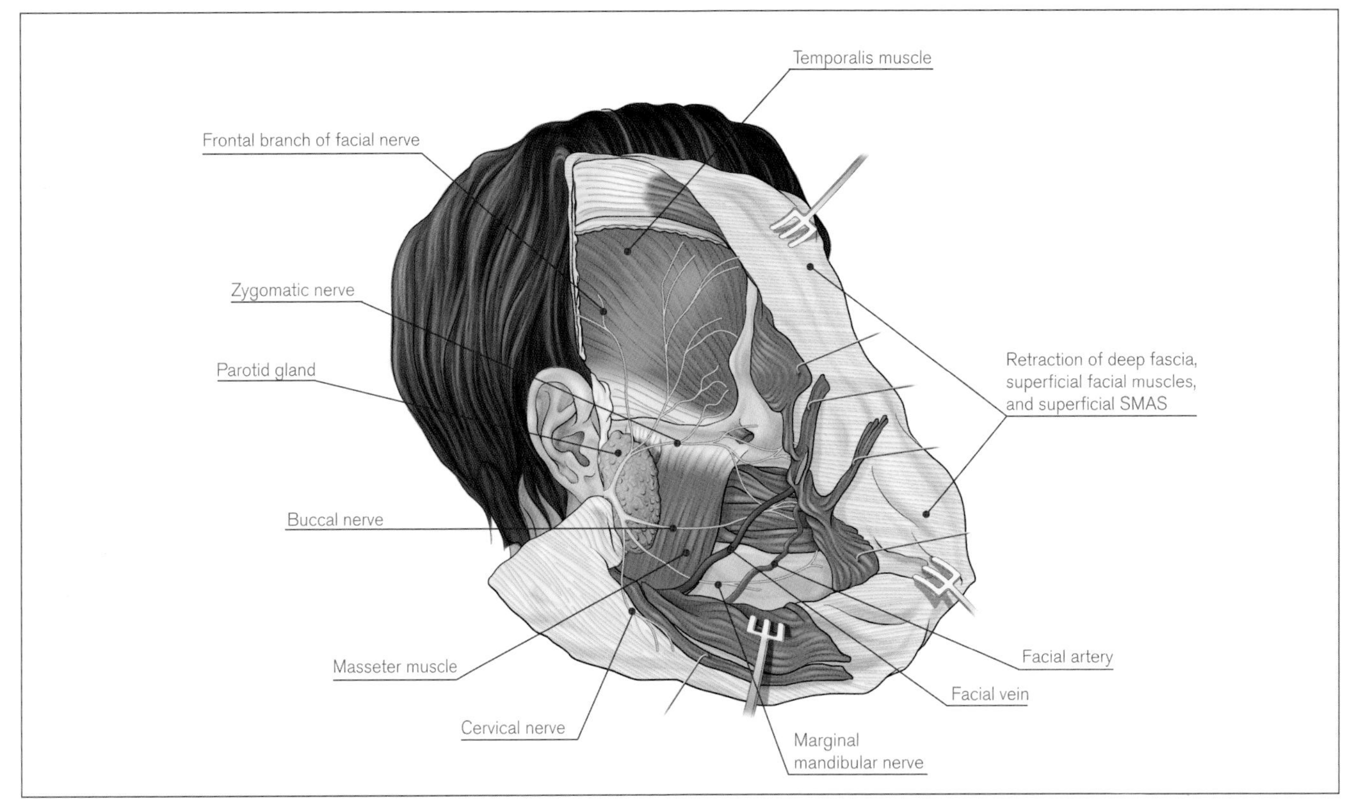

Fig 6-2 **Nerve distribution to facial musculature.**

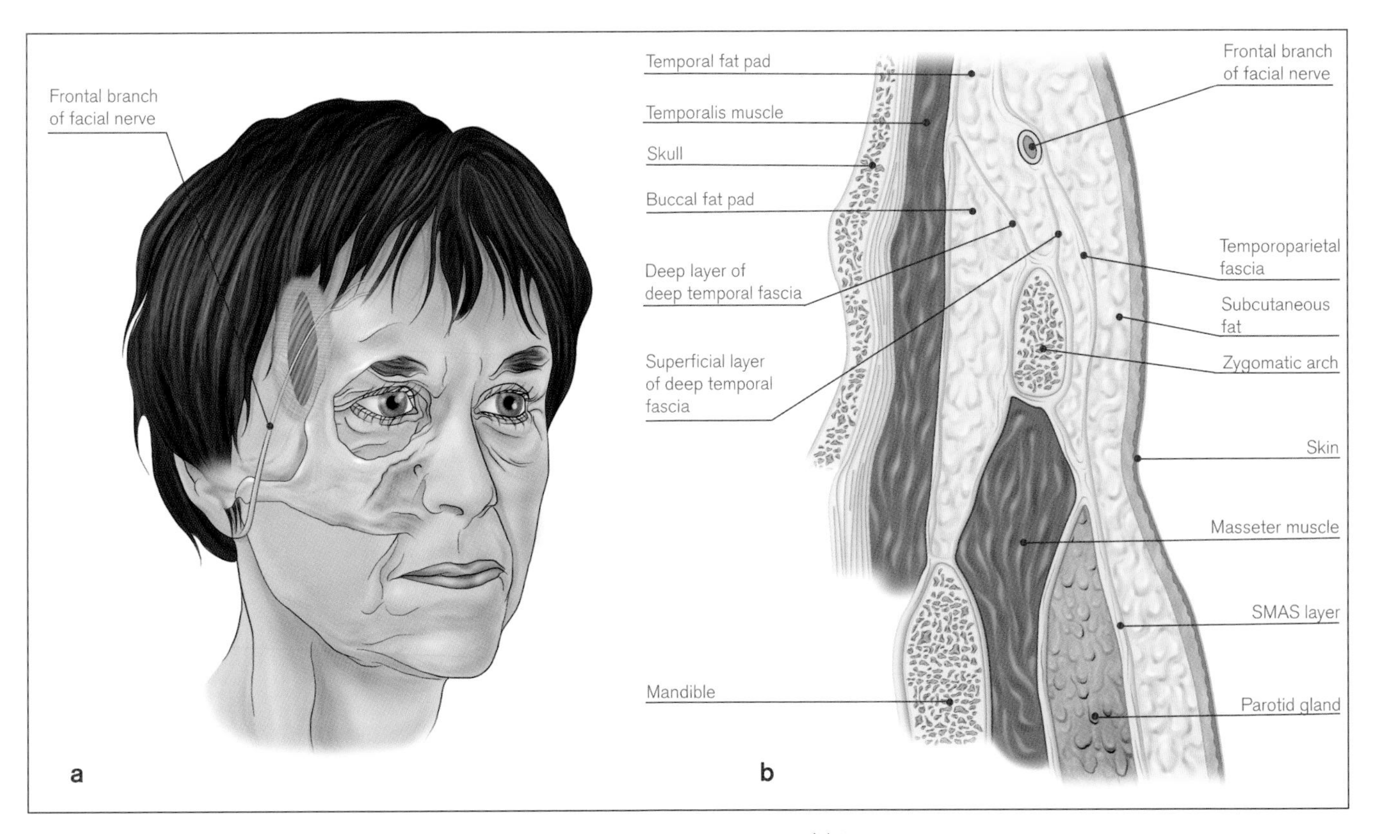

Fig 6-3 ***(a)*** **Path of frontal branch of facial nerve as it crosses the zygomatic arch.** ***(b)*** **Cross-section view.**

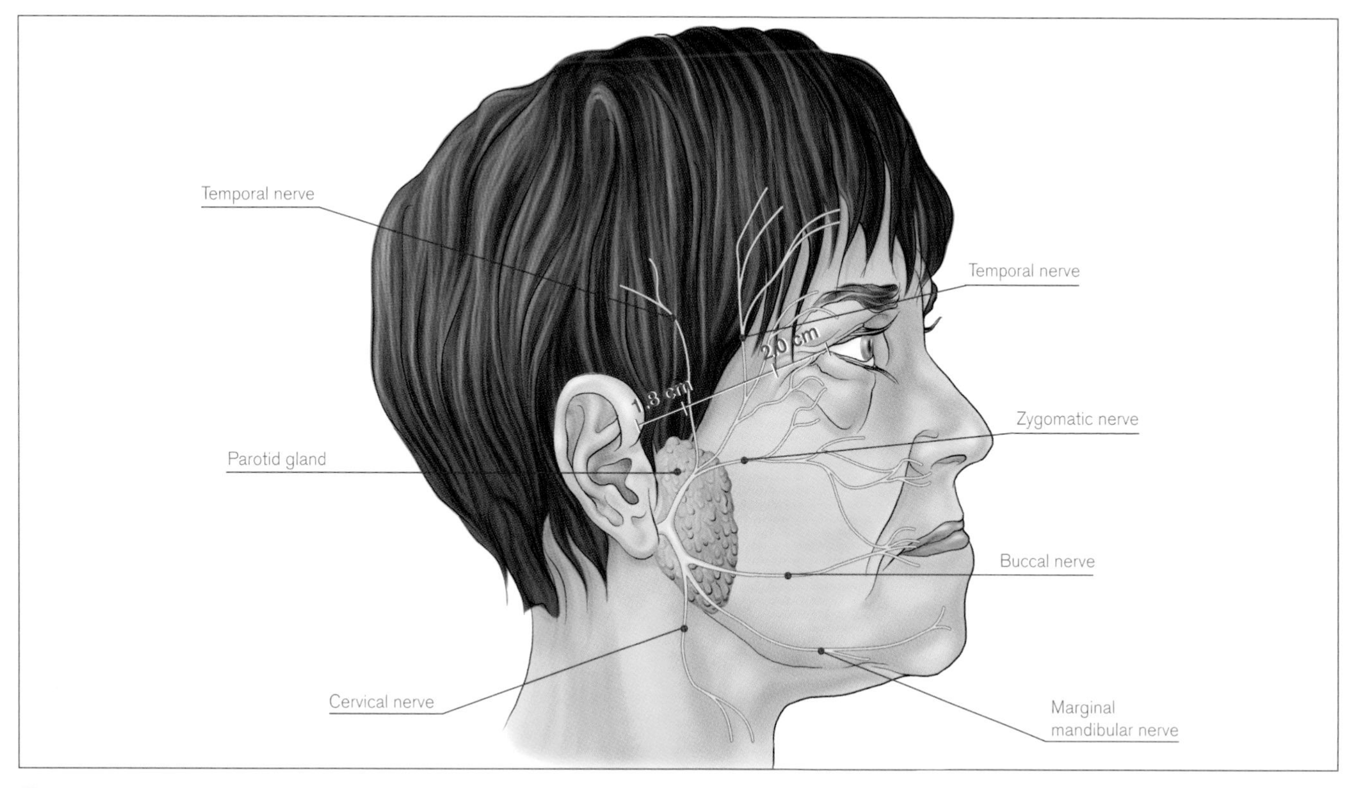

Fig 6-4 Area encompassing the zygomatic arch requiring careful attention and meticulous dissection. The practitioner must exercise caution when dissecting the area, starting 1.8 cm from the ear and continuing until 2.0 cm from the eye *(pink line)*. This area is where the temporal branch of the facial nerve is present.

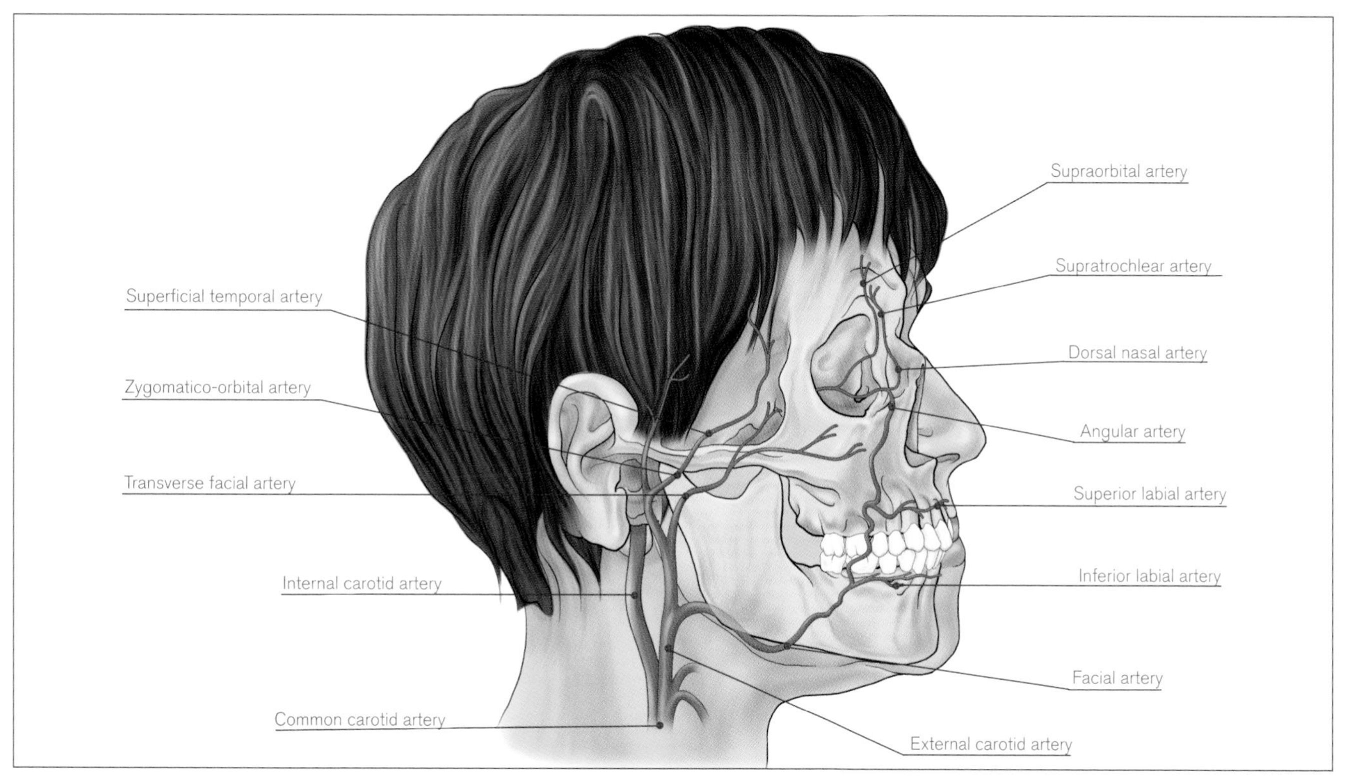

Fig 6-5 Arterial supply to the face.

Blood supply and lymphatic drainage

The blood supply to the superficial structures of the face stems from the external carotid artery. At the anterior edge of the masseter muscle, the facial artery crosses the mandible and courses superiorly toward the lateral nose. After imparting the first two branches—the superior and inferior labial arteries—the facial artery becomes the angular artery at the lateral nose. At this point, there is a significant anastomosis between the facial artery with branches of the infraorbital artery, a branch of the internal maxillary artery. A branch from here is further formed, called the *transverse nasal artery*, which supplies the lateral nose. The majority of the superficial facial structures are supplied directly by the facial and infraorbital arteries. The subdermal plexus, which is paramount in maintaining flap viability, emanates from these two arteries (Fig 6-5). The venous drainage system of the face is named corresponding with the arterial names. The facial vein runs parallel with the facial artery and empties into the internal jugular vein. The infraorbital vein drains into the pterygoid plexus, which drains the deeper structures of the face. The pterygoid plexus drains into the maxillary vein and then joins the superficial temporal vein to become the retromandibular vein. The retromandibular vein drains the parotid region and joins the posterior auricular vein to become the external jugular vein, which empties into the subclavian vein.

Lymphatic fluid from the midface drains into the parotid lymph nodes. Drainage of the lower face occurs via the submental and submandibular lymph nodes. Drainage of the temporal and infratemporal region empties into the upper cervical lymph node chain (level II nodes).

Aging face changes

It is important to critically evaluate each patient on an individual basis. Patients who have undergone aging face changes have essentially experienced a natural process in human life. Gradual changes in the facial structures begin in the third decade, with a descent of the eyebrows, excess eyelid skin laxity, psuedoherniation of orbital fat, and formation of glabellar frown lines and prominent nasolabial folds.[7,8] These changes become accentuated in the fifth and sixth decades. In addition, the midface begins to descend, wrinkles appear in the perioral region, and submental fat begins to accumulate; in the lower face, platysma banding and jowling occur. In the seventh and eighth decades, the skin becomes thinner, subcutaneous fat diminishes, and wrinkling is more exaggerated (Fig 6-6).

The force of gravity over a lifetime imparts a gradual drooping of all soft tissue components of the face including the muscles, SMAS, and skin (see Fig 4-1). Nasolabial folds become accentuated as the malar fat pad, nasolabial fat pad, and suborbicularis oculi fat descend.[2,9,10] The drooping facial musculature and subcutaneous fat atrophy lead to an overall loss of facial contour.[9] Rhytidosis of the skin occurs because of the lack of organization of elastic fibers and collagen of the skin, in conjunction with weakening of the facial musculature.[7,11] Jowling is thought to occur from the accumulation of subcutaneous fat in the neck and mandibular body areas and may be accentuated from ptosis of the skin and the SMAS layer, caused by the

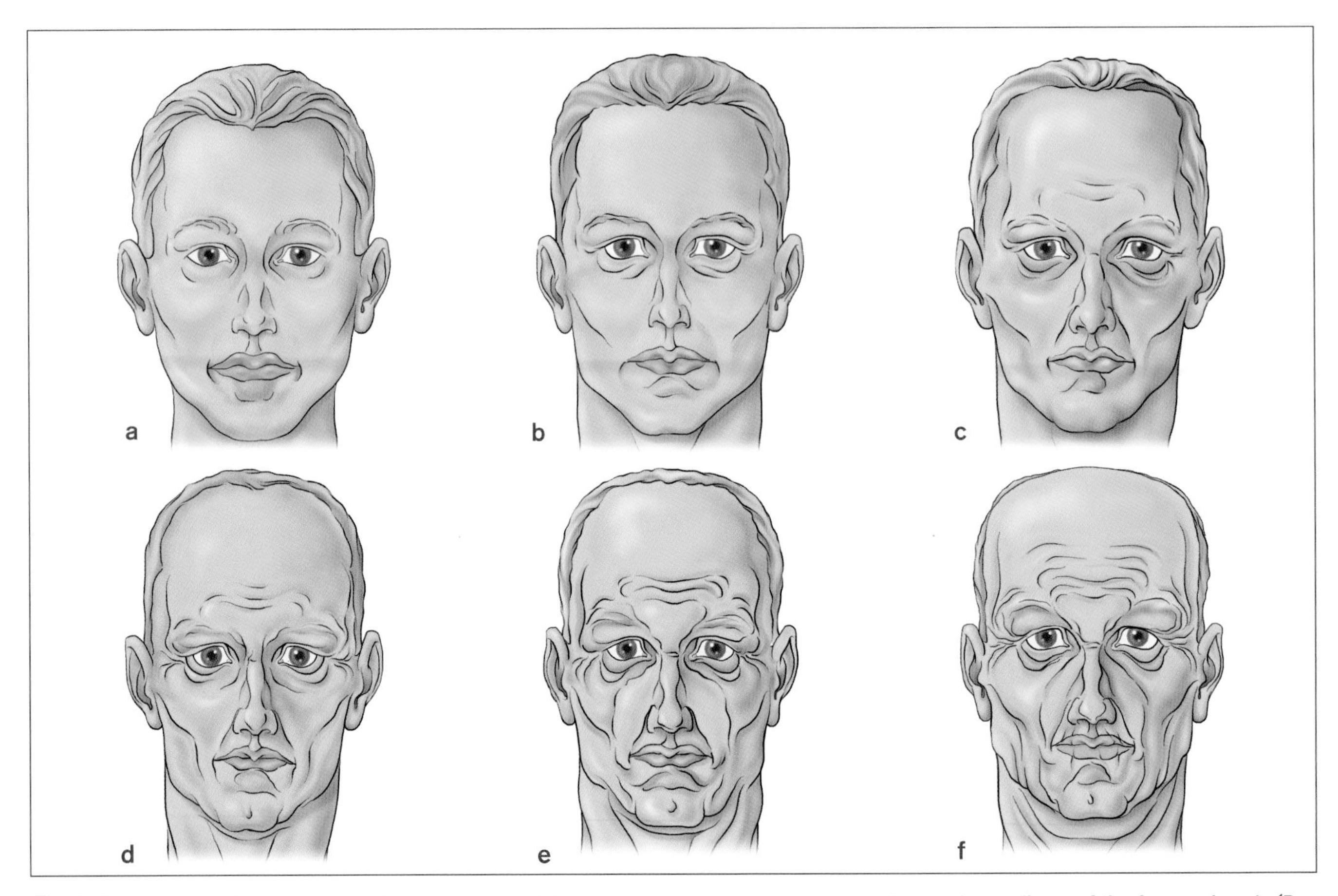

Fig 6-6 *(a to f)* **Effects of the gradual aging process. Note the increase in rhytids, ptosis, jowling, and overall sag of the face and neck. (Redrawn based on Friedman[7] with permission.)**

descent of the malar fat pad as a consequence of gravity.[7,12–14] Mandibular resorption at the anterior mandibular groove in edentulous patients can exaggerate the jowling appearance.[15]

Excess laxity in the platysma muscle may create two oblique vertical bands in the neck area that extend from the clavicle to the submental musculature, making an opening, or dehiscence, between the bands. Because of this platysmal banding, subplatysmal fat and soft tissue can herniate through the dehiscence, leading to neck fullness and submental lipodystrophy and creating the appearance of an obtuse cervicomental angle. The addition of environmental factors such as smoking and sun exposure may accelerate the aging appearance of the face by damaging the skin and creating a rough skin surface and coarse wrinkles.[7,16]

Patient Selection

Many patients seen in consultation are not sure what they need; they simply desire a fresher, more youthful appearance. Some of these patients may be young—in their 40s or 50s—and present with minimal to moderate signs of facial aging. These patients exhibit a minimal amount of skin laxity and jowling and little soft tissue ptosis. Different options can be explained to these patients, but the minimal incision facelift should be considered. This abbreviated rhytidectomy procedure offers several benefits in comparison to the full cervicofacial rhytidectomy, including shorter operating time and cost, decreased tissue trauma, diminished recovery period, greater range of surgical candidates, and increased margin of safety.[17] All of these points should be addressed during the consultation. Patients who present with a significant amount of facial jowling, skin laxity, soft tissue ptosis, and rhytidosis are not candidates for the minimal incision facelift procedure and should possibly be considered for the full facelift and necklift (see chapters 4 and 5).

Preoperative Evaluation

Another important part of preoperative planning is taking good photographs to compare with the final postoperative result. Frontal view photographs document the overall appearance of the face and the degree of aging. Left and right lateral views show the amount of lipodystrophy and skin laxity in the neck area. Should the patient require attention to the neck, these views will be important in helping the practitioner consider the different options needed to provide comprehensive treatment. For example, a mini-facelift can be performed in conjunction with a separate submental liposuction and/or platysmaplasty procedure to address minimal to moderate facial aging with lipodystrophy of the neck region. In a situation where the face and neck show more extensive aging and moderate to severe submental lipodystropy and platysmal banding, the decision may call for a full facelift with submental lipectomy, midline platysmal plication, and platysmal suspension.

Patients who are deemed good candidates for minimal incision rhytidectomy are prepared preoperatively. Those who smoke cigarettes are strongly urged to quit smoking 2 weeks prior to the procedure and to refrain from smoking for 2 weeks following the procedure. Cigarette smoke creates an unfavorable vascular flap, and those who continue to smoke may develop a dreaded flap necrosis after surgery. In addition, patients taking anticoagulants, including herbs and vitamins, are asked to discontinue their supplements 2 weeks prior to the procedure to avoid hematoma and hemorrhaging during surgery.

The minimal incision facelift is planned for either intravenous sedation or general anesthesia. The majority of cases can be performed in the office setting. Those requiring hospitalization due to a medically compromised status can be planned for the hospital operating room accordingly. It is advisable that either a certified registered nurse anesthetist or anesthesiologist be present on the day of surgery to enable the surgeon to focus solely on the procedure without being distracted by other concerns. Performing these procedures under local anesthesia is possible but not recommended because of patient discomfort and possible patient dissatisfaction.

Surgical Procedures

Incision design and hydrodissection

After the patient is brought to a proper plane of anesthesia, the incision markings are drawn in the preauricular crease anterior to the auricle (Fig 6-7a). The oblique incision overlying the temporal tuft of hair should be in hair only and should end just prior to where the hairline stops. The posterior portion of the incision begins at the inferior attachment of the ear lobule and extends up the posterior conchal wall to the level of the external auditory meatus, where the incision makes a gradual turn posteriorly and obliquely to end in the skin overlying the mastoid region (Fig 6-7b). The surgical marker is then used to delineate the extent of the dissection anteriorly, inferiorly, and posteriorly. A dotted line is placed 5 cm anterior to the incision line and continues inferiorly in a curvilinear direction all the way behind the ear (Fig 6-7c).

The incision lines are then infiltrated with local anesthetic solution containing epinephrine. Following placement of local anesthetic, hydrodissection with tumescent solution is performed to provide a clean plane of dissection. The tumescent solution is composed of the following: 10 mL of 2% lidocaine, 0.5 mg of epinephrine, and 5 mg of triamcinolone mixed with 250 mL of 0.9% normal saline. The 10-mL syringes connected to 18-gauge needles are of adequate size to perform hydrodissection; however, larger syringes can be used. The plane of hydrodissection is between the dermis and the SMAS layer, and the fibrous attachments located there either separate or expand as the tumescent solution is injected (Figs 6-7d to 6-7f). Clinically, a ballooning effect of the outer skin can be visualized. It is important to note that the hydrodissection must be thorough. The solution should be injected underneath the entire planned flap and just slightly beyond the planned dissection plane to create an environment for a safe and smooth dissection. It is equally important to refrain from overzealous stabbing of the tumescent syringe into the patient. The technique should reflect a gliding, controlled movement. The solution is injected into the desired plane and the needle partially withdrawn (but not out of the patient). Then, the needle is again gently but deliberately inserted, and solution is injected into another area. One puncture through the skin with the tumescent needle should be sufficient for three or four sweeps of hydrodissection. Puncturing the skin, tumescing, withdrawing the needle out of the body, and then puncturing the skin again repeatedly is not recommended and reflects poor technique.

Dissection

After making the entire rhytidectomy incision in front of and behind the ear, the facelift scissors are used for dissection in the supra-SMAS plane to create a flap. The tips of the scissors should be placed upward, toward the skin side, to prevent a deep dissection. Careful technique should be used here, and the flap thickness should be evaluated to ensure viability of the flap and dissection in the correct plane. If the flap feels thin, the viability of the flap diminishes, and the chance of undesirably perforating the skin increases. Conversely, if the flap feels too thick, the dissection may be too deep, and the risk of facial nerve injury and hemorrhaging escalates. The flap continues to develop as the fibrous attachments between the dermis and SMAS are

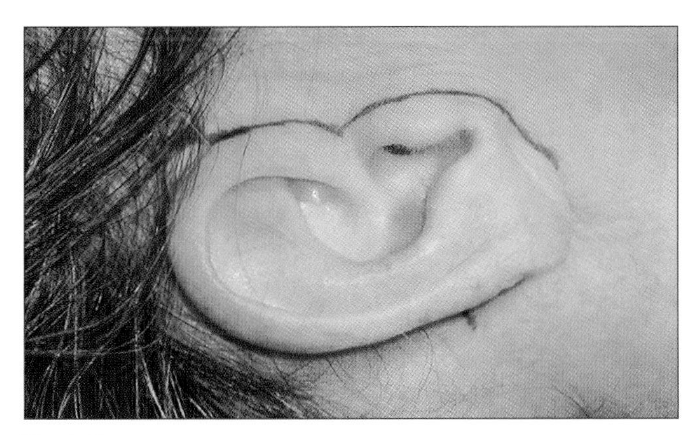

Fig 6-7a Incision marking in the preauricular crease and temporal hair tuft.

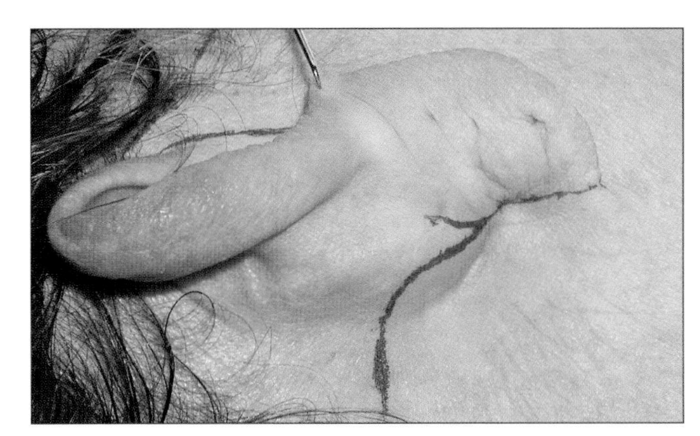

Fig 6-7b Incision marking behind the ear connecting the anterior incision and following it up the posterior conchal bowl, then making a gradual curve to end in the mastoid region.

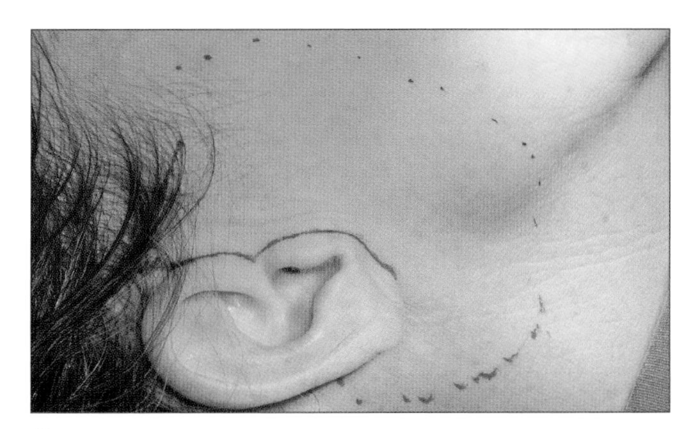

Fig 6-7c Dotted line representing the anterior limit of supra-SMAS dissection.

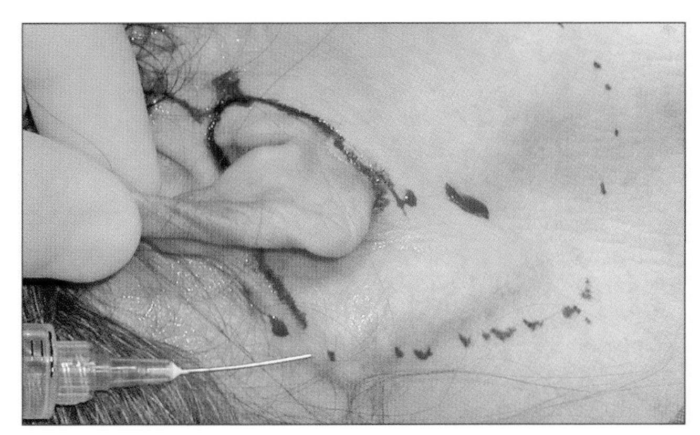

Fig 6-7d Hydrodissection behind the ear. It is important to avoid inadvertent dissection deep into this area. The skin behind the ear is thinner than that in front of the ear.

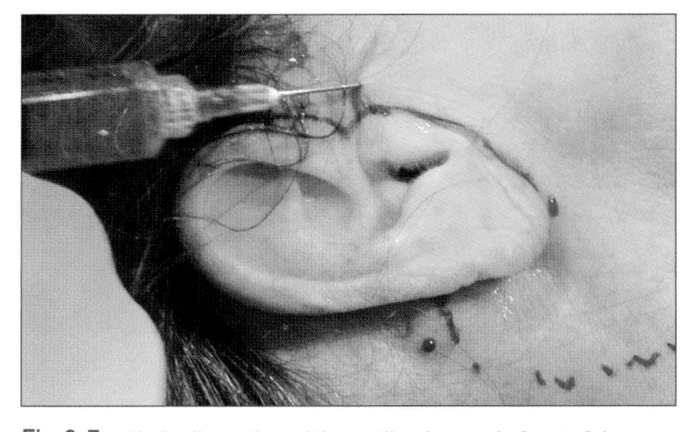

Fig 6-7e Hydrodissection of the outlined areas in front of the ear.

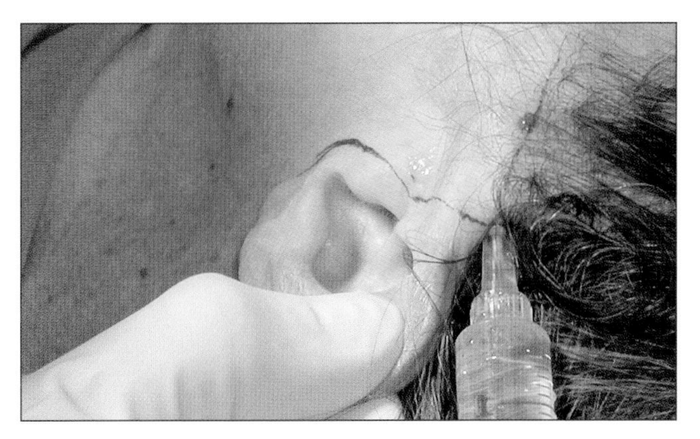

Fig 6-7f Hydrodissection along the temporal hair tuft.

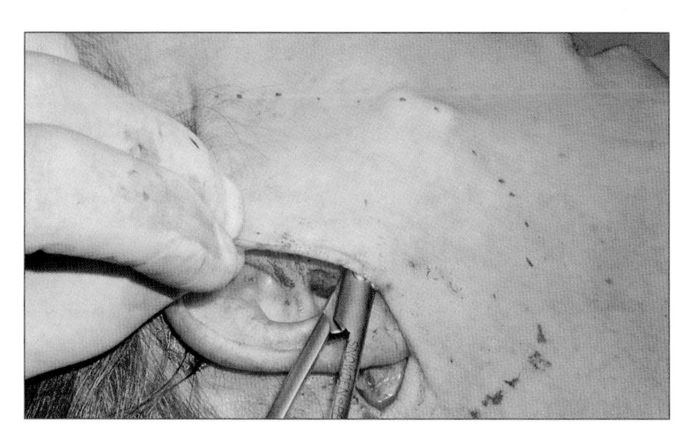

Fig 6-7g Keeping the facelift scissor tips pointed upward allows the surgeon to better visualize the anterior boundary of the dissection.

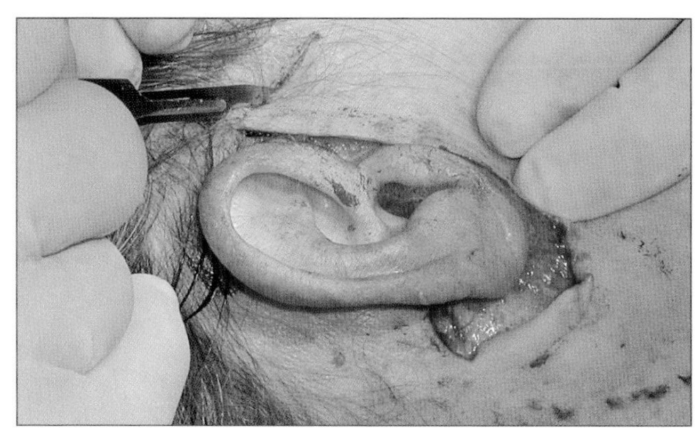

Fig 6-7h Bevelled incision at the temporal hair tuft is made as parallel as possible to the hair shafts.

cut in a plane already created by the hydrodissection, if it was performed correctly. Placing the tips of the scissors in an upward direction facilitates seeing the instrument on the outer skin to ensure the proper extent of the dissection (Fig 6-7g). Careful dissection should be exercised in the malar area near the McGregor patch, and dissection beyond the planned dotted markings on the face may lead to hemorrhaging, which is difficult to control. The vascular plexus will likely be encountered if the surgeon is not aware of the anterior extent of the dissection. In the temporal region, the dissection is performed slightly beyond the incision marking superiorly, posteriorly, and anteriorly. Because the skin in the posterior auricular region is much thinner than that on the face, careful attention should be paid to avoid making the flap too thin and perforating it externally. In addition, meticulous undermining must be performed as the surgeon dissects inferiorly in the posterior auricular area, because the risk of hemorrhaging increases due to the rich vascular bed. The posterior undermining is then continued anteriorly around the ear to connect to the facial portion of the dissection to make one large skin flap extending from the temporal tuft to the mastoid area. At this point, the forefinger can be swept back and forth underneath the flap in a semicircular pattern to ascertain the removal of all subdermal attachments.

After the dissection is completed to the extent of the dotted lines marked preoperatively, an oblique incision is made in the temporal tuft of hair. It is important to place the scalpel blade at an acute angle to the scalp, paralleling the root of the hair to keep the hair follicles viable (Fig 6-7h). It will be readily apparent that after making this temporal incision, the flap opens up tremendously, thereby facilitating retraction of the skin flap and better visualization of the SMAS and dermal layers from underneath. The sequence of placing this incision after the subdermal dissection is crucial to achieve maximum undermining of the flap.

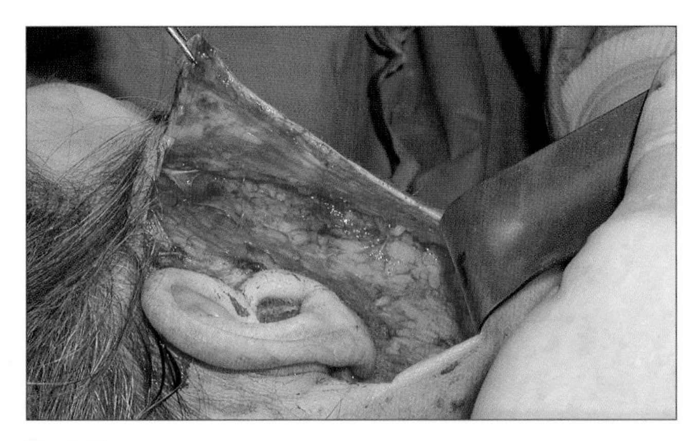

Fig 6-7i Elevation of the anterior portion of the flap and visualization of the SMAS layer.

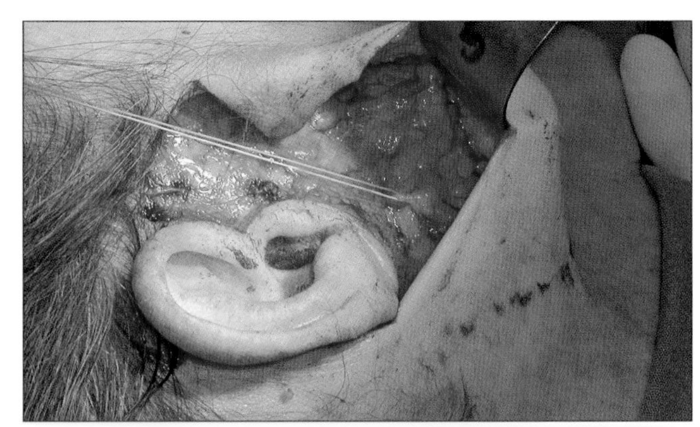

Fig 6-7j Elevation of the SMAS near the angle of the mandible after placing a suspension suture.

Once the flap is completely freed from the subdermal attachments, it can be elevated (Fig 6-7i). At this point, the dissection can be checked for precision and the presence of hemostasis. Bleeding vessels can be cauterized with a monopolar or bipolar electrocautery device. In addition, the placement of the SMAS suspension can be identified. The SMAS is a mobile unit and is not tightly bound to the underlying muscle. Therefore, it can be grasped with an instrument (such as an Adson-Brown forceps) and manipulated freely to evaluate the best place for suspension.

Suspension and skin redraping

The first suspension suture is placed in the SMAS overlying the area of the mandibular angle. In our experience, the most desirable spot is found by palpating the angle of the mandible with the forefinger and placing the suture in the SMAS just slightly superior to it. A large bite of SMAS is engaged with a 2-0 Vicryl suture (Johnson & Johnson) on a large, noncutting needle and lifted superiorly (Fig 6-7j). To evaluate the amount of lift the patient will get clinically, the suture can be pulled in the superoposterior vector, with the skin being redraped and pulled in the same vector. If done correctly, any jowling in this area can be seen being lifted up by the suture pull. The suture is then tied down to the fascia overlying the zygomatic arch. The anatomical location of the arch is first palpated, and the needle is placed to grab a large bite of tissue in the inferosuperior direction, 1 cm anterior to the skin margin of the ear. This suture is not tied firmly to the tissues, because the suture will press against the SMAS, leaving an undesirable, uneven appearance. In addition, the patient will likely complain of postoperative pain from a firmly bound suture.

The second area of suspension lies in the SMAS overlying the zygomatic prominence. There is no absolute, objective manner to identify the location of the next suture, but suffice it to say that the SMAS layer is loose tissue and exhibits laxity when

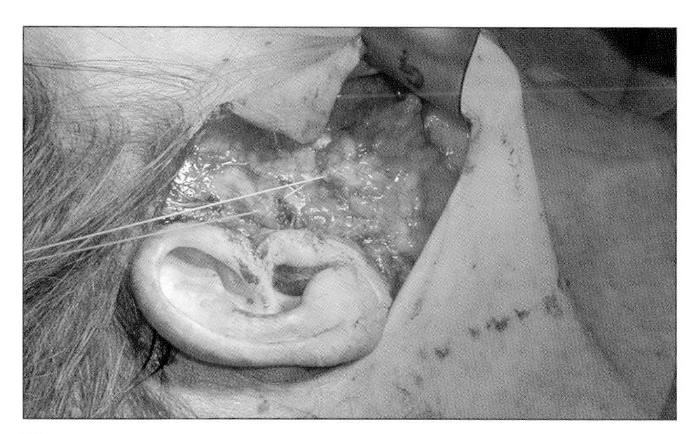

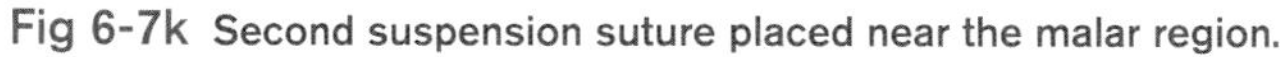

Fig 6-7k Second suspension suture placed near the malar region.

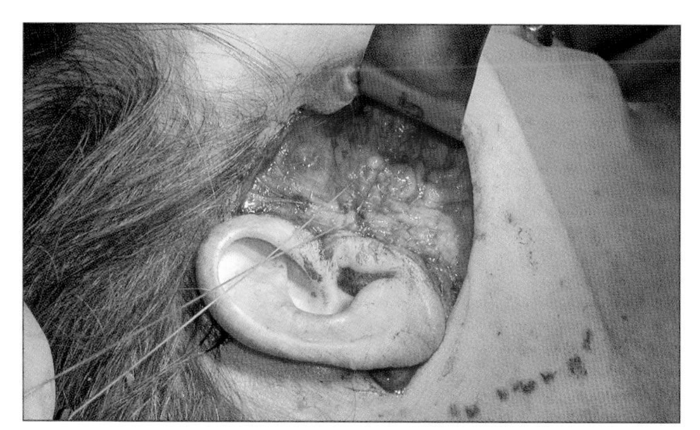

Fig 6-7l Third suture placed in the SMAS to flatten any irregular areas created by the second suspension suture.

manipulated with an instrument. The 2-0 Vicryl suture is again placed through the SMAS, where it must grab a large bite of tissue. Then, it is once more pulled in the same vector as the preceding suspension suture (Fig 6-7k). The skin is redraped over the SMAS to check for adequacy of SMAS lift. There is no cause for concern if the skin dimples when the suture is pulled. Dimpling simply indicates that the dermal attachments are also being pulled by the suture and either that the anterior extent of the facelift dissection was not sufficient or the suspension suture was placed too close to the anterior extent of the dissection. This effect can be eliminated by using the facelift scissors to carefully dissect under the skin flap, superficial to the suture, in the area of the dimples. The suture is again tied down in the fascia overlying the zygomatic arch in the same area as the preceding suspension suture. The suture must not be fastened so tight as to gouge into the SMAS and create an undesirable result.

After placement of the second suspension suture, bunching of the SMAS (visible as a bulge through the skin) can be seen just anterior to the ear, which is essentially created by the previous two suspension sutures. Bunching will produce unacceptable results. The solution is to place a third 2-0 Vicryl suture in a horizontal mattress fashion, engaging the anterior redundant SMAS and securing it to the posterior area of redundant or bunched-up SMAS to pull the suture in the same vector as the previous two sutures (Fig 6-7l). After placement of this third suture, the entire SMAS bed under the skin flap should be smooth, with no crevices created by overly tight sutures. Redraping the skin and pulling in the same posterosuperior vector should be performed as a means of checking for dimpling or unwanted uneven areas. It is common to remove undesired suspension sutures and place others to facilitate a better outcome.

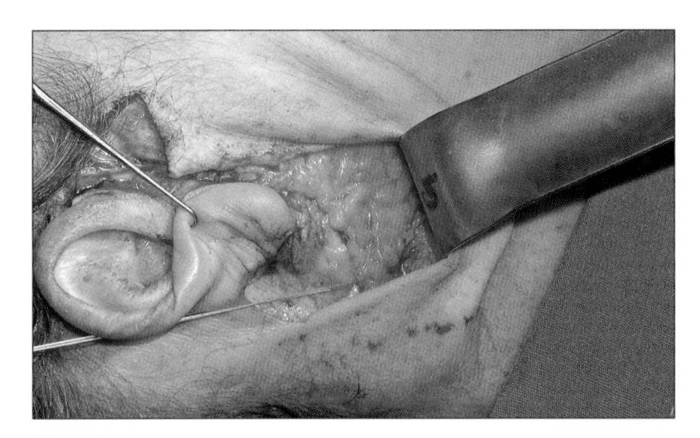

Fig 6-7m Suspension suture near the angle of the mandible will be secured to the mastoid fascia.

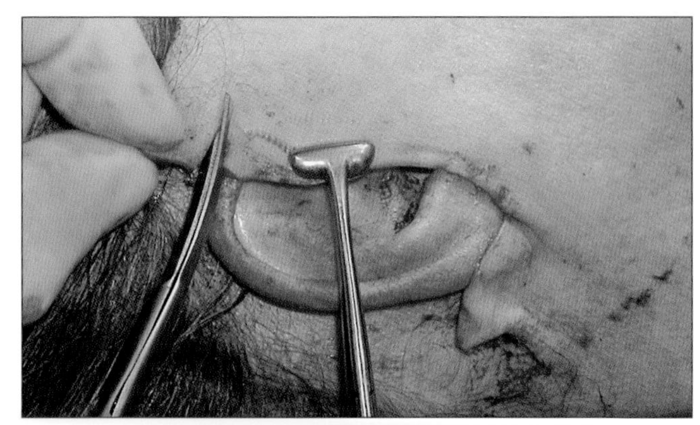

Fig 6-7n Prior to placing the first key suture, the flap is grabbed and pulled in a posterosuperior direction. A cut is then placed in the flap, tangential to the top of the auricle, so as to remove the excess skin.

The fourth and final suspension suture is placed with the same 2-0 Vicryl suture, grabbing a bite of SMAS near the angle of the mandible and suspending it to the mastoid fascia (Fig 6-7m). Again, careful attention to the posterosuperior vector is observed when pulling the SMAS layer to produce the most desirable appearance. After securing this suspension suture to the mastoid area with the same tension as the previous sutures, a final check beneath the skin flap is performed to verify hemostasis as well as to check for acceptable contouring of the entire SMAS layer. In addition, the skin is also redraped and pulled posterosuperiorly to assess the amount of skin excision that will take place and to confirm a smooth, even appearance of the face.

Securing the skin flap

Upon completion of the dissection, suspension, and redraping of the skin, attention is turned toward placing key external sutures at the skin level to secure the skin flap that is under tension in the posterosuperior vector. When pulling the skin flap, it is recommended that facelift clamps be used near the skin flap margin to avoid slippage and to execute adequate pull on the flap. Marks placed on the skin from the teeth of the clamps should not worry the practitioner because this redundant skin will be excised later.

The first key suture is planned where the posterior margin of the flap meets the anterior corner. Prior to placing this key suture, the facelift scissors are used to make a cut tangent to the superior helical rim of the ear to expose the top portion of the ear (Fig 6-7n). Continued pull on the flap is desired to tighten the outer skin. Then the suture is positioned using 3-0 silk on a large cutting needle on an imaginary line tangent to the superior helical rim of the ear, just anterior to the helix (Fig 6-7o).

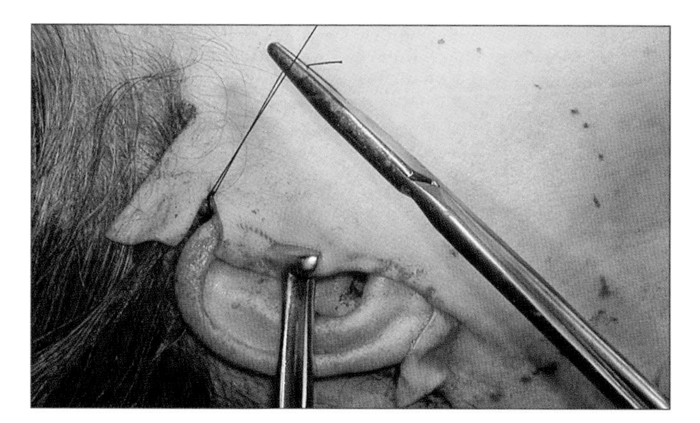

Fig 6-7o First key suture intact at the posterior edge of the temporal hair tuft.

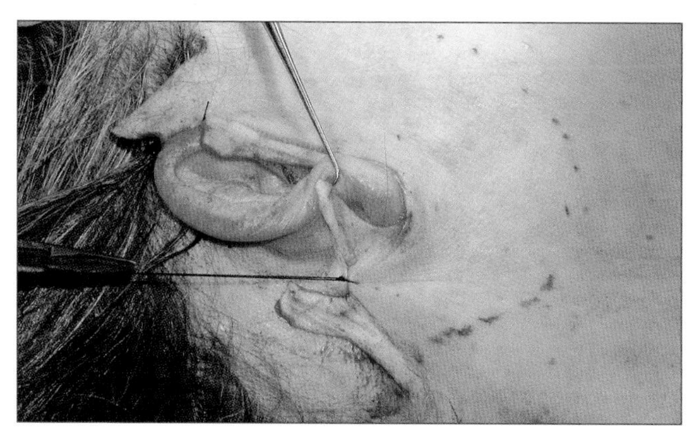

Fig 6-7p Placing the second key suture behind the ear while placing the same posterior and superior traction on the flap. Once again, a cut is made in the flap so there is no overlap between the skin edges prior to suturing.

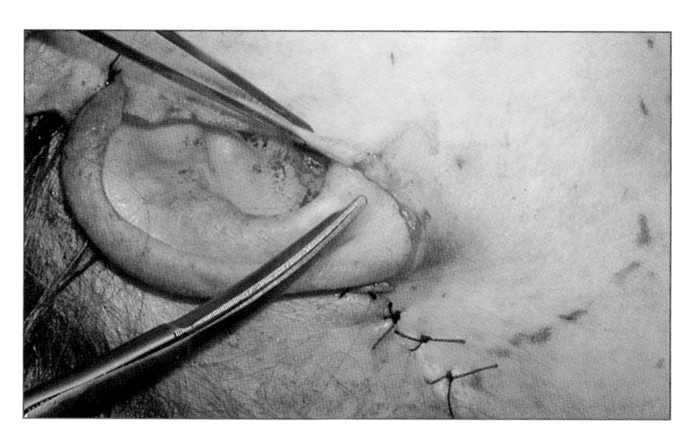

Fig 6-7q Prior to placing the third key suture, facelift scissors are used to follow the contour of the outer edge of the lobule.

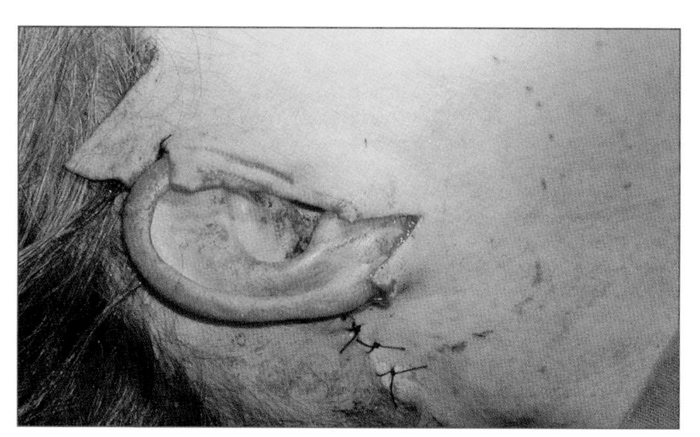

Fig 6-7r A cut is made with the facelift scissors into the flap to create room for the lobule to rest. If the cut is made too long, excessive tension will be placed near the skin of the lobule, and a pixie ear deformity may result.

The second key suture is placed behind the ear at the approximate midpoint of the posterior auricular incision while simultaneously holding traction on the skin flap in the same vector previously mentioned (Fig 6-7p). After placing this suture, obvious excess skin is trimmed with the facelift scissors so as to align the two skin edges passively. After removing the skin and adapting the skin edges, the closure of the posterior auricular area is performed with 3-0 silk sutures in an interrupted fashion.

The next step of the procedure is vital to the cosmesis of the ear lobule. While traction is pulled on the skin flap, facelift scissors are used to cut the skin around the inferior auricle obliquely in an inferomedial direction to facilitate the exposure and proper positioning of the ear lobule (Figs 6-7q and 6-7r). There is no predetermined, designated

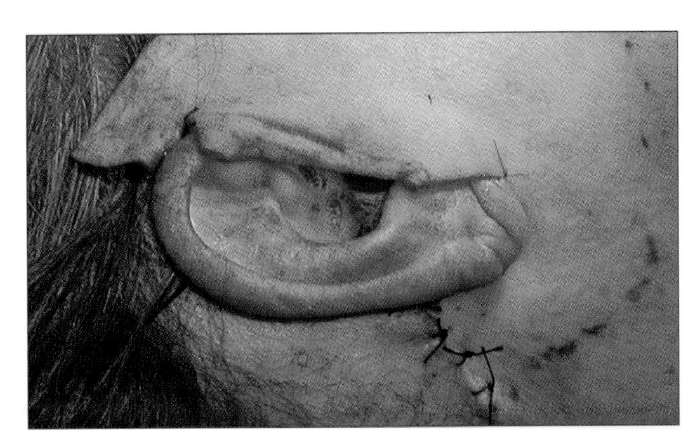

Fig 6-7s Third key suture placed at inferior part of initial incision, near base of the ear lobule.

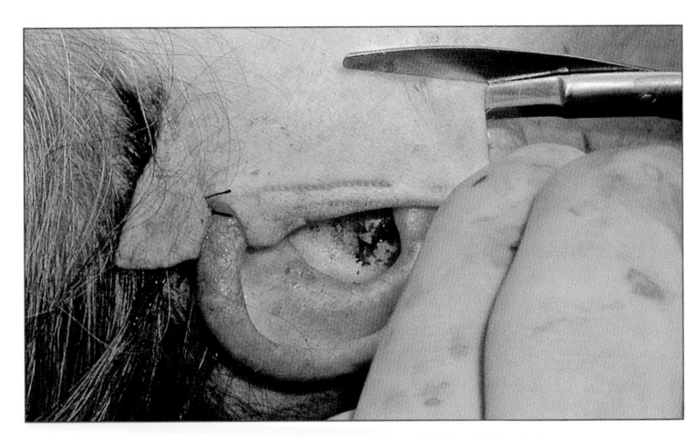

Fig 6-7t Excision of excess skin after pulling posterosuperior traction on the flap. There will be two C-shaped cuts made in this portion of the flap.

amount to cut. It is advisable, however, to err on the conservative side, because excessive cutting of this area of the skin flap causes tension at the inferior ear. When the ear lobule is tugged inferiorly by the cheek skin, the result is a pixie ear deformity. After uncovering the ear from underneath the flap, a third key suture consisting of 6-0 nylon on a small cutting needle can be placed at the junction of the superoanterior earlobe skin and cheek skin at the inferior preauricular incision (Fig 6-7s).

Skin excision and flap closure

After placing these three key sutures, the practitioner can take a breath and be relieved, because the skin flap has essentially been set to its new position on the face. The excess skin in the preauricular area is removed first with facelift scissors. After traction is placed on the flap edge in the same posterosuperior vector, the cut is started inferiorly and continued superiorly in a curvilinear fashion, mimicking the outline of the initial incision (Fig 6-7t). Two cuts are needed to properly excise this area because there are two separate curves in the incision pattern (see Fig 6-7a). It is important that upon completion of the skin excision, the two skin margins are passive to avoid placing tension on the wound and subsequent unesthetic scarring.

Once a passive alignment of the preauricular skin edges has been established, the excess skin found in the hair-bearing area of the temporal tuft can be excised with the facelift scissors (Fig 6-7u). Again, the skin to be removed is held under traction while it is being cut. After cutting the superfluous skin, the skin margins should passively adapt such that the wound will be under minimal tension. The temporal area is then closed with 3-0 silk sutures in an interrupted fashion, followed by su-

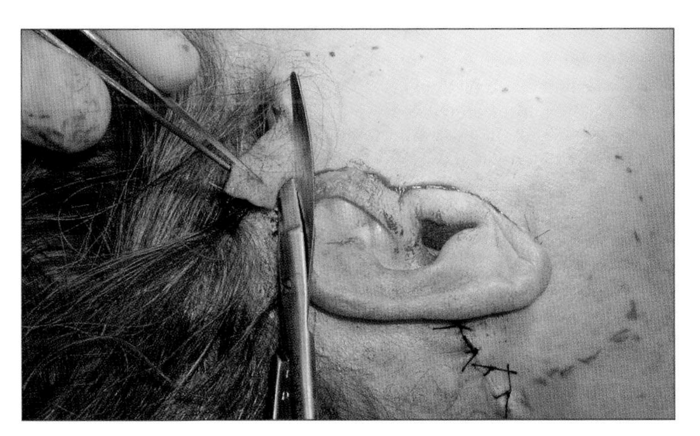

Fig 6-7u Excising excess skin at the temporal hair tuft.

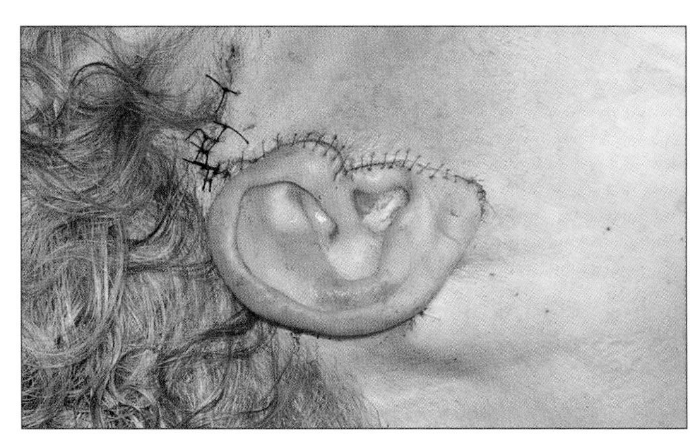

Fig 6-7v Final closure of the flap.

Fig 6-7w Occlusive head wrap placed immediately postoperatively.

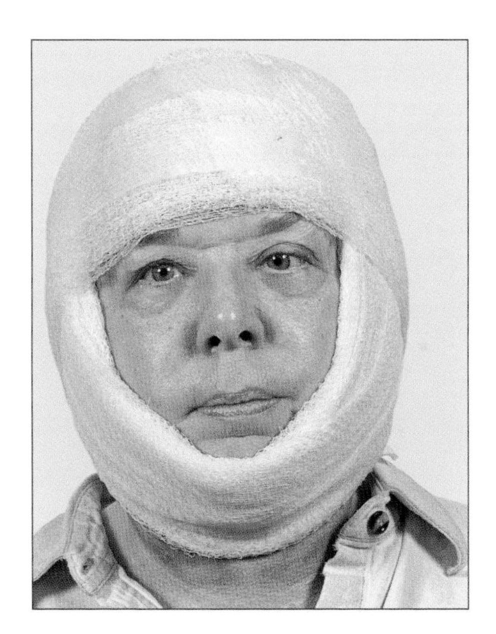

turing of the preauricular skin with running 6-0 nylon sutures on a small cutting needle (Fig 6-7v). When closing the incisions, surgeons should handle "dog ear" tags with precision and a conservative technique with only minimal amounts of skin snipping. Overzealous snipping of these redundant areas of skin results in a much longer scar after healing has occurred.

After all closures are completed and the patient is thoroughly cleaned off, antimicrobial ointment is applied over the wounds, and 4-inch^2 gauze packs are stacked and placed in front of and behind the ear. Next, a head wrap is placed around the chin and head, covering the ears and effectively applying pressure over the surgical sites (Fig 6-7w), which helps adapt the new skin to the underlying tissues as well as minimize the risk of hematoma.

Postoperative Care

After surgery is completed, it is important to keep the patient from gagging, wretching, or vomiting. Any of these actions may induce bleeding in the operated areas. Care must be taken to eliminate factors that promote bleeding in order to prevent hematoma underneath the skin. If a hematoma does develop, it may expand and may need to be drained shortly after surgery. It is therefore wise for the surgeon or the anesthetist to administer an antiemetic intravenously, intramuscularly, or via a patch. The scopolamine patch, placed behind the ear, is effective along with a possible adjunctive dose of intravenous promethazine or ondansetron. After it is determined that the patient is stable, discharge instructions and appropriate antibiotic and analgesic prescriptions are given, and the patient is discharged.

The patient is instructed to wear the compressive head dressing for 24 hours and then return to the office for a dressing change. The head is rewrapped, this time with a lighter facial compressive band head wrap (eg, Veronique Compression Wear) or something similar. The patient's wounds and face are checked for dehiscence, hematoma, symmetry, and facial nerve function. The patient is then discharged and asked to return in 2 days for another dressing change. After the second head dressing change, the patient is scheduled for a postsurgical follow-up visit a week later, where the head dressing is not replaced and all sutures are removed. Subsequent follow-up visits are planned as needed, and postoperative photographs are taken after 6 to 8 weeks.

Demonstration of pre- and postoperative photographs to the patient is very important. Often, patients do not remember their appearance prior to the procedure and thus may not be impressed with the results. Therefore, it is crucial to keep good photographic records for each patient to compare the final product to the initial presentation (Figs 6-8 to 6-10). Those patients who receive a subtle but improved change may be especially disappointed if a photographic comparison cannot be made.

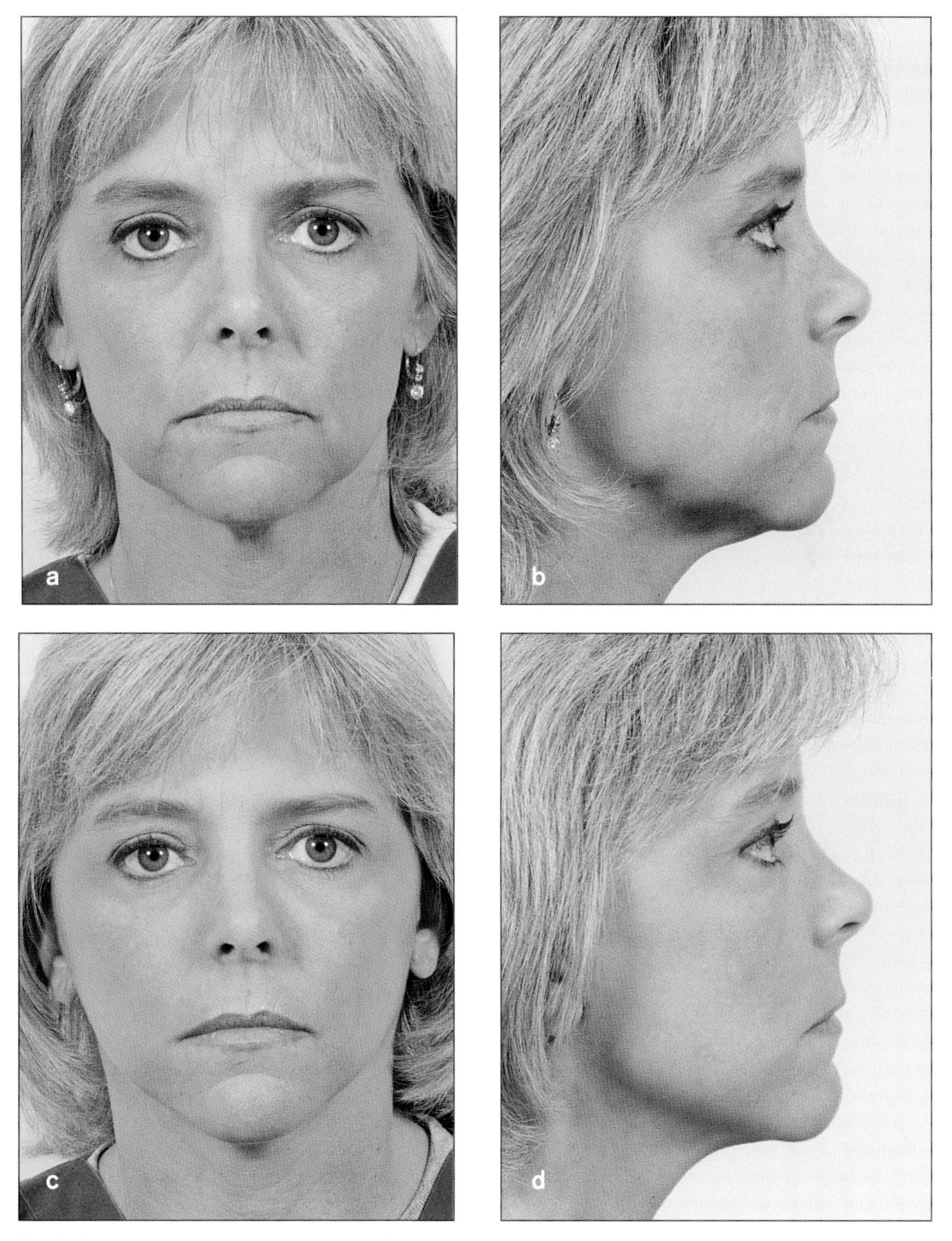

Fig 6-8 *(a and b)* Preoperative views. *(c and d)* Postoperative views.

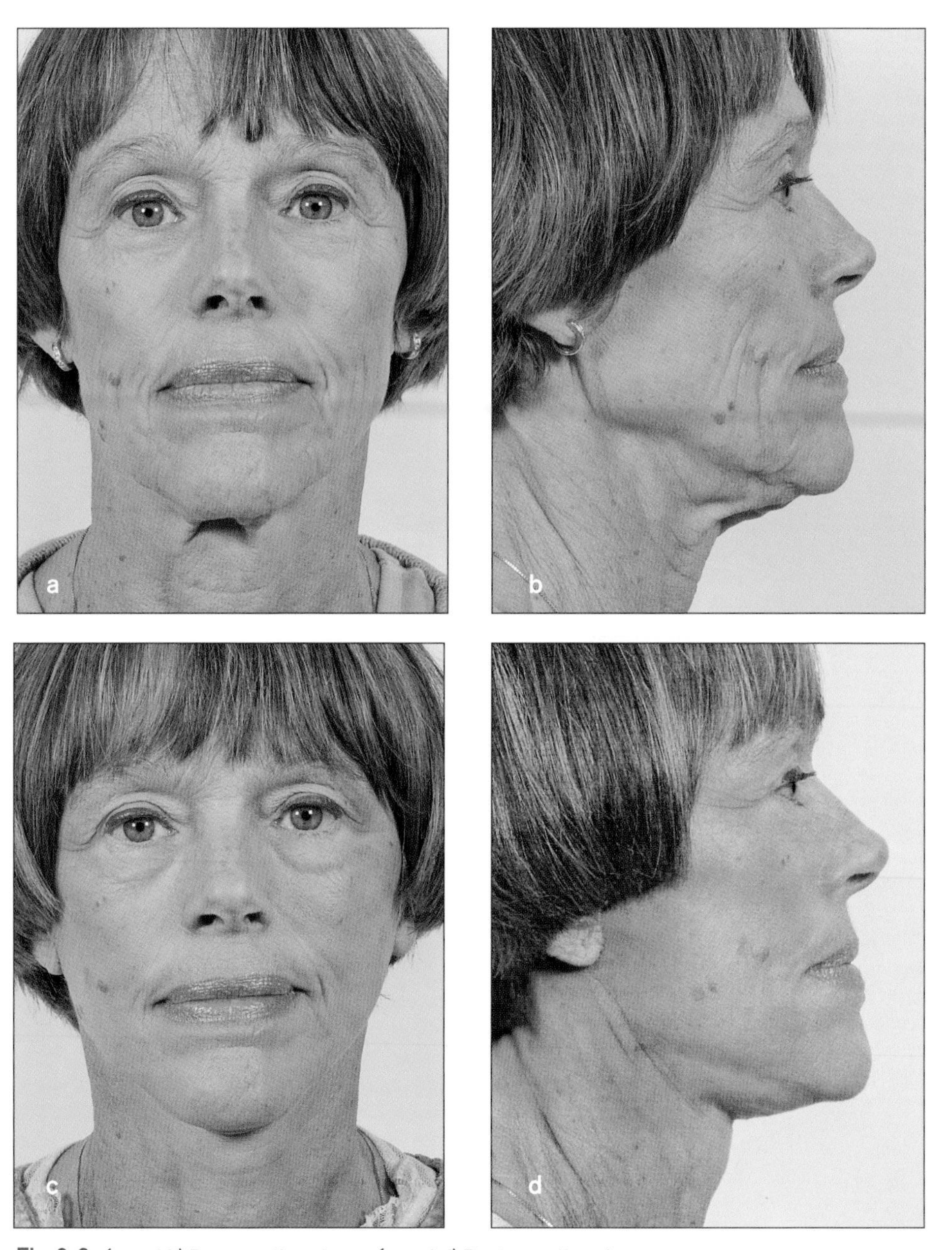

Fig 6-9 *(a and b)* Preoperative views. *(c and d)* Postoperative views.

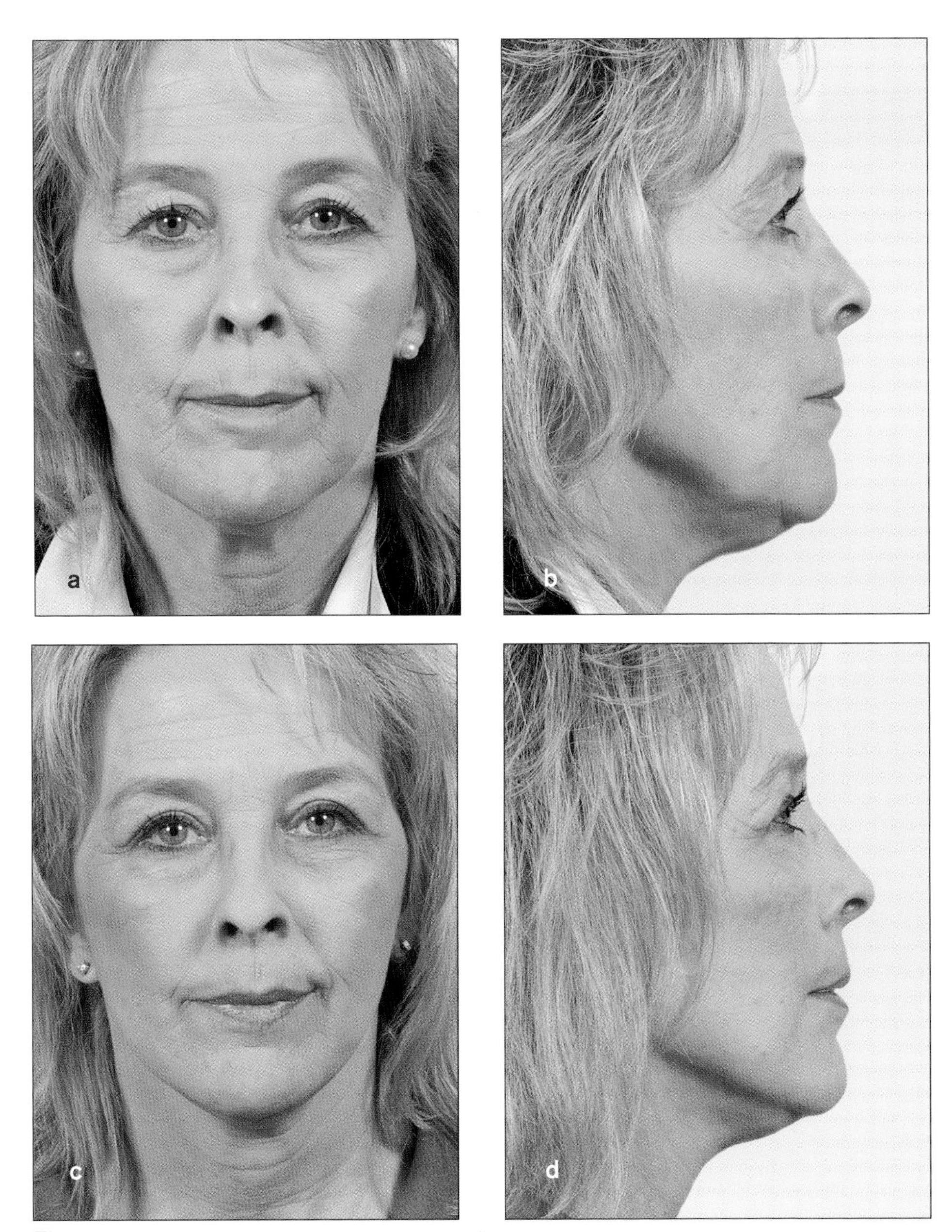

Fig 6-10 *(a and b)* Preoperative views. *(c and d)* Postoperative views.

Complications

Complications that exist in minimal incision facelift are the same as those that occur in standard rhytidectomy procedures. Please refer to chapter 4 for a discussion of the complications associated with this procedure.

Summary

The minimal incision facelift can be an excellent procedure to use in the oral and maxillofacial surgeon's practice. It is simpler than the conventional full facelift, requires less operative time, and is well suited for many patients with a mild to moderate amount of facial aging who desire a rejuvenated appearance. A good set of pre- and postoperative photographs is necessary to demonstrate the positive changes in each patient and are a part of good record keeping. With careful attention to the details presented in this chapter, a high degree of patient satisfaction is obtainable.

References

1. La Trenta GS. The aesthetic anatomy of the face. In: La Trenta GS (ed). Atlas of Aesthetic Face and Neck Surgery. Philadelphia: Saunders, 2004:2–45.
2. Honrado CP, Bradley DT, Larrabee WF. Facial embryology and anatomy. In: Azizzadeh B, Murphy MR, Johnson CM Jr (eds). Master Techniques in Facial Rejuvenation. Philadelphia: Saunders, 2007:17–32.
3. Dingman RO, Grabb WC. Surgical anatomy of the mandibular ramus of the facial nerve based on the dissection of 100 facial halves. Plast Reconstr Surg 1962;29:266–272.
4. Adamson PA, Moran ML. Complications of cervicofacial rhytidectomy. Facial Plast Surg Clin North Am 1993;1:257–271.
5. Rees TD, Aston SJ. Complications of rhytidectomy. Clin Plast Surg 1978;5:109–119.
6. Baker DC. Complications of cervicofacial rhytidectomy. Clin Plast Surg 1983;10:543–562.
7. Friedman O. Changes associated with the aging face. Facial Plast Surg Clin North Am 2005;13: 371–380.
8. Larrabee WF, Makielski KH, Henderson JL. Surgical Anatomy of the Face. Philadelphia: Lippincott, Williams & Wilkins, 2004.
9. Azizzadeh B, Hadlock TA, Cheney ML. Short-flap SMAS rhytidectomy. In: Azizzadeh B, Murphy MR, Johnson CM Jr (eds). Master Techniques in Facial Rejuvenation. Philadelphia: Saunders, 2007:153–172.
10. Yousif NJ, Gosain A, Matloub HS, Sanger JR, Madiedo G, Larson DL. The nasolabial fold: An anatomic and histologic reappraisal. Plast Reconstr Surg 1994;93:60–69.
11. Montagna W, Carlisle K. Structural changes in ageing skin. Br J Dermatol 1990;122(suppl 35): 61–70.
12. Byrd HS. The extended browlift. Clin Plast Surg 1997;24:233–246.
13. Hamra ST. The deep plane rhytidectomy. Plast Reconstr Surg 1990;86:53–61.
14. Wang TD. Rhytidectomy for treatment of the aging face. Mayo Clin Proc 1989; 64:780–790.
15. Murphy MR, Johnson CM Jr, Azizzadeh B. The aging face consultation. In: Azizzadeh B, Murphy MR, Johnson CM Jr (eds). Master Techniques in Facial Rejuvenation. Philadelphia: Saunders, 2007:1–16.
16. Bolgnia JL. Dermatologic and cosmetic concerns of the older woman. Clin Geriatr Med 1993;9: 209–229.
17. Adamson PA, Litner JA. Evolution of rhytidectomy techniques. Facial Plast Surg Clin North Am 2005;13:383–391.

7

Blepharoplasty

TAYLOR P. MCGUIRE, BSc, DDS, MSc, FRCD(C)

Across many surgical disciplines, blepharoplasty remains one of the most requested facial cosmetic procedures. The history and evolution of this procedure are well documented and extensive.[1–4] Blepharoplasty is performed routinely for both cosmetic and functional reasons, but it is estimated that more than 100,000 people every year have this procedure performed for cosmetic purposes alone. The eyes, more than any other facial feature, are a focus of attention for both patients and observers—hence the common metaphor, "the eyes are the window to the soul." Changes in the face, whether due to aging or genetics, seem paramount when they take place in the orbital region.

Blepharoplasty carries with it the potential for a high degree of patient and surgeon satisfaction. Successful outcomes arise most predictably when sound surgical skill and judgment are coupled with informed consent and realistic patient expectations. It behooves the surgeon to have a complete understanding of the technical aspects of upper and lower eyelid blepharoplasty and a complete grasp of how to manage minor and major complications that may occur. This chapter will help "open your eyes" to the beauty that is blepharoplasty through a comprehensive review of orbital anatomy, patient selection criteria, pathways for diagnosis, upper and lower eyelid techniques, and case presentations.

Applied Anatomy

The eye and surrounding orbital contents are undoubtedly some of the most intricate and complex structures found in the human body. Advanced, applied surgical knowledge of the anatomy of this region is mandatory for the practicing oral and maxillofacial surgeon. As with orbital trauma, cosmetic blepharoplasty begins with a systematic evaluation of the external anatomy of each of the patient's eyes in the rest, or *primary gaze*, position. This allows for the identification and analysis of key anatomical structures such as the skin, sclera, conjunctiva, cornea, iris, limbus, lacrimal caruncle, punctum, upper and lower tarsal plates, upper and lower eyelid creases, grey line, palpebral fissure, and medial and lateral canthi (Fig 7-1).

There are many important anatomical relationships that the cosmetic blepharoplasty surgeon must be able to recognize (Fig 7-2). The adult palpebral fissure averages 28 to 30 mm in width and 10 to 12 mm in height. This height constitutes *eye opening at rest* and can be divided into the mean reflex distance (MRD) 1 and 2. When examining the eye at rest, the MRD1 represents the vertical distance from the inferior edge of the upper eyelid down to the center of the pupil (the point at which

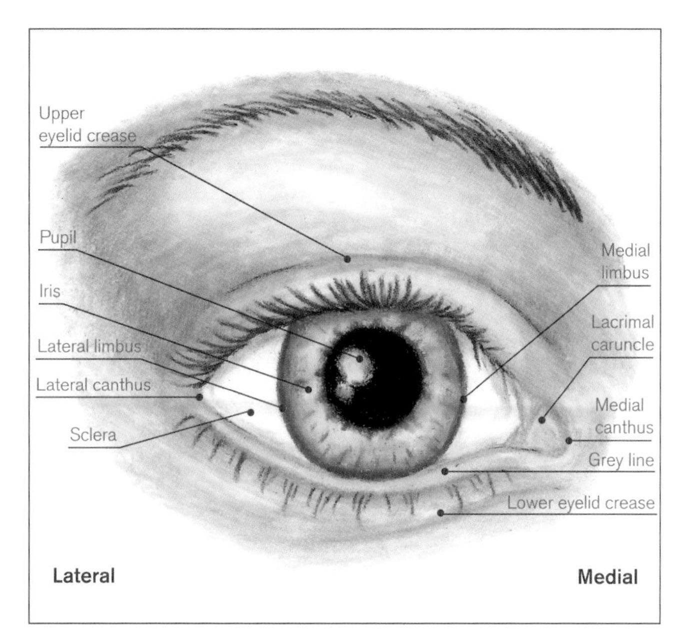

Fig 7-1 External anatomy of the eye. *Sclera:* white of the eyes covering posterior ⅚ of the globe. *Conjunctiva:* clear mucous membrane covering anterior ⅙ of the globe; does not cover the cornea and is not depicted here. There are two types—*bulbar,* which covers the sclera, and *palpebral,* which lines the eyelids. *Cornea:* anterior transparent five-layered aspect of the eye that covers the iris, pupil, and anterior chamber (not depicted here); it is confluent with the sclera. *Limbus:* corneoscleral junction at the edge of the iris. *Iris:* colored fibrovascular pupillary sphincter; posterior to cornea, anterior to lens. *Pupil:* ocular aperture located at the center of the iris. Other important landmarks include the lacrimal caruncle, the upper and lower eyelid creases, and the medial and lateral canthi.

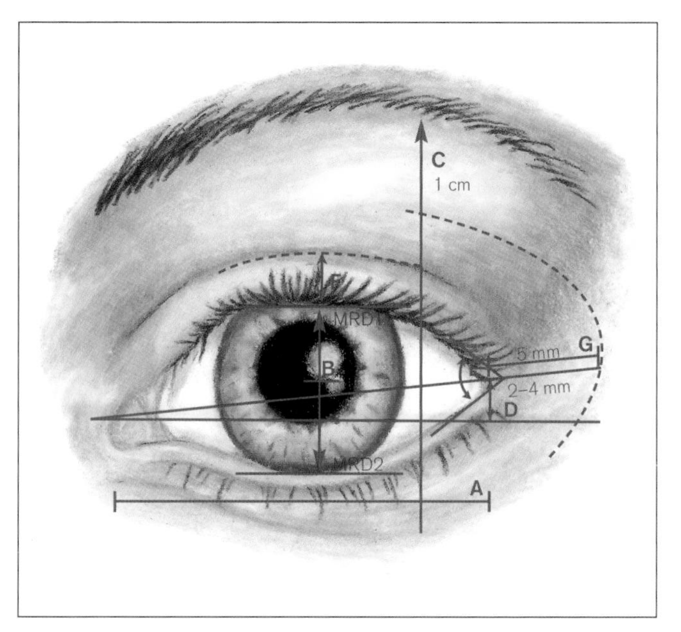

Fig 7-2 Superficial topography of the eye. (A) *Palpebral width:* 28 to 30 mm; distance between the medial and lateral canthi. (B) *Mean reflex distances* (MRD1 and MRD2); *palpebral height:* 10 to 12 mm; MRD1 + MRD2. (C) Highest point of brow corresponds to tangent vertical to the lateral limbus and inferior aspect of brow along line C sits about 1 cm superior to the supraorbital rim. (D) *Intercanthal axis:* Lateral canthus sits 2 to 4 mm superior to the medial canthus. (E) *Lateral canthal angle:* 30 to 40 degrees. (F) *Margin crease distance* (MCD): men, 7 to 9 mm and women, 9 to 12 mm. (G) Distance from lateral canthus to lateral orbital rim is about 5 mm.

maximal light reflection may be observed). Similarly, the MRD2 is the vertical distance from the center of the pupil down to the superior edge of the inferior eyelid. Subtle decreases in the MRD1 may be seen with true upper eyelid ptosis, while increases in the MRD2 may occur with ectropion or lower eyelid retraction. As such, regular attempts to measure the MRD1 and MRD2 to the nearest 0.5 mm significantly help with diagnosis and allow for better communication among surgeons.[1,5] The lower lid margin has a tangential relationship to the lower limbus, with the lowest point being found just lateral to the pupil. Seldom does the lower lid cover the corneal margin by more than 1 mm. The upper lid margin is positioned at 1 to 2 mm below the upper limbus, with its highest point just nasal to a vertical line drawn through the center of the pupil. These lid margins meet laterally at a 30- to 40-degree angle at the lateral canthus. The lateral canthus itself is located 5 mm inside the lateral orbital rim and approximately 1 cm below the zygomaticofrontal suture at a slightly superior position (2 to 4 mm) with respect to the medial canthus. Together, the medial and lateral canthi delineate the horizontal palpebral aperture.

The superior palpebral sulcus, also known as the *upper lid crease,* results from the insertion of the levator aponeurosis into the skin of the upper eyelid. It can be easily located with repetitive eye opening. Its location is measured from the central aspect of the upper eyelid margin up to the deepest dominant fold, or sulcus, found in the upper

Fig 7-3 Cross-sectional anatomy of the upper and lower eyelids. Note the relationship of the orbital septum to the upper and lower eyelid retractors. The orbital septum is a robust anatomical barrier. The levator aponeurosis sits superficial to the Müller muscle and inserts onto the anterior surface of the superior tarsal plate and directly into the skin.

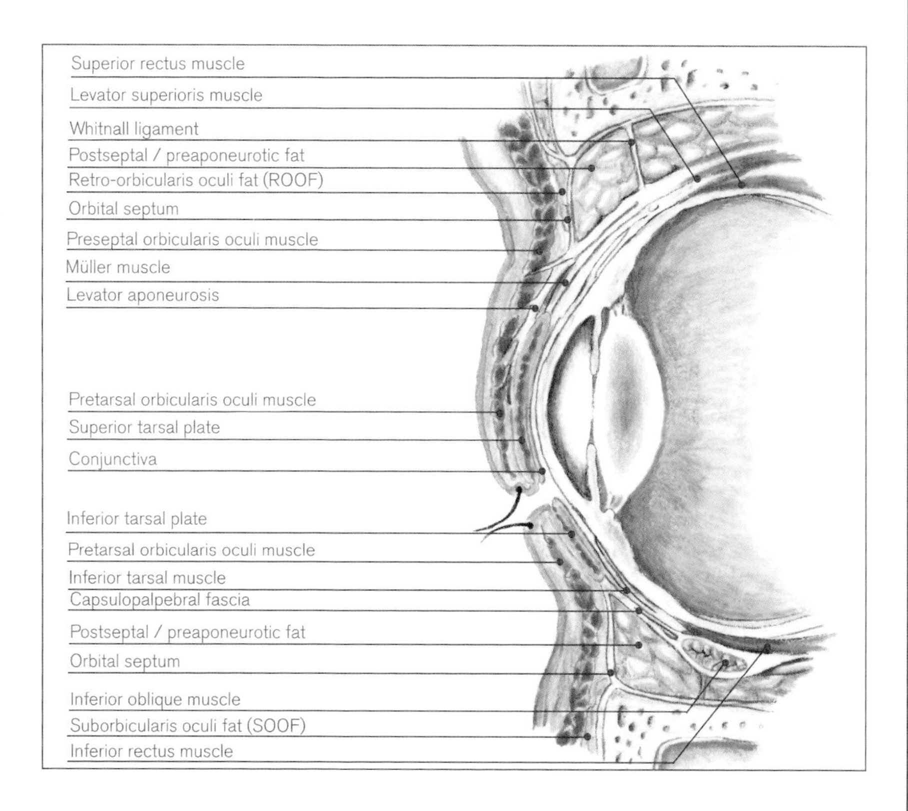

eyelid; this distance is typically termed the *margin crease distance* (MCD). The MCD ranges from 7 to 9 mm in men and from 9 to 12 mm in women.[6] This measurement varies considerably with ethnicity, so the upper lid crease may be located more superiorly in eyes that have a prominent supraorbital rim with little fat, or it may be completely absent, as is the case in 50% of the Asian population.[7] When present, the upper eyelid crease creates the false illusion of a larger, more open eye. In actuality, most palpebral fissures are of the same dimension, regardless of sex or ethnicity.

The inferior palpebral sulcus, more commonly called the *lower lid crease*, marks the lower margin of the tarsal plate of the inferior eyelid. It is found approximately 3 to 4 mm below the margin of the lower eyelid. The malar sulcus, also known as the *nasojugal groove*, is much more variable in its position and depth and is formed by subcutaneous insertion of the orbitomalar ligament, which arises from the arcus marginalis of the inferior orbital rim and represents a unique bony attachment of the orbicularis oculi.

Eyelid Skin

The composition, or layering, of the cross-sectional anatomy of the human eyelid varies slightly, depending on whether one is looking at the pretarsal or preseptal region. In general, the layers to be aware of—in order from superficial to deep—include skin, subcutaneous tissue, orbicularis oculi muscle, tarsal plates/orbital septum, postseptal fat, upper and lower eyelid retractors, and the tarsal/palpebral conjunctiva (Fig 7-3). The average skin thickness of the human eyelid is equal to that of a split-thickness skin graft (0.008 to 0.015 inch) and, with the exception of the prepuce and the labia minora, the eyelid represents the thinnest skin in the body.[1,2,8,9] The eyelid skin is firmly attached over the tarsal plates. It is nearly devoid of subcutaneous fat and quickly transitions to underlying muscle with increasing depth. In all age groups, the eyelid skin becomes thicker, coarser, and oilier as it travels over the bony orbital rims.[10] The appearance of periorbital youthfulness, however, is heralded by skin that is uniform in color and texture, free of contour defects such as rhytids and folds, and smooth in transition zones with surrounding facial subunits.

Orbicularis oculi muscle and canthal ligaments

The orbicularis oculi muscle and associated canthal tendons are important, inseparable anatomical structures. The orbicularis oculi is a large, striated skeletal muscle that receives its motor innervation from cranial nerve (CN) VII via its inferior surface. It is most often described as having three distinct yet conjoined muscular bands: orbital, preseptal, and pretarsal[1,2,5,9] (Fig 7-4). The medial canthal tendon (MCT) is formed by the condensation of all three portions of this muscle. It is reliably found to have a larger, more dominant anterior head that inserts directly into the anterior lacrimal crest of the maxilla and a smaller, more posteriorly situated head that inserts into the posterior lacrimal crest of the lacrimal bone. The larger, more powerful orbital aspect of this muscle has the MCT as its origin and insertion. It thus encircles and overlies the bony orbital rims, blends with the frontalis muscle superiorly and the corrugator supercilii medially, and is responsible for the lateral crow's feet wrinkling seen with forceful closure of the eyes. It occupies a more superficial plane with respect to its deeper palpebral counterpart.

The palpebral portion of the orbicularis oculi is subdivided into pretarsal and preseptal regions. Each upper and lower eyelid possesses a superficial and a deep "head," or band, that contributes to the anterior and posterior limbs of the MCT, respectively (Fig 7-5). The superficial limbs of the pretarsal and preseptal muscles both attach to and form a portion of the anterior limb of the MCT, while the anatomy of the deep heads is slightly more intricate. The deep heads of the pretarsal portion that arise off the medial aspect of the upper and lower eyelid tarsus (the Horner muscle) each insert into the posterior lacrimal crest, just behind the lacrimal sac. Similarly, the deep heads of the preseptal muscles both insert just anterior to their deep pretarsal counterparts by attaching directly to the fascia overlying the lacrimal sac and the medial orbital wall above and below the Horner muscle.[5,9]

The lateral edge of the superficial preseptal orbicularis oculi fibers form an indistinct raphe that attaches to the lateral orbital rim and the overlying skin. The upper and lower deeper lateral aspects of the pretarsal orbicularis oculi fibers fuse to form the more posterior, dominant head of the lateral canthal tendon (LCT), which in turn inserts directly onto the Whitnall ligament. There is a vascular space between the attachment of the LCT and the more superficial raphe. Unlike the pretarsal and preseptal muscles, the more superficial orbital muscle has no firm lateral attachment except to the skin lateral to the LCT.[9]

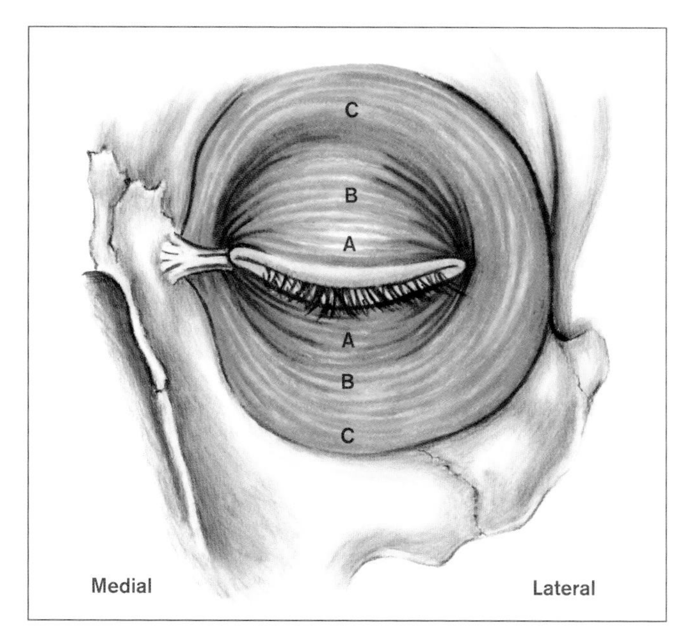

Fig 7-4 The three muscular bands of the orbicularis oculi muscle: (A) pretarsal, (B) preseptal, and (C) orbital.

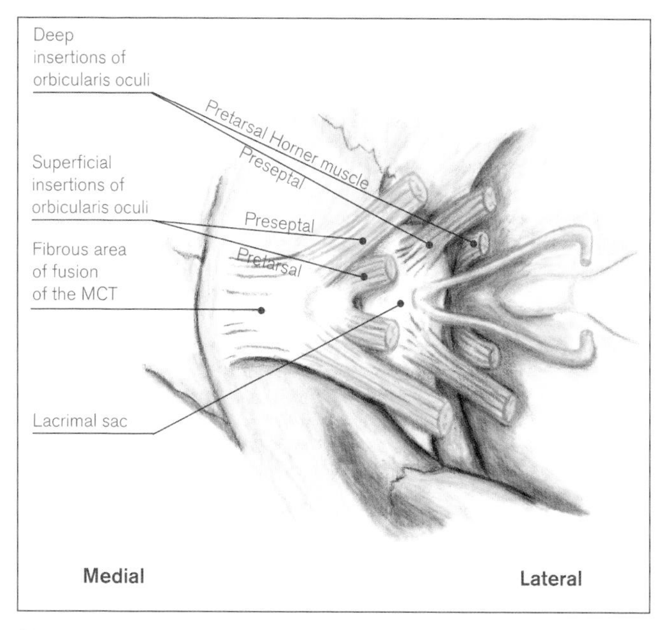

Fig 7-5 Components of the medial canthus. The anatomical relationships existing between the preseptal and pretarsal aspects of the MCT are displayed.

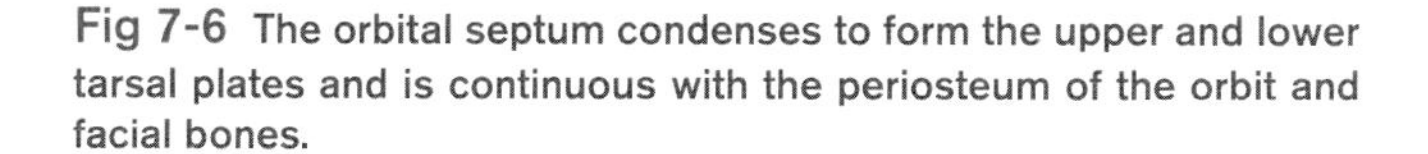

Fig 7-6 The orbital septum condenses to form the upper and lower tarsal plates and is continuous with the periosteum of the orbit and facial bones.

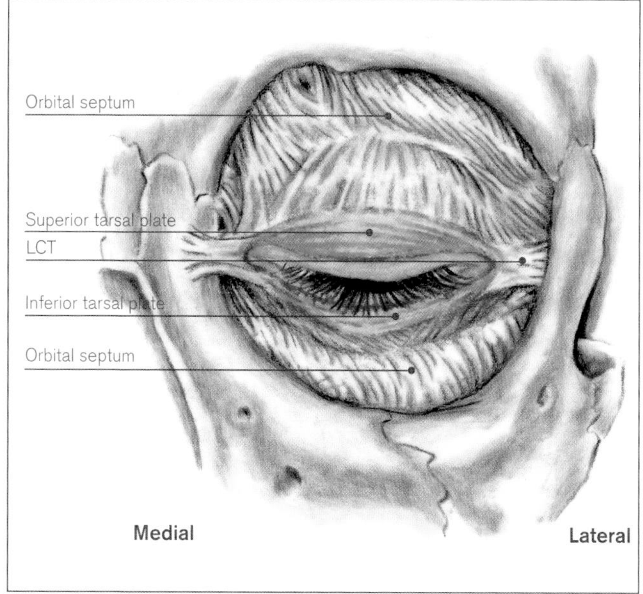

Orbital septum and tarsal plates

The orbital septum lies deep to the orbicularis oculi muscle. It serves as the dominant structural framework of the eyelids and is responsible for separating the orbital contents (postseptal) from the external (preseptal) structures[2] (Fig 7-6). It is anatomically continuous with the orbital periosteum and the periosteum of the facial bones overlying the orbital rims. These two periosteal layers fuse circumferentially 1 to 2 mm inside the orbital rims to form the *arcus marginalis*. The septum arises from the arcus marginalis and extends into the eyelids to form the upper and lower tarsal plates.[5,9]

The tarsal plates anatomically and conceptually resemble cartilage. In actuality, however, they are fibrous tissue formed from the condensation and thickening of the orbital septum. The tarsal border parallels the free margin of the eyelids and is responsible for giving the lids their convex shape. They both are approximately 30 mm in length, with the average height of the upper tarsal plate measuring 10 to 12 mm and that of the lower tarsal plate measuring 4 mm. Each tarsal plate is attached by dense fibrous tissue both medially and laterally to the MCT and LCT.[5]

In the upper eyelid, the orbital septum fuses with the underlying levator aponeurosis at a variable distance from the superior edge of the upper tarsal plate. This point of fusion in Caucasians takes place approximately 8 to 10 mm above the superior tarsal border. It not only limits the downward extent of the postseptal fat pads but also allows for the terminal interdigitations of the aponeurosis to insert into the subdermal aspect of the pretarsal upper eyelid skin. Contraction of the levator consequently pulls the upper eyelid open and forms the supratarsal upper eyelid crease. Those lacking an upper eyelid crease generally exhibit a lower point of fusion of the orbital septum with the levator aponeurosis.[7] This in turn leads to a lack of attachment of the terminal levator strands into the subdermal skin. When coupled with the increased ability of the postseptal fat pads to descend downward, such eyelids can appear fuller or puffier, with an ill-defined or absent upper eyelid crease. In the lower lid, the orbital septum fuses with the capsulopalpebral fascia approximately 5 mm inferior to the inferior tarsal plate.

Orbital fat

Fat exists in abundance in the orbital region and is best thought of in terms of preseptal and postseptal fat. Preseptal fat consists of subcutaneous fat (sparse to nonexistent in the eyelids) and the retro-orbicularis oculi fat (ROOF) pad and the suborbicularis oculi fat (SOOF) pads (see Fig 7-3). The ROOF pad is a submuscular fat pad located deep to the interdigitation of the frontalis and upper aspect of the orbicularis oculi muscle.[5,9] It is also known as the *sub-brow fat pad*, and while still a consideration in periorbital esthetic procedures, it more often is encountered with endoscopic forehead lifting and upper third facial rejuvenation procedures. The SOOF pads may be found as a thin layer of fat located deep to the orbicularis oculi muscle within the lower eyelids. Repositioning of this fat has been described as an adjunctive procedure performed in certain instances with lower eyelid rejuvenation.

Postseptal, or *preaponeurotic*, fat is much more abundant and better described than preseptal fat.[5,9] This extraconal fat surrounds vital structures in the posterior orbit including vessels, nerves, and muscles. In this capacity, it functions to cushion and envelop the globe and its attached musculature, thereby aiding with stabilization while simultaneously providing for frictionless movement.[2] Postseptal fat is located just posterior to the orbital septum and may be found as three distinct compartments in the lower lid and two in the upper lid (Fig 7-7). In the lower lid, the medial and central fat pads are separated by the inferior oblique muscle. The lower lateral fat pad is really con-

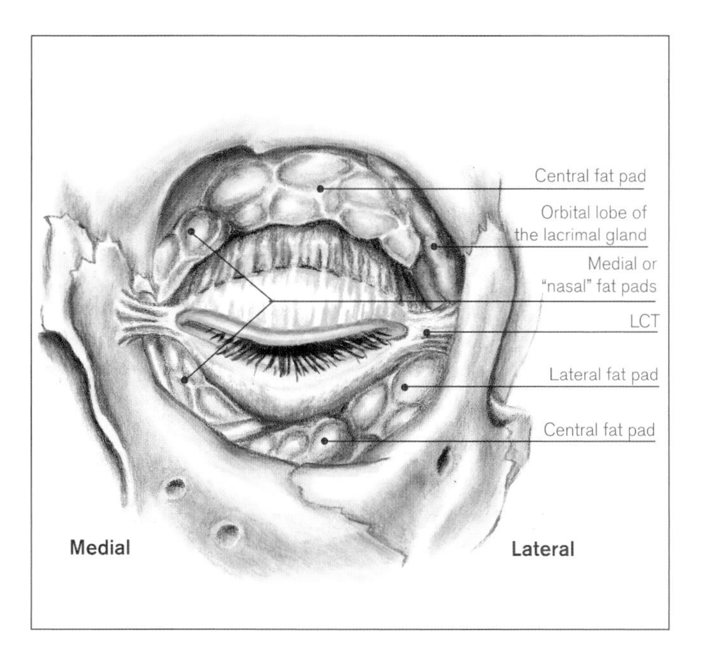

Fig 7-7 **Postseptal orbital fat compartments. The orbital septum has been removed to yield the upper and lower eyelid fat pads. Note that the inferior oblique muscle separates the medial and central fat pads of the lower eyelid.**

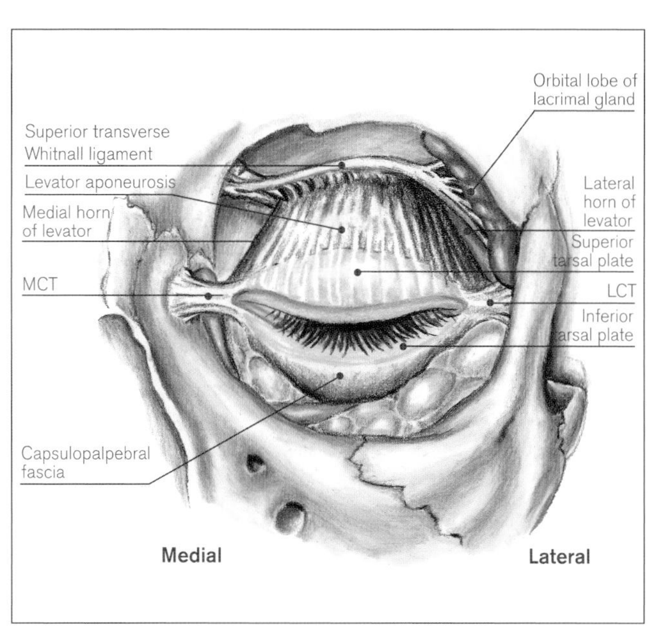

Fig 7-8 **Upper and lower eyelid retractors. The orbital septum and upper eyelid fat pads have been removed. Observe the Whitnall ligament and the medial and lateral horns of the levator aponeurosis.**

tinuous with the central fat pad, separated anteriorly only by thin fascial extensions of the lateral and inferior rectus muscles. The medial fat pad of the upper lid is similarly isolated from the upper central fat pad by the trochlea of the superior oblique muscle. Both the upper and lower medial fat pads are paler, firmer, and more fibrous than the central and lateral (lower only) fat pads. The lacrimal gland occupies the most lateral postseptal position within the upper eyelid and looks entirely different in appearance and consistency. It should never be mistaken for the upper eyelid central fat pad.[1,5]

Upper and lower eyelid retractors

The levator palpebrae superioris is the main retractor, or principal elevator, of the upper eyelid. It is made up of a proximal, posterior muscular section innervated by CN III and a distal, anterior tendinous portion, better known as the *levator aponeurosis* (Fig 7-8). The muscular component is composed of striated muscle that arises from the lesser wing of the sphenoid deep in the superior orbital apex. It travels anterosuperiorly above the globe and superior to the superior rectus muscle for approximately 4 cm before it begins to flatten out to form the aponeurosis. This transition takes place in the region of the Whitnall ligament, just above the insertion point of the superior rectus into the globe. The Whitnall ligament functions as a superior transverse or mediolateral check ligament for the globe. It is formed from the condensation of the superior sheath of the levator muscle.[1,5,9] The central aspect of the tendinous levator aponeurosis continues anteriorly to the Whitnall ligament for 15 to 20 mm before it fuses with the orbital septum and inserts into the anterior surface of the tarsal plate and eyelid skin, as described previously. The medial horn of this aponeurosis simply fuses with the posterior head of the MCT while the lateral horn helps to simultaneously support and divide the lacrimal gland into a deep orbital and superficial palpebral portion before it ultimately fuses with the LCT. Traumatic or hereditary disinsertion of the levator aponeurosis results in the condition known as *blepharoptosis*.[10]

The other less powerful but equally important upper eyelid retractor is the Müller muscle. This small retractor is composed of involuntary smooth muscle that is sympathetically innervated. It lies deep to the levator and is extremely adherent to the palpebral conjunctiva on its deep surface. Daily sustained contraction of this muscle contributes up to 2 mm of overall upper eyelid retraction;[5] therefore, it plays an important role in the overall diagnosis of patients presenting with eyelid asymmetry and/or unilateral upper eyelid ptosis.

The lower eyelid retractors function in much the same way as their upper eyelid counterparts. The main lower eyelid retractor is known as the *capsulopalpebral fascia*. It arises as a peripheral extension of condensed fascia from the sheath of the inferior rectus muscle. As it proceeds anteriorly, it splits to simultaneously envelop the inferior oblique muscle and form the inferior suspensory transverse or mediolateral check ligament, termed the *Lockwood ligament*.[1,5,9] Eventually, the capsulopalpebral fascia inserts into the inferior border of the inferior tarsal plate (see Fig 7-3). Its intimate origin with the inferior rectus muscle serves to directly transmit the action of this muscle onto the lower tarsus. The other lower eyelid retractor that is analogous to the Müller muscle is the inferior tarsal muscle. It too lies deep to the capsulopalpebral fascia and is composed of smooth muscle that is innervated by the sympathetic nervous system. Unlike the upper eyelid retractors, however, incision of or damage to the lower retractors rarely contributes as heavily to postoperative eyelid asymmetries or esthetic issues.

Preoperative Evaluation

Proper preoperative evaluation of prospective blepharoplasty patients is paramount. It offers surgeons the best chance to choose both their patients and the appropriate corresponding procedure(s) based on patient histories, pertinent clinical findings, and mutually agreed upon surgical goals.

Chief complaint

The initial blepharoplasty consultation begins with the surgical team's attempt to elicit the patient's primary request for wanting the procedure. This task can be adequately accomplished by properly trained assistants, nurses, or residents. At least 30 minutes in a relaxed, warm, properly equipped cosmetic consultation room is needed for most thorough consultations and evaluations. Initially, each patient's chief complaint, medical history, and major pertinent clinical findings are summarized by the staff and/or residents. Then each patient is asked to verbalize and simultaneously demonstrate in a properly lit mirror his or her chief request or issue(s) for the surgeon. By far, the most common complaint or blepharoplasty request is the desire to have excess, baggy skin removed from the upper eyelids. Eyelids that are drooping or bulging may project a look of fatigue and a lack of vigor despite adequate rest and good health. Other common presenting complaints include protruding, puffy, or large fat bags in the lower eyelids, persistent dark circles, and generalized periorbital wrinkling. Some patients present with a laundry list of facial esthetic requests, whereas others are unable to pinpoint the source of the problem and simply express a desire for rejuvenation of the tired, aged look they feel they exhibit. In any event, it is important to establish that a reasonable and rational motivation exists for the procedure before any physical evaluation is begun. Surgeons must keep in mind that not all requests are surgically correctable or attainable, so the initial discussion and examination are designed to identify which cosmetic problems are correctable so that they can then be compared with the patient's expectations.

Medical and ophthalmologic history

Specific questions aimed at the patient's past medical, surgical, and ophthalmologic history, along with specific risk factors for bleeding and dry eyes in particular, are important aspects of selecting blepharoplasty candidates with minimal to low risks for postoperative complications. Adhering to rational patient selection based on medical management betters the chances for both a happy patient and a happy surgeon. Medical emphasis is on identifying people with untreated or unstable thyroid, cardiovascular, hypertensive, or liver disease. In addition, those with acquired or congenital coagulopathies, a history of abusive alcohol or cigarette consumption, or unusual edema should be identified. Patients' use of commonly prescribed medications capable of causing unwanted intra- or postoperative bleeding with blepharoplasty procedures (eg, aspirin, nonsteroidal anti-inflammatory drugs, clopidogrel bisulfate, warfarin, and steroids) must also be assessed. Certain herbal medications and vitamins, such as ginseng, ginko, garlic, St John's wort, and vitamin E, are also capable of significantly affecting the coagulation cascade and prolonging bleeding.[11] They all should be stopped at least 2 weeks prior to surgery.[6]

The ophthalmologic history must identify any visual problems, history of conjunctivitis, sties, ocular herpes, or chalazion, along with the need for and/or use of cosmetic or corrective lenses.[2] A history of prior facial trauma and facial cosmetic or other ophthalmologic surgical procedures should also be investigated. Although commonplace and often omitted by patients on their health histories, laser-assisted in situ keratomileusis (Lasik) eye surgery is still significant. There is, unfortunately, no consensus on the time period that should be observed between Lasik eye surgery and cosmetic blepharoplasty.[1] In these instances, it is best to consult directly with the ophthalmologist who performed the surgery.

Finally, special emphasis must be placed on investigating prospective patients for a history of or propensity for dry eyes. The risk for prolonged postoperative dry eyes is greatest in patients who have a history of dry eyes preoperatively, and it is worse with upper blepharoplasty procedures.[11] If a patient has a history of frequent blinking, tearing, burning, eye sensitivity, ocular foreign body sensation, or regular use of lubricating eye drops, the surgeon should question whether the patient is a good candidate for blepharoplasty. In addition, patients with a history of any signifi-

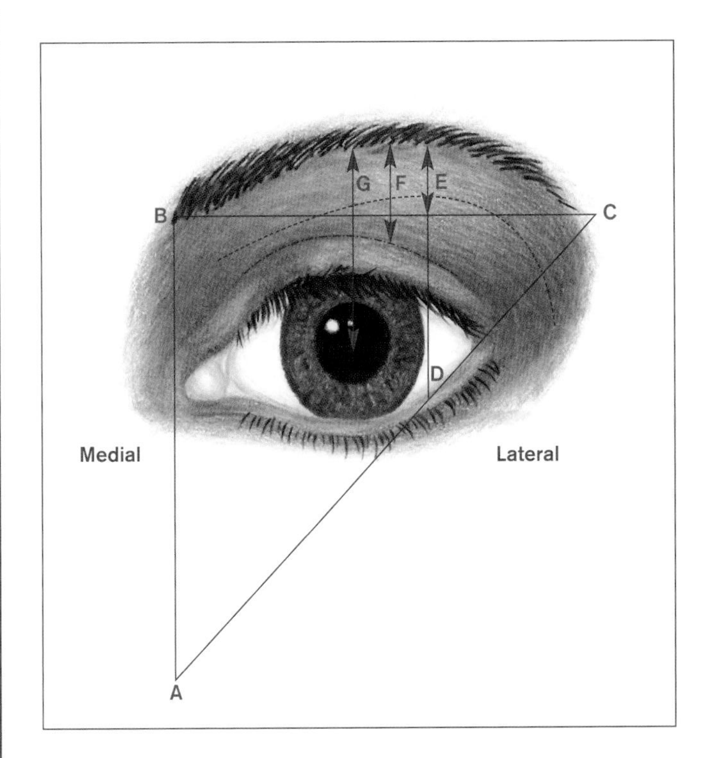

Fig 7-9 **Geometric relationships and measurements of the esthetic brow. Line A-B: The medial brow falls vertically in line with the medial canthus and the ipsilateral nasal ala (not depicted). Line B-C: The medial and lateral brow fall either on the same plane or the lateral brow sits slightly superior (females). Line A-C: The lateral brow terminates on an oblique line connecting the lateral canthus, lateral brow, and ipsilateral nasal ala. (D) Highest point of the brow corresponds to tangent vertical to the lateral limbus. (E) Inferior aspect of the brow sits about 1 cm superior to the supraorbital rim. (F) Brow to upper eyelid crease measures about 1.6 cm. (G) Brow to midpupil measures about 2.5 cm.**

cant systemic collagen vascular diseases, including rheumatoid arthritis, scleroderma, systemic lupus erythematosus, Sjögren syndrome, Wegener granulomatosis, and polyarteritis nodosa, or a history of heavy smoking also pose a high risk of associated dry eye syndrome.[2] The threshold for obtaining a preoperative ophthalmologic consultation in the context of elective blepharoplasty should be low.[11]

Clinical examination

Forehead and eyebrows

The eyebrows and lower forehead form an important esthetic, expressive, and structural foundation that has profound effects on the overall appearance of the eyes. Varying subjective and objective thoughts exist as to what constitutes ideal brow esthetics. Subjectively, most surgeons agree that attractive and youthful-appearing brows have *(1)* a gentle arch along a curve that is harmonious and continuous with the dorsal line of the nose; *(2)* a medial brow start-point that is thicker than the lateral brow and is usually vertically coincident with the medial canthus; *(3)* a tapered lateral tail that ends on a line drawn tangent through the ala of the nose and the lateral canthus; *(4)* a medial brow height vertically coincident with or just inferior to the vertical height of the lateral brow; and *(5)* a brow peak or point of maximal brow height located along a vertical line drawn tangentially to the lateral limbus of the eye[6,8,10] (Fig 7-9).

When examining the forehead and eyebrows, the cosmetic surgeon is primarily assessing the patient for the presence or absence of brow ptosis and brow asymmetry. Brow ptosis occurs to varying degrees in individuals as a normal part of the facial aging process. It can contribute significantly to excessive upper eyelid folds and so can make the actual quantification of excessive upper eyelid skin, termed *dermatochalasis*, difficult. In cases where brow ptosis is not properly identified or corrected and upper eyelid blepharoplasty alone is performed, the thicker brow skin gets transferred incorrectly onto the upper eyelid.[10] This, in turn, leads to further brow descent and unesthetic results. There are a number of objective measurements that may be used as guidelines for the determination of brow ptosis.[6,8,10] Perhaps the most common objective guideline is that the brow peak usually sits approximately 1 cm superior to the supraorbital rim in females and more directly over the supraorbital rim in males. When determining the amount of brow ptosis, the clinician should manually elevate the patient's brow to a cosmetically acceptable level, and the amount of elevation should be quantified and then compared with the opposite brow for symmetry. Symmetric brows, much like symmetric eyelids, improve the esthetic quality of the face. For the purposes of this chapter, it is assumed that the brow is properly positioned and symmetric; however, it is most important always to remember that decisions regarding upper eyelid blepharoplasty must be made with the brows properly positioned.

Midface

Historically, periorbital and midfacial rejuvenation procedures were treated as separate entities. The evolution of surgical techniques, materials, and multidisciplinary collaboration has, however, allowed for the realization that these areas are interdependent anatomical and surgical regions, especially at the lower eyelid–upper cheek junction. Consequently, any esthetic evaluation of the lower eyelids should also include an assessment of the midface.[9] Specifically, it should be assessed for ptosis, volume, and symmetry. Significant ptosis is often accompanied by deep nasolabial folds and prominent nasojugal or "tear-trough" deformities. The inferior orbital rims should also be palpated and assessed, because hollowing and flattening of the cheeks in combination with tear-trough deformities can be additional signs of midface ptosis. Midface ptosis is addressed via a number of different techniques, some of which can be performed simultaneously with lower eyelid blepharoplasty. In general, the esthetically pleasing lower eyelid has smooth skin that blends into the upper cheek, malar, and midface regions with little to no contour irregularities. Volume deficiency and contour irregularities can be corrected via adjunctive rejuvenation procedures, including autologous fat grafting, injectable fillers (see chapter 8), and alloplastic midface implants.

Ophthalmologic examination

Mandatory ophthalmologic tests include visual acuity, cranial nerves, extraocular muscle movements, and pupillary light reflexes.[1,2,8] In most instances, the standard 20-foot distance test for visual acuity is not feasible, but a mini–Snellen chart test is much more practical. Results should be recorded and documented for both eyes. A full cranial nerve examination (excluding the olfactory nerve) is routinely performed along with an assessment of the patient's extraocular movements and pupillary light reflex responses. Abnormal, unexplainable findings are noted and investigated with advanced testing or referral, when required.

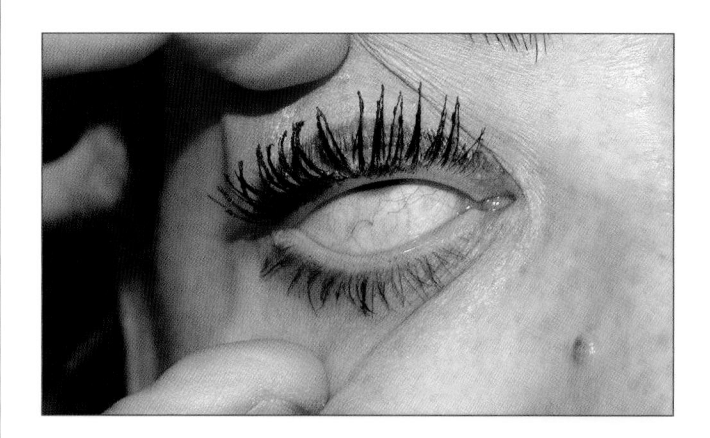

Fig 7-10 The Bell phenomenon is a protective reflex that involves involuntary rolling upward of the eyes upon closure of the lids. Only the sclera should be visible when the eyelid is forcefully opened with an intact Bell reflex.

Other adjunctive and occasionally required preoperative blepharoplasty tests include the Schirmer test for dry eye syndrome, visual field testing, and the corneal slit-lamp and fundoscopic examinations. The Schirmer test evaluates basic tear secretion or lacrimal gland function and is performed by placing a Schirmer adsorbent strip in the temporal aspect of the conjunctival folds in both lower eyelids. The patient is asked to look upward, and the amount of wetting is measured over a 5-minute period. Less than 10 mm of wetting is considered abnormal. Patients with moderate to severe dry eye syndrome are not good candidates for cosmetic blepharoplasty, whereas those with mild symptoms are referred for definitive ophthalmologic management.[1,6,8] Visual field testing is performed on patients in whom there is a question of peripheral visual field obstruction secondary to upper eyelid dermatochalasis and/or brow ptosis.[6] These fields are customarily assessed with and without the brow elevated by an independent, qualified examiner.

Upper eyelid

The upper eyelid is evaluated for *(1)* lid protective mechanisms, *(2)* excess skin and MCD, *(3)* palpebral fissure relationships and ptosis, and *(4)* orbital fat and prolapse of the lacrimal gland.

Protective mechanisms

The upper eyelid protective mechanisms are responsible for ensuring corneal coverage. Loss of or damage to these mechanisms places patients at a higher risk for dry eye syndrome. The practitioner should therefore be aware of and know how to test for *(1)* the Bell phenomenon, *(2)* CN VII function, *(3)* lagophthalmos, *(4)* corneal sensation, and *(5)* decreased blinking. Both the Bell phenomenon and CN VII function are simultaneously assessed by forcefully prying the eye open against the patient's voluntary resistance[2,8] (Fig 7-10). Adequate CN VII function or orbicularis muscle resistance is somewhat subjective, but it should at least be equal in both eyes. When forcefully opened, only the sclera of the eye and not the iris should be visible because of a reflexive upward rotation of the eye termed the *Bell phenomenon.* Absence of this reflex predisposes patients to an increased risk of ocular irritation and keratosis. Lagophthalmos is determined by having the patient extend the neck while gazing downward maximally. More than 2 mm of opening of the palpebral fissure(s) or an inability of the upper eyelid to almost completely cover the cornea is considered abnormal. Corneal sensation is assessed by gently passing a piece of cotton across the sclera. This test is usually performed in selected patients displaying corneal staining, as viewed with fluorescein dye and the cobalt blue light of a slit lamp. Decreased blinking is assessed by direct observation. The normal blinking process takes place at a rate of 10 to 12 blinks per minute,[2,8] and the palpebral fissures should close completely with each blink. A decreased blink rate or inadequate or improper eyelid closure can predispose patients to ocular irritation and dry eye syndrome.

Excess upper eyelid skin and MCD

The amount of excess upper eyelid skin is determined with the patient sitting in the upright position with the eyes closed. The skin is gently grasped with a nontoothed forceps from medial to lateral. The more skin grasped, the more the upper eyelid will elevate and evert, leading to palpebral fissure opening. Generally, minimal lagophthalmos with this pinching corresponds to the maximal limit for excess skin removal. The extent of redundant skin lateral to the orbital rim is also evaluated. Most if not all upper eyelid blepharoplasty incisions terminate lateral to the lateral canthus so as to incorporate the excess skin that exists in the lateral orbital rim. All too often, redundant skin exists in the lateral region, and if not adequately removed, the resulting accentuation in lateral hooding will impede any attempts to achieve a good esthetic result. It is this lateral area of skin that is most commonly grabbed and pinned by patients in consultations, so there is little difficulty in explaining to patients that they will have a redder, longer-lasting scar in this area during the healing process compared with the area more directly above the upper eyelid. This again is attributable to the differing properties of the thicker, oilier, lateral orbital skin versus the very thin eyelid skin. The opposite eye should undergo the same pinch test and the overall symmetry should be evaluated. Never assume that symmetric-appearing eyes require equal amounts of tissue excision. Lastly, as mentioned previously, it has been assumed for the purpose of this chapter that the brow is in an ideal position, not requiring any concomitant brow elevation as part of the blepharoplasty. However, the concepts associated with assessment of the brow and the extent of upper eyelid skin should be thought of as inseparable.

Following the assessment of excess skin, the upper eyelid crease, or MCD, is next determined and compared in both eyes (see Fig 7-2). If the determined MCD is significantly larger than 9 to 12 mm in women or 7 to 9 mm in men and differs significantly from that of the opposing eye, then it is highly probable that a unilateral levator aponeurosis disinsertion exists. If the MCD is much lower than the expected range, reconstruction or reestablishment of a new MCD should be discussed with the patient to prevent suboptimal esthetic results.[6,10] For simplicity, this chapter assumes that the patient's preexisting MCD is at an acceptable esthetic location and is symmetric with the opposing eye.

Palpebral fissure relationships

Specific topographic relationships must be determined when assessing the palpebral fissures for blepharoplasty (see Fig 7-2). Measurements to objectively determine in each eye include the *(1)* palpebral fissure width (28 to 30 mm), *(2)* palpebral fissure height (10 to 12 mm), *(3)* MRD1, and *(4)* MRD2. As previously mentioned, subtle decreases in the MRD1 may be seen with true upper lid ptosis, and increases in the MRD2 may occur with ectropion. Subjective relationships and questions to address include the following:

- *Overall impression of symmetry:* Are the palpebral fissures symmetric or asymmetric?
- *Upper eyelid–to-limbus relationship:* Is the upper lid margin positioned at, or 1 to 2 mm below, the upper limbus, with its highest point just nasal to a vertical line drawn through the center of the pupil?
- *Lower eyelid–to-limbus relationship:* Does the lower lid margin have a tangential relationship to the lower limbus, with the lowest point just lateral to the pupil?
- *Intercanthal axis:* Is the lateral canthus located in its ideal position, 2 to 4 mm superior to the medial canthus?
- *Lateral canthal angle:* Do the lateral palpebral margins meet at a 30- to 40-degree angle?

These objective and subjective findings are important because subtle preexisting palpebral fissure inequalities often exist without patients even being aware of them. These inequalities should be pointed out and corrected where possible because an unnoticed asymmetry undoubtedly becomes more readily apparent following blepharoplasty as patients and their families closely scrutinize the surgical result.

Ptosis assessment

Investigations for upper eyelid ptosis are based on subjective feelings of asymmetry and objective MRD1 findings. The levator excursion test measures the distance from extreme upgaze to downgaze with the patient's brow immobilized. It is the best clinical test of levator function.[1] A result of 10 to 12 mm or greater is considered good; 5 to 9 mm is fair; and 4 mm or less is poor. In patients with minimal ptosis (ie, 2 mm or less), a phenylephrine test is customarily performed in the involved eye under examination by an ophthalmologist. Two phenylephrine drops (2.5%) are placed in the affected eye, and the MRD1 is reassessed 5 minutes later. Upper eyelid elevation of 1.5 mm or greater is considered a positive test. In these patients, a Müller muscle conjunctival resection (MMCR) is indicated for ptosis repair.[12] If the phenylephrine drops do not correct the ptosis, corrective repair must proceed via levator aponeurotic surgery. In the author's practice, patients requiring ptosis repair are identified and referred for definitive management by an occuloplastic colleague (Fig 7-11).

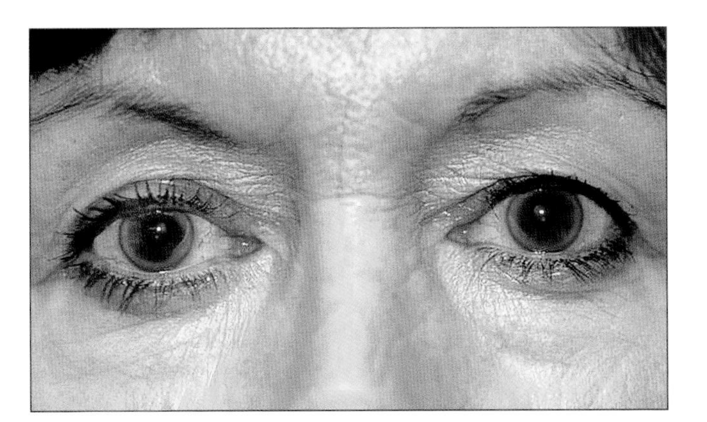

Fig 7-11a Patient presented for upper blepharoplasty and facelift consultation with complaint of excess skin, worse on the left eyelid. Clinical examination revealed reduced MRD1 consistent with asymptomatic and unrecognized ptosis of the right eye with bilateral upper eyelid dermatochalasis.

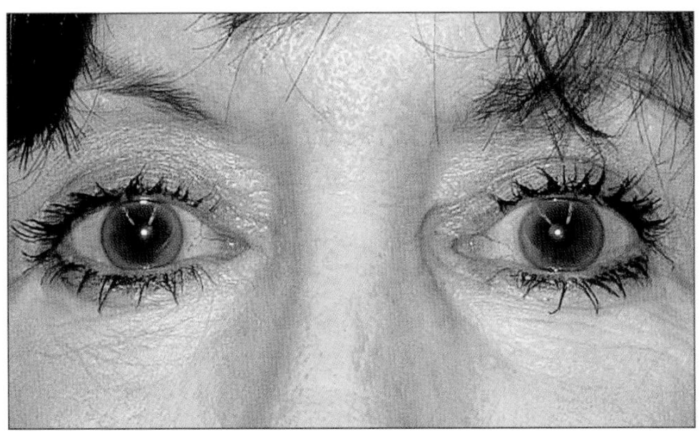

Fig 7-11b Patient 5 months post-MMCR and bilateral upper eyelid blepharoplasty. Interdisciplinary collaboration allowed for simultaneous right MMCR, left upper blepharoplasty (both performed by an oculoplastic surgeon), and facelift (performed by the author of this chapter). A delayed, isolated right upper blepharoplasty was performed 8 weeks after the MMCR to correct residual dermatochalasis.

Orbital fat

Large or puffy fat bags known as *steatoblepharon* are common blepharoplasty complaints. As with other facial structures in the body, most clinicians agree that the orbital septum weakens with age. Although true herniation of the postseptal/ preaponeurotic orbital fat pads through the orbital septum can take place, it is more common in clinical practice to observe pseudoherniated fat pads. Degrees of orbital fat pseudoherniation may be evident in a wide age range starting in the late teens; however, pseudoherniation is frequently familial or hereditary, worsens with age, and does not correlate in severity with overall body form or obesity. These fat pads are readily sensitive to fluid shifts and water accumulation secondary to positional changes and gravity and so often appear worse in affected individuals on awakening in the morning. Many patients with lower eyelid fat pseudoherniation also complain of dark circles around their eyes. Where as a darker complexion of the lower eyelid is more evident in certain people, the appearance of dark circles can be accentuated with overhead lighting, because shadows are cast by the protruding fat bags.

The definition of what constitutes excessive orbital fat is subjective. It is generally more difficult to assess the degree of fat pad pseudoherniation for the upper eyelid than it is for the lower eyelid. Furthermore, the medial compartments within each eyelid are generally less herniated and harder to assess clinically than their central (or lateral in the lower eyelid) counterparts. Pseudoherniation of the lower fat pads is accentuated when patients look in an upward gaze[6] as gentle pressure is applied to the globe while the eyelids are closed, a maneuver termed *retropulsion.*[8] The increase in intraorbital pressure leads to exaggerated fat pad pseudoherniation. These maneuvers aid the clinician preoperatively by demonstrating the problem areas to prospective patients and intraoperatively by helping with fat pad resection. The routine removal of fat from the upper eyelids is no longer commonplace. Through experience, cosmetic blepharoplasty surgeons have discovered that the removal of too much orbital fat from these compartments can make the eye look gaunt and hollowed out postoperatively. With this in mind, apparent fullness of the temporal aspect of the upper eyelid without large amounts of medial and central fat should make the examiner suspicious of lacrimal gland prolapse or ptosis. Lacrimal gland ptosis can be assessed clinically by gently pulling upward on the upper eyelid skin. When lacrimal gland ptosis exists, the elevation of this skin will demonstrate a small nodule showing beneath the lateral orbital rim. This nodule is the palpebral portion of the lacrimal gland. If the gland is ptotic, the surgeon should plan to suspend it behind the orbital rim at the time of surgery.

Lower eyelid

The lower eyelid is evaluated for *(1)* excess skin, *(2)* orbicularis hypertrophy, *(3)* palpebral fissure relationships and lower eyelid retraction, *(4)* lower eyelid laxity, *(5)* orbital fat, and *(6)* midface considerations.[11,13,14] The palpebral fissure relationships, assessment of lower eyelid orbital fat, and midface considerations have been previously discussed.

Excess lower eyelid skin and orbicularis hypertrophy

Excess skin in the lower eyelid is assessed with the patient looking upward. This upward gaze places the lower eyelid skin under the greatest tension, so excess skin as determined via pinching with fine, nontoothed pickups is potentially associated with less chance of postoperative cicatricial retraction or ectropion. When incorrectly assessed with the patient in primary gaze, too much skin may potentially be removed. The room for error with skin excision is much smaller in the lower eyelids than it is in the upper ones. To that end, preoperative skin condition regimens, trichloroacetic acid *(TCA)* facial peels, and fraxel laser resurfacing are helpful adjunctive skin resurfacing and tightening techniques that complement lower eyelid blepharoplasty.[8] When properly used, these techniques can reduce the amount of skin that would otherwise be removed from conventional transcutaneous approaches. This in turn enhances facial esthetics and reduces the chances of postoperative retraction and ectropion.

Orbicularis hypertrophy presents as thickened lower preseptal eyelid bulges in patients while squinting[8,14] (Fig 7-12). These bulges add unesthetic convexities to the lower eyelid region that, when combined with lower eyelid fat pseudoherniation, result in additional shadowing, contour irregularities, and a potentially tumultuous transition down into the midface. The hypertrophic muscle is surgically trimmed and smoothed through a transcutaneous approach, when required.

Lower eyelid retraction

Lower eyelid retraction arises for many reasons and is evident by increased scleral show. As mentioned above, the normal lower eyelid has a tangential relationship with the lower limbus. Retraction can be quantitatively assessed by determining both the MRD2 and the distances from the inferior limbus to the lower eyelid nasally, centrally, and temporally.

Lower eyelid laxity

Testing the lower eyelid for tone and laxity is an important part of the blepharoplasty examination. Most patients will be severely distressed with postoperative inferior

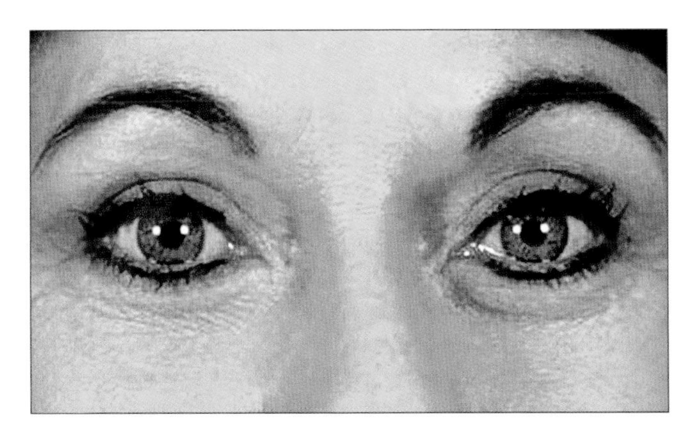

Fig 7-12 A patient with orbicularis hypertrophy presenting with thickened preseptal eye bulges and contour irregularities of the lower eyelids.

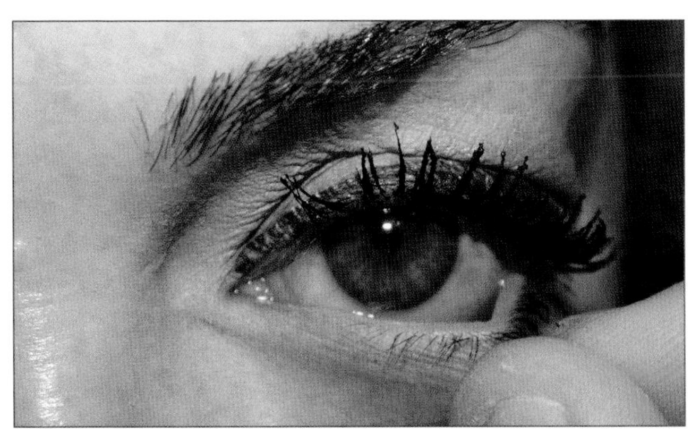

Fig 7-13 The snap test is important in revealing lower eyelid tone and laxity. The eyelid is pulled away from the globe and released. Lower eyelids with normal tone snap back against the globe almost immediately.

repositioning of the lower eyelid because it will lead to increased scleral show, lateral "hound dogging," or ectropion. Simple initial observation of preexisting palpebral relationships often provides accurate insight into the overall lower eyelid strength. Scleral show prior to lower eyelid blepharoplasty may become worse postoperatively if not simultaneously addressed surgically via lid-tightening procedures. There are three tests for lower eyelid laxity that the cosmetic blepharoplasty surgeon must perform preoperatively: *(1)* the snap test, *(2)* the inferior retraction test, and *(3)* the lateral and medial "bowstring" tests.[2,4,11]

A simple snap test reveals the lower eyelid tone and laxity (Fig 7-13). The lower eyelid is grasped gently with the thumb and forefinger and is pulled away from the globe in a horizontal plane and released. Lower eyelids with normal tone snap back to contact the globe almost immediately. The ability to distract the lid greater than 8 mm away from the globe or failure of the lid to return to direct contact with the globe in less than 5 seconds indicates poor tone. The inferior retraction test is similar to the snap test, except the lid is simply distracted inferiorly as opposed to out and away from the globe. Lower eyelids with normal tone should not be able to be retracted inferiorly any more than 10 mm. Again, the lower eyelid should return quickly to its normal position. Blinking during these tests can lead to false negative results because the act of blinking automatically returns the lids to their normal position. Lateral and medial bowstring tests commonly performed with naso-orbital-ethmoidal fractures can quickly be performed on both eyes. Any appreciable movement of the medial or lateral canthal ligaments with this test indicates an abnormal finding suggestive of increased lid or canthal laxity.

Photographic documentation

Photographic documentation performed in a standard, reproducible fashion is highly recommended for all phases of esthetic surgery. Most clinicians have or are migrating to digital cameras and esthetic software programs, but these are not essential. The advantages of photographs are obvious as they provide visual documentation of preexisting cosmetic issues and allow for pre- and postoperative comparisons to be objectively made. They also provide another diagnostic avenue for the surgeon; subtle nuances of perceived problem areas can often be missed clinically but can later be noticed and better appreciated on the photograph. Preoperative photographs that should be obtained for blepharoplasty include *(1)* full face (1:10 ratio) with frontal, right and left profile, and right and left oblique views, all in primary gaze; and *(2)* close-up of the eyes (1:5 ratio) with frontal and right and left oblique views in primary gaze along with frontal views in up and down gazes. Older personal photographs of high-enough quality brought in by patients can also be of diagnostic help. They offer the surgeon the chance to comprehend the effects of aging on the patient's periorbital region and so help to delineate what can and cannot be surgically addressed with an attempted blepharoplasty.

Surgical Procedures

Skin marking and incision design

Upper eyelid

Marking the upper eyelid incision takes place under good lighting with the patient awake and sitting upright. Unwanted running or spreading of the ink is minimized by first cleansing the skin gently with an alcohol wipe. A fine-tipped surgical marker should be selected to ensure that the final incision design remains as delicate and accurate as possible. Major discrepancies in final skin excision can arise as a result of seemingly small errors due in part to skin markings that are thick and not crisp. Preoperative details from the initial consultation, including the MCD, quantity of skin to be excised, and overall surgical plan, should once again be reviewed prior to initiating sedation or beginning surgery.

First, the upper eyelid crease is identified as described previously, and a thin curvilinear line is drawn parallel to and just below the upper eyelid crease. The MCD is then measured with calipers (Fig 7-14a). By marking and incising the inferior limb of the skin excision slightly below, as opposed to directly within, the upper eyelid crease, final scars are better camouflaged because the actual incision will settle slightly superiorly to rest in the natural upper eyelid crease following suturing. The opposing upper eyelid crease is similarly marked, and the MCDs are evaluated and compared (Fig 7-14b). For the purpose of this chapter, all patients demonstrated esthetic upper eyelid crease positions heralded by MCD values in acceptable and symmetric ranges. Consequently, no reconstruction of or alteration to the position of their preexisting upper eyelid creases was required. The medial aspect of the planned inferior incision line is carried parallel and slightly inferior to the natural upper eyelid crease until approximately 1 to 2 mm medial to the puncta. It stops at this point, and surgeons should avoid continuing farther medially into the nasal concavity because unesthetic webbing and increased scarring can occur. The lateral aspect of this inferior line similarly continues parallel and slightly inferior to the upper eyelid crease until just before the lateral canthal region of the upper eyelid. At this point, it becomes increasingly more horizontal and then curves slightly superiorly, ending approximately 1 cm lateral to the lateral canthus (Fig 7-14c). It seems intuitive to extend the incision inferolaterally along a dominant natural crow's foot rhytid out into the lat-

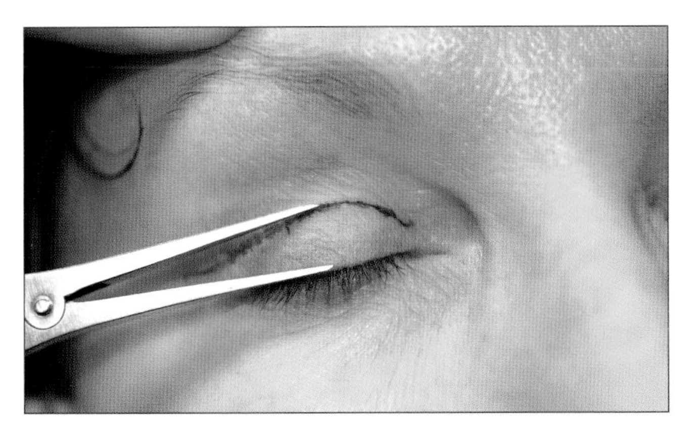

Fig 7-14a The natural upper eyelid crease is assessed and marked, and then the MCD is determined with calipers and recorded.

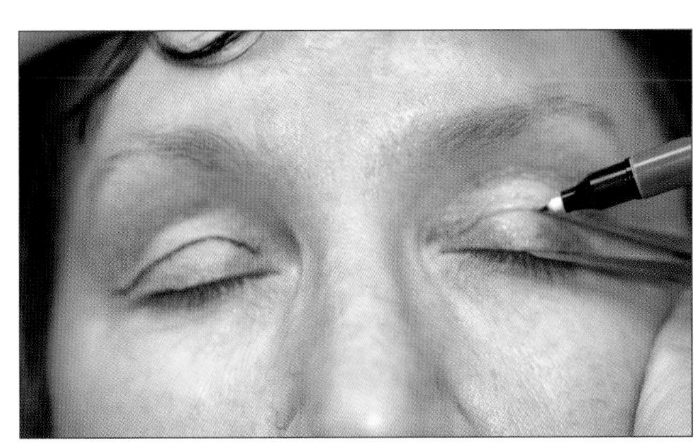

Fig 7-14b The opposing natural upper eyelid crease is assessed and marked. In the absence of planned or required upper eyelid reconstruction, the MCDs should be very similar and symmetric to each other.

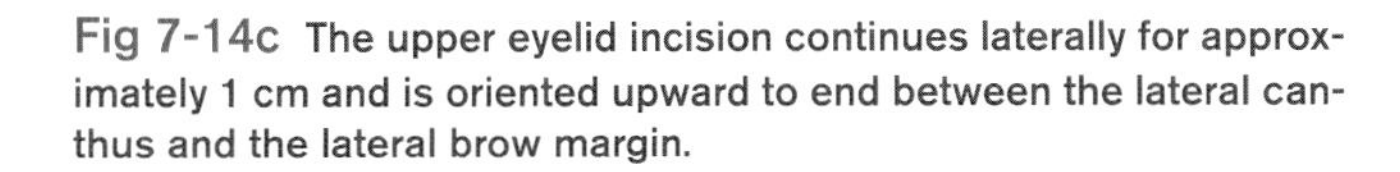

Fig 7-14c The upper eyelid incision continues laterally for approximately 1 cm and is oriented upward to end between the lateral canthus and the lateral brow margin.

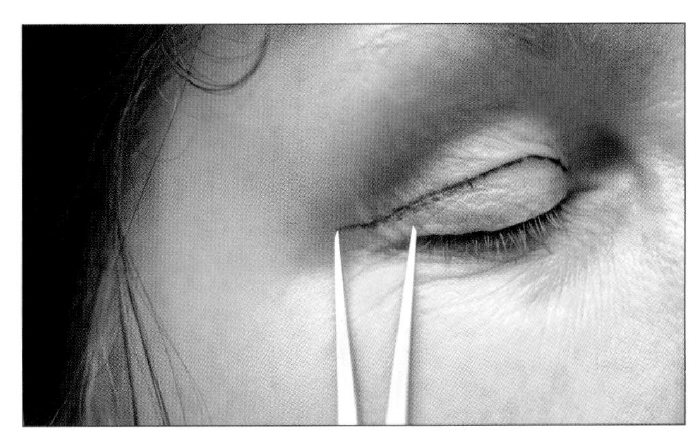

eral orbital skin, but this should be avoided. Low incisions here will pull the tail of the brow downward following suturing, leading to persistent lateral hooding. In addition, incisions placed this low are more obvious and difficult to hide with makeup. Rather, an incision that is properly oriented more upward, to end between the lateral canthus and the lateral brow margin, will properly deal with unwanted lateral hooding. This type of incision placement directly removes excess skin and purposefully elevates the skin inferior to the incision, thereby making it more readily camouflaged by makeup. Lateral extension beyond the orbital rim is very rarely required or performed. Remember to inform patients that the incision in this region will be more visible and redder in the first few postoperative months compared with that directly above the eyelid. Reassure them that with time, it too will fade to become less perceptible.

The upper limb of the eyelid marking is designed to encompass all redundant skin that is safely removable. While the patient's eyes are closed, the redundant skin is gently grasped with a nontoothed forceps to estimate the amount to be removed. One blade of the forceps is placed at the central aspect of the lower lid mark, while

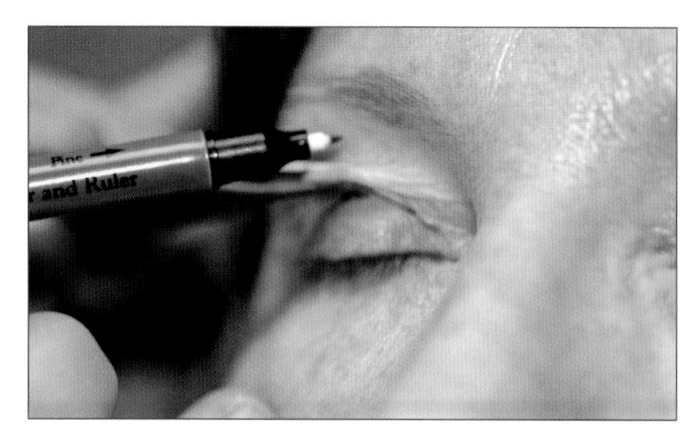

Fig 7-14d The redundant skin of the upper eyelid is gently grasped with a nontoothed forceps to estimate the amount to be removed. One blade of the forceps is placed at the central aspect of the lower lid mark, while the other blade is used to gather as much skin as possible without causing the palpebral fissure to open.

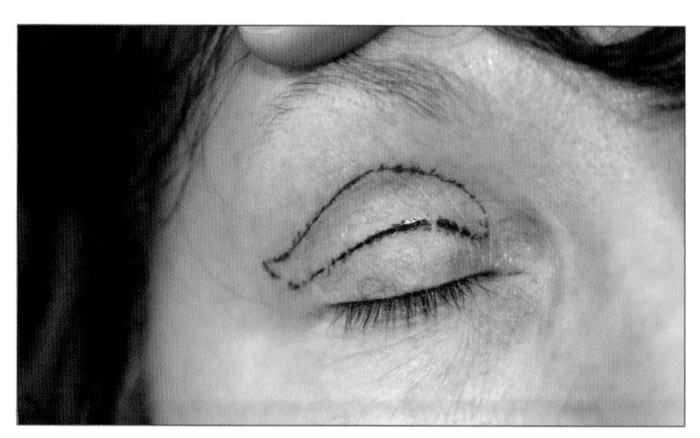

Fig 7-14e When finished marking, the planned incision lines should be thin and crisp with the upper and lower limb markings meeting laterally at a 30- to 40-degree angle.

the other blade is used to gather as much skin as possible without elevating the upper lid margin away from the lower lid margin, so that the eye does not open (Fig 7-14d). The goal is to avoid iatrogenic opening of the palpebral fissure, thereby controlling the amount of skin excised so as to prevent unwanted lagophthalmos. Surgeons should remember that some intraoperative tissue contracture is to be expected when the skin, orbicularis muscle, and orbital septum are incised and cauterized with a CO_2 laser. This combined with the scar maturation and wound contracture that takes place as part of normal healing can contribute to lagophthalmos and should be factored into the overall incision design. In general, 7 to 10 mm of skin is removed, with relatively more removed lateral to the midpupillary line than medial to it. When marking has been finished, the lateral aspect of the upper and lower limb markings should meet at a 30- to 40-degree angle to help prevent any "dog-ear" formation that can arise during suturing (Fig 7-14e).

Lower eyelid

The technique chosen for lower eyelid blepharoplasty deserves special attention. Lower eyelid blepharoplasty can be performed through transcutaneous or transconjunctival approaches. Each technique has its inherent indications and contraindications, advantages and disadvantages, and enthusiasts and opponents. Although different subtypes of transcutaneous approaches exist, the standard skin-muscle flap (SMF) is described in this chapter. The transconjunctival approach is also discussed, along with an adjunctive skin pinch technique (SPT) often used with it.

Transcutaneous SMF approach

The SMF lower eyelid blepharoplasty technique dates back to 1960, when it was first described by Reidy.[4,11] The main advantage of the SMF for lower eyelid blepharoplasty lies with its ability to alter skin (excess and tightness), muscle (excess and tone), and fat (volume and repositioning). The major disadvantages are associ-

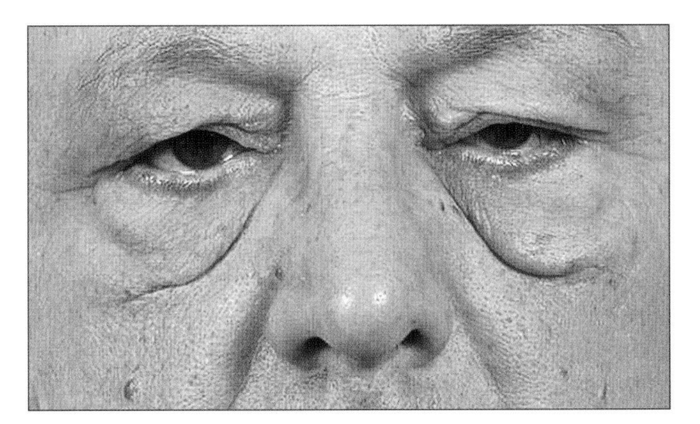

Fig 7-15 Man in primary gaze presenting with severe bilateral lower dermatochalasis and orbital fat pseudoherniation. Note how prolapsed lower orbital fat has led to festoons and deep nasojugal grooves.

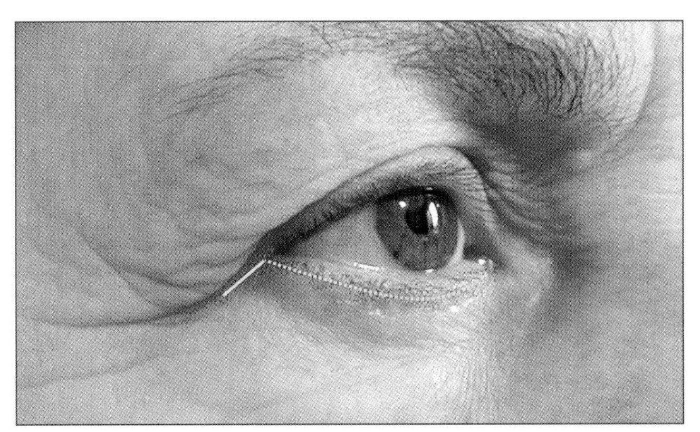

Fig 7-16 SMF lower eyelid marking depicting a 1-cm horizontal extension at the level of the lateral canthus. The subciliary aspect of the planned incision sits 2 to 3 mm inferior to the lashes and is not customarily marked. It is dotted here for demonstration purposes.

ated with higher rates of postoperative complications such as lid retraction and ectropion.[14] The SMF approach for lower eyelid blepharoplasty should be limited to selected patients presenting with excessive lower eyelid skin and muscle.[11,14] These are usually older patients who present with significant lid-to-cheek contour irregularities, festoons, and deep nasojugal folds (Fig 7-15).

For the SMF approach, the skin is marked starting with a line drawn at the lateral canthus. This line extends horizontally for approximately 1 cm. It can be incorporated into an existing crow's foot rhytid, but it should not drop inferiorly just to stay in one. It rarely extends out farther laterally than the orbital rim and should never be any closer vertically than 5 mm to the more superiorly placed upper blepharoplasty incision when both eyelids are being operated on. It is possible to mark only the lateral extension portion of the SMF, because the subciliary component of the incision is more easily appreciated without a surgical marking on it. The subciliary component of the SMF approach sits 2 to 3 mm inferior to the cilia and travels parallel to the lower lid margin, ending medially no farther than the inferior lid puncta (Fig 7-16).

Transconjunctival approach in combination with SPT

The transconjunctival blepharoplasty (TCB) approach for lower eyelid blepharoplasty was first described in 1924 by Julian Bourget.[4,11] Although chronologically much older than the trancutaneous SMF approach, the TCB more recently became popular and accepted again among cosmetic surgeons when it was reintroduced in 1989 by Baylis as a safe approach with minimal risks and complications.[4] The major advantage of the TCB over the SMF is that it avoids the need to incise the orbicularis oculi or the orbital septum, thereby dramatically reducing the postoperative risk of lower eyelid retraction and ectropion. It is usually less bloody (because no muscle is cut) and almost always faster. Canthopexy and canthoplasty via a tarsal strip procedure for treatment of excessive lower lid laxity are well suited to the TCB approach, when indicated.[14]

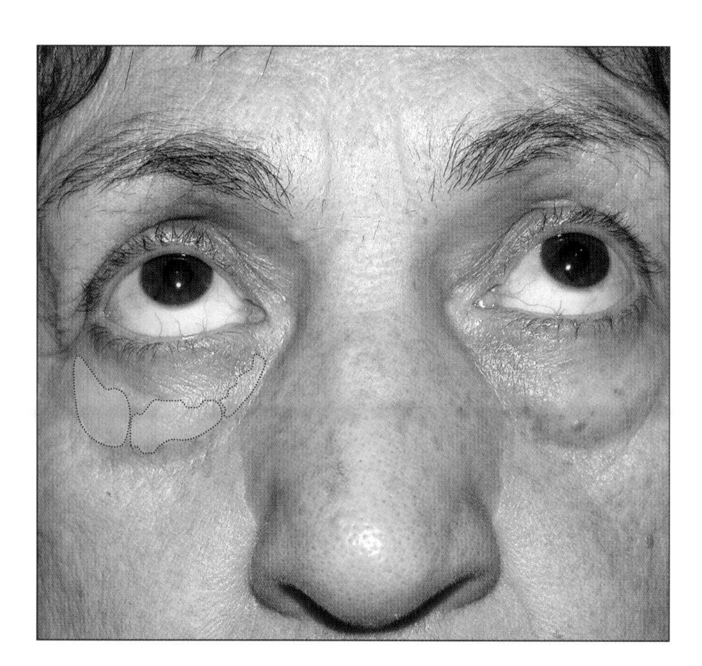

Fig 7-17 The lower eyelid fat pads can be better visualized when patients take an upward gaze. The borders of these fat pads can be marked to help delineate them intraoperatively.

The TCB technique for blepharoplasty is most reliably indicated for the removal of herniated orbital fat in patients with excellent skin, muscle, and tendon tone (ie, younger patients) who have minimal to no evidence of dermatochalasis or orbicularis oculi hypertrophy. It is also advantageous for patients with prior lower eyelid surgery at risk for retraction or ectropion and patients with minimally wrinkled skin in whom a SPT or chemical or laser resurfacing of the lower eyelid skin is useful.[4,13] With this technique, no skin marking is required other than a subtle demarcation of the outlines of the lower fat pads that the surgeon wishes to address (Fig 7-17). This TCB technique is not well suited for patients presenting with orbicularis hypertrophy, inferior orbital rim or nasojugal hollowing and depression, or severe orbital festoons.

During the 1970s, Parkes described the SPT for the treatment of excess skin of the lower eyelid.[4] It is a relatively simple technique that complements the TCB approach. It is used in patients with minimal lower eyelid skin (less than 5 mm) and is especially useful for candidates in whom skin resurfacing procedures are not recommended (either chemical or laser) because of increased risk of prolonged erythema or hyperpigmentation (ie, Fitzpatrick IV to VI individuals). As with TCB, there is no formal skin marking that takes place with a surgical marker.

Anesthesia

Many oral and maxillofacial surgeons provide both intravenous and general anesthesia for a number of different outpatient procedures. Although an isolated blepharoplasty up to a formal facelift can be accomplished using local anesthesia alone, intravenous sedation provides for optimal patient and doctor comfort, whenever feasible. If the blepharoplasty is being completed simultaneously with other, more involved procedures such as a facelift, the surgeon will select a route of anesthesia from deep intravenous sedation to general anesthesia. General anesthesia alone is rarely indicated for blepharoplasty.

As with standard oral surgical procedures, intravenous sedation is no substitute for good local anesthesia. Local anesthesia for blepharoplasty proceeds after intravenous sedation and prior to sterile preparation. Standard dental carpules containing 2% lidocaine with epinephrine (1:100,000) are used to perform both infiltrations and regional periorbital blocks. For infiltrations, a 27-gauge long (1.5-inch) needle is inserted in the subcuticular plane at the lateral aspect of the upper or lower blepharoplasty incision. For upper blepharoplasty, the needle is advanced in this plane in a horizontal fashion along the upper and lower limbs to their medial extents, and then upon withdrawal, a controlled amount of local anesthesia totaling no more than one carpule (1.8 mL) per eye is slowly deposited (Fig 7-18a). An identical technique is used for the lower SMF blepharoplasty technique with no more than 1.8 mL being used. Additional infiltration above this quantity along planned markings does not contribute to improved anesthesia or significantly enhanced vasoconstriction but rather leads to increased tissue distortion and skin excision errors.

Attempts to minimize additional puncture and entry points along the lid markings should be made because the unnecessary tissue trauma can lead to unwanted bleeding and hematomas within the underlying muscle layer. Furthermore, the needle should not be oriented perpendicularly to the skin nor should there be any attempt at injection of the orbital fat in the upper or lower lids during initial injections. Perpendicular orientation of the needle may inadvertently result in penetration of the orbital septum, whereas injection into orbital fat by definition involves penetration of the orbital septum, which can damage delicate postseptal blood vessels, thereby leading to secondary bleeding and possible intraorbital hematoma formation. Topical anesthesia is administered because it increases patient comfort and allows for the diminution of involuntary reflexive blinking, which arises as a result of direct corneal stimulation. Within 25 seconds, two drops of 0.5% tetracaine hydrochloride placed into the palpebral conjunctiva in each eye will provide anywhere from 15 to 45 minutes of profound anesthesia (Fig 7-18b).

The ophthalmic division of the trigeminal nerve, or fifth cranial nerve (CN V_1), is responsible for the sensory innervation of the upper eyelid. This innervation is specifically provided via four distinct branches. The extreme medial aspect of the upper eyelid receives its sensory innervation from the supratrochlear and infratrochlear nerves. These nerves pierce the orbital septum above and below the trochlea of the superior oblique muscle and may be anesthetized in a regional fashion with a single injection of 0.5 mL of local anesthetic (Fig 7-18c). The supraorbital nerve emerges through a groove or canal at the superomedial aspect of the supraorbital rim to supply the central and medial components of the upper eyelid. It can likewise be regionally anesthetized using 0.5 mL of local anesthesia (Fig 7-18d). The fourth and final nerve, the lacrimal nerve, supplies the more lateral aspect of the upper eyelid. It is not routinely anesthetized in a regional manner.

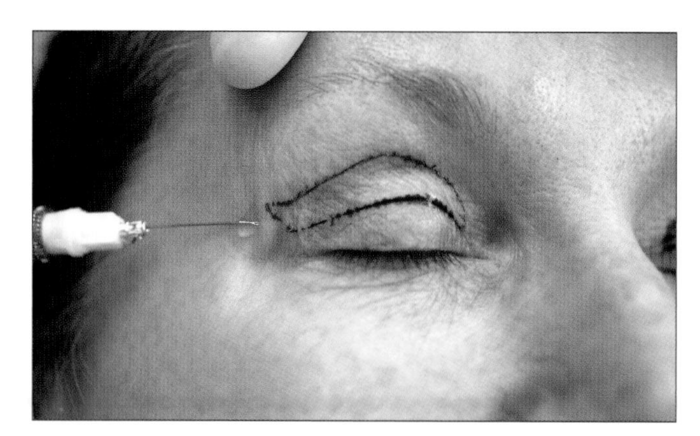

Fig 7-18a Local infiltration using a syringe containing 1.8 mL of 2% lidocaine with epinephrine (1:100,000) with a 27-gauge long (1.5-inch) needle inserted in the subcuticular plane at the lateral aspect of the upper blepharoplasty incision.

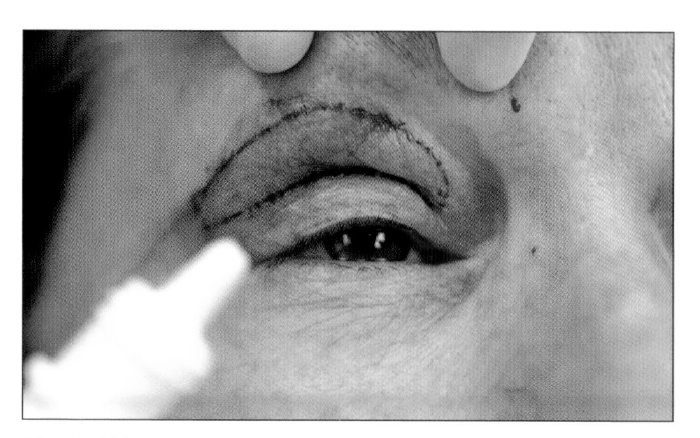

Fig 7-18b Two drops of topical anesthetic (0.5% tetracaine hydrochloride) are placed into each eye.

The maxillary division of the trigeminal nerve (CN V_2) supplies the lower eyelid sensation via the zygomaticofacial branch and terminal palpebral branches of the infraorbital nerve. These nerves emerge via their respective lateral and medial foramina. Extraoral infraorbital block for lower eyelid blepharoplasty can be performed again using 0.5 mL of local anesthesia.

Regional anesthesia for blepharoplasty is not mandatory. These blocks by definition pierce the orbital septum near the orbital rims, and while they are located outside the surgical incision zones, they theoretically can be associated with unwanted postseptal bleeding. Therefore, they are used in selected cases in which enhanced anesthesia is required above and beyond local infiltration.

Local anesthesia for a planned TCB is accomplished with the same local anesthesia and needle as described above. For this technique, one carpule (1.8 mL) of local anesthesia is injected directly into the postseptal orbital fat in each lower eyelid transconjunctivally at the level of the fornix (Fig 7-18e). Gentle pressure applied to the lower eyelid helps to facilitate diffusion of the fluid within the postseptal fat.

Maximum epinephrine-induced vasoconstriction occurs 10 to 15 minutes following injection. This added hemostasis is very valuable when operating in this vascular area. Consequently, the full time required for its efficacy should be allotted prior to incision. The eyelids maintain anesthesia after infiltration, as described above, for approximately 1 hour. This is a shorter time frame than is experienced with local anesthesia in other areas of facial skin. As a result, the timing of the injections depends on the speed and experience of the surgeon. The length of time needed for a simultaneous upper and lower eyelid blepharoplasty can vary from less than 1 hour to as long as 3 hours. When performing simultaneous upper and lower blepharoplasty, the upper eyelids are anesthetized at the outset and then, just before beginning the skin incision on the second upper eyelid, both lower eyelids are infiltrated. If all eyelids are anesthetized at the beginning of the procedure, it is commonly necessary to reinfiltrate the second lower eyelid. This reinfiltration can make precise skin and fat removal unnecessarily difficult.

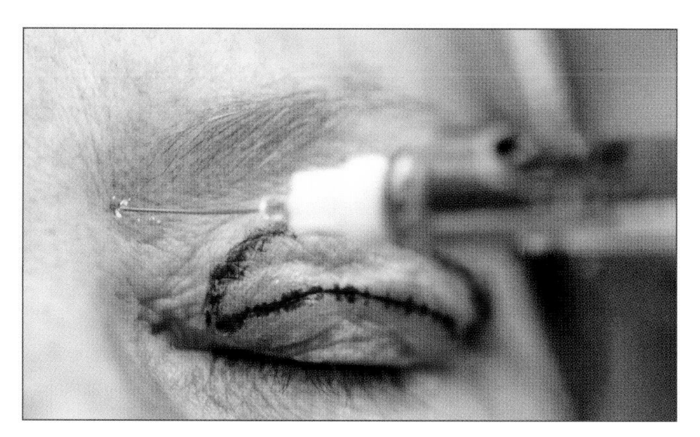

Fig 7-18c **Regional supratrochlear nerve block is performed using 0.5 mL of 2% lidocaine with epinephrine (1:100,000).**

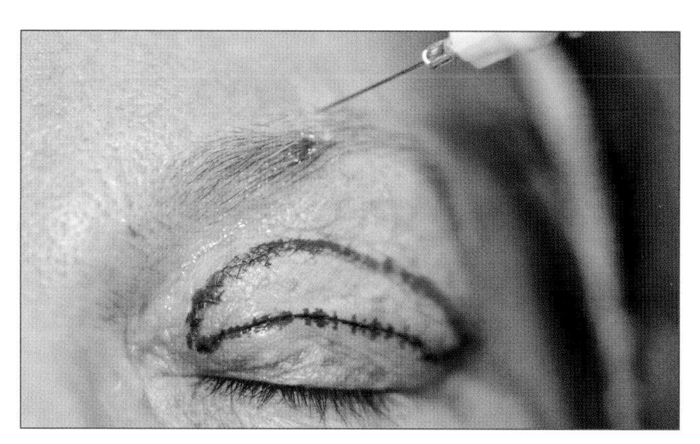

Fig 7-18d **Regional supraorbital nerve block is performed using 0.5 mL of 2% lidocaine with epinephrine (1:100,000).**

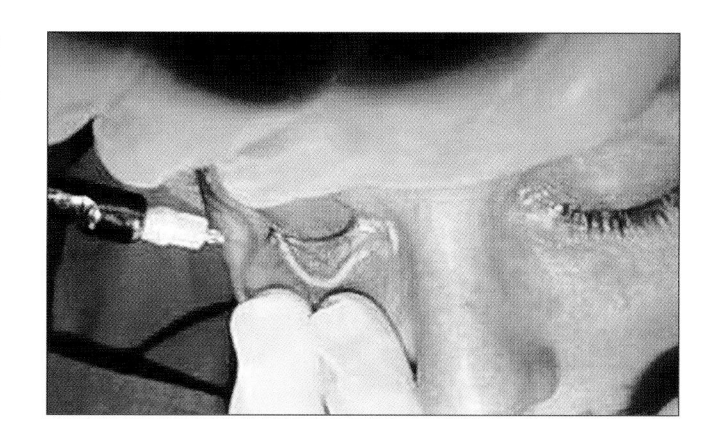

Fig 7-18e **Local transconjunctival infiltration into the postseptal fat using 1.8 mL of 2% lidocaine with epinephrine (1:100,000). Gentle pressure applied to the lower eyelid helps facilitate diffusion of the fluid within the postseptal fat.**

Method of incision

There are many different ways to complete a blepharoplasty incision. Many surgeons prefer to use a scalpel and scissors when performing upper and lower blepharoplasty. Although these "cold steel" techniques are efficient, proven esthetic modalities that have been used for hundreds of years, they are associated with increased intraoperative bleeding. Bleeding is always problematic with surgery, but it can be even more so with blepharoplasty because structures are extremely delicate and thus can be easily obscured when saturated with blood. Some surgeons also think that excessive bleeding can lead to increased swelling, bruising, and even pain. Although this has yet to be objectively established with blepharoplasty, bloodless modalities for performing these procedures include electrocautery, radiowave surgery, and CO_2 laser technology. The main advantage of these procedures over conventional scalpel techniques is that they provide a dry, bloodless surgical field and therefore reduce operative time.

Electrocautery was first used for surgery in 1923 by Wyeth and then again in 1924 by the famous neurosurgeon Dr Harvey Cushing.[3] William Bovie, a Harvard physicist, aided Dr Cushing in the development of the first electrosurgery units capable of cutting and coagulation modes. Use of this technology in blepharoplasty surgery for removal of herniated fat with superior hemostasis was reported by various authors in the 1980s.[3,7] Most blepharoplasty surgeons never make a *skin* incision with electrocautery. This is because traditional electrosurgery devices cut skin tissue by passing an electric current through the patient using an electrode tip to provide resistance. This effectively causes high temperature heating of the electrode tip and excessive lateral tissue damage, which in turn can result in increased swelling, pain, and scarring. Although electrocautery is effective at coagulating blood vessels, there is always the potential risk of shock, burn, and irreversible neural damage to the patient.

Radiofrequency (RF) surgery is a relatively new technology that is capable of cutting and coagulating tissues using a high-frequency (4.0 MHz) alternating current. This surgical modality is very different from traditional electrosurgery and other forms of electrocautery because it can simultaneously cut and coagulate tissues without applying pressure. Most important is the fact that there is controlled and minimal lateral tissue damage with the 4.0-MHz high-frequency, low-temperature RF surgery. RF surgery differs from electrosurgery in that the water in the tissue serves as the resistance instead of the electrode. This means there is no heating of the RF electrode tip. Instead, intracellular water in the tissue provides the resistance. When exposed to the RF current, the water vaporizes without the lateral thermal damage observed with electrosurgery. This RF tissue vaporization is capable of significant hemostasis and esthetic healing, without any risk of electric shock or burn to the patient.[15]

Laser technology has been used by ophthalmologists for almost 30 years to treat diseases of the retina. Its application in medicine and surgery has expanded exponentially in recent years. The first laser to be used widely in blepharoplasty was the neodymium-doped yttrium aluminum garnet (Nd:YAG) laser. With these initial Nd:YAG units, laser power was transmitted through a fiberoptic coil to a probe that was applied directly to the skin. Dr S. Baker and coworkers first introduced the carbon dioxide (CO_2) laser for use in blepharoplasty in 1984.[7,16] Much like RF instruments, CO_2 lasers are capable of precise tissue cutting and coagulation, and CO_2 laser incisions tend to bleed less. Also, with laser blepharoplasty, eyelid fat can be removed without first clamping to prevent bleeding, a step that may eliminate some patient discomfort. Major disadvantages associated with this procedure are increased equipment costs and loss of tactile sense because CO_2 lasers do not directly contact the skin as scalpels and RF electrodes do.

Overall, most unbiased studies have shown that there are no significant long-term esthetic differences in healing when comparing blepharoplasty incisions made with either the scalpel versus the CO_2 laser or RF surgery versus the CO_2 laser.[15] In reality, the differences between laser, RF surgery, and conventional scalpel blepharoplasty are so slight and insignificant that they do not really matter. To achieve a good result in blepharoplasty requires that a surgeon possess a thorough understanding of eyelid anatomy and adequate training and experience. The chosen method of incision is merely preference. The author's preference is the CO_2 surgical laser (Fig 7-18f).

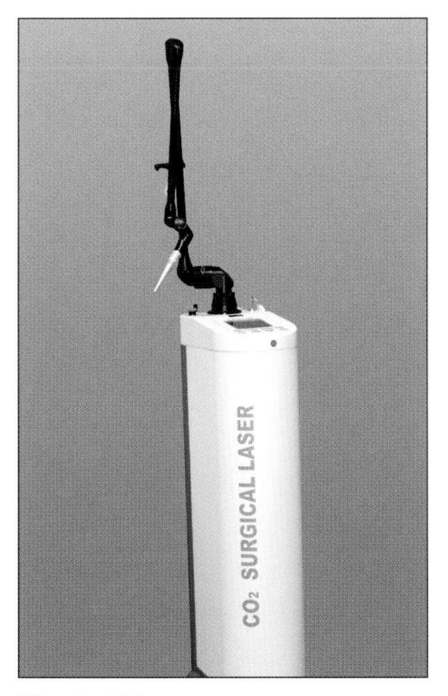

Fig 7-18f Superpulse CO_2 surgical laser, model L5-25 (Sandstone Medical Technologies).

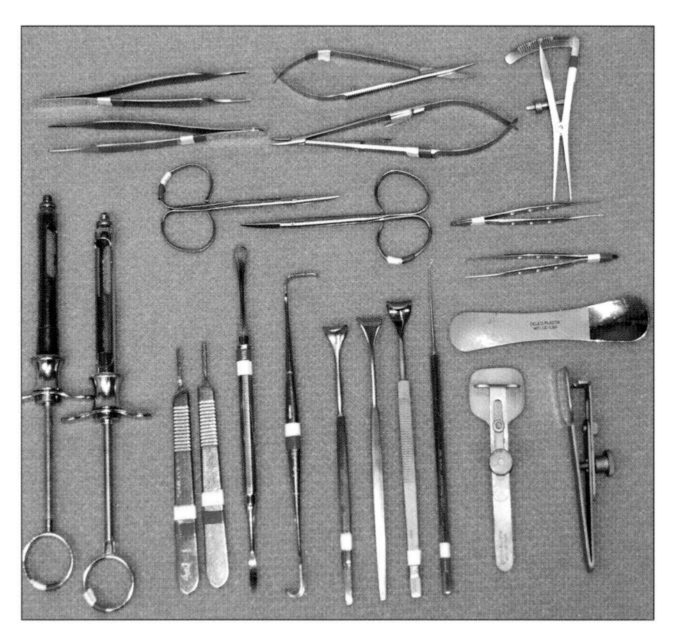

Fig 7-18g Standard blepharoplasty tray. Bottom, left to right: dental syringes (2); no. 15 scalpel handles (2); no. 9 periosteal elevator; Senn retractor (dull); Desmarres lid retractors (10, 12, and 14 mm); single skin hook; David Baker lid clamps (small: 24 mm; large: 32 mm); Jaeger lid plate. Top, left to right: Adson-Brown forceps (2); Castro-Viejo needle driver and scissors; strabismus scissors; Kaye-Tieman scissors; 0.5-mm toothed and nontoothed fine forceps.

Upper eyelid blepharoplasty

Following eyelid marking and injection, the patient's periorbital region is prepared with Betadine (Purdue Pharma) and then draped "sterilely." Blepharoplasty, by nature, is not a sterile procedure, so while all attempts to maintain sterility should be undertaken, it is most often safely carried out in a clean or antiseptic fashion. Instrumentation is highly variable among blepharoplasty surgeons, and there are a multitude of specialized blepharoplasty instruments available. The author has attempted to keep his blepharoplasty instrument tray simple and functional (Fig 7-18g).

The procedure begins by inserting the David Baker upper eyelid retractor, which features a simple, curved clamping mechanism to gently retract the upper eyelid while protecting sensitive scleral membranes. The retractor is clamped to the superior tarsal plate just inferior to the inferior limb of the planned incision. With tension now applied to the upper eyelid via the retractor, the incision is made with the CO_2 laser at predetermined power settings of 5 W in continuous pulse mode

(Fig 7-18h). The laser offers no tactile feedback, so it must be advanced along the incision marking at a constant speed and distance from the skin to ensure a uniform depth through the skin only. The incision begins medially and continues laterally in two separate single strokes (one for each limb). The lateral angle must be very crisp at 30 degrees (Fig 7-18i). The upper eyelid skin is then removed using the CO_2 laser from lateral to medial in a plane superficial to the orbicularis oculi (Fig 7-18j). Use of a presterilized tongue depressor placed medially inside the wound edge helps prevent "overshoot" of the CO_2 laser onto medial orbital and nasal skin outside the planned zone of skin excision (Fig 7-18k). A decision is then made about whether to remove the orbicularis oculi muscle.

Removal of a portion of this muscle allows for greater definition of the upper eyelid crease, which in turn creates a sculpted appearance of the upper lid. The surgeon must consider the fact that the muscle is present in varying degrees in different individuals. Therefore, muscle removal in some will effect subtle esthetic changes with little to no significant alteration in overall orbicularis oculi function. The same procedure poorly applied to older, thin-skinned patients presenting with scant orbicularis muscle volume may, however, result in compromised esthetics and an inability to properly close the affected eye. Compromised esthetics arise in these patients because a deeply sculptured eyelid crease may impose an aged look (especially when combined with fat removal in patients with prominent supraorbital rims) or may impart a more feminine look in male upper eyelid blepharoplasty patients. The author of this chapter routinely excises a very thin strip of this muscle from lateral to medial using a pair of strabismus or tenotomy (Stevens) scissors in the majority of his patients. Care is taken to ensure that the excised strip of muscle remains thin and is taken from the midsection of the wound without violation of the underlying orbital septum. Some muscular bleeding is to be expected, and hemostasis is achieved at this stage using the CO_2 laser at a defocused, or increased, distance (Fig 7-18l).

Following removal of the redundant skin and any indicated orbicularis muscle, the medial and central fat pads are addressed. Unlike the approach to the orbicularis oculi, it is rarely necessary to excise fat when performing an upper eyelid blepharoplasty. Fat pad removal is often a major goal with lower eyelid blepharoplasty; however, the philosophy "less is more" is a good approach when dealing with upper eyelids, beecause conservation of tissue and dissection yields better esthetic results. Many experienced clinicians who originally recommended subtractive techniques many years ago now favor a conservative approach. In upper eyelid blepharoplasty, the overresection of upper eyelid fat, especially when combined with aggressive orbicularis resection, can leave patients with a hollowed-out, aged, cadaveric look. Nevertheless, when indicated, the medial and central fat pads are addressed. Small buttonholes are made over top of these fat pads by gently spreading the orbital septum with a Steven scissors or a fine hemostat. As mentioned, the medial fat will appear paler and more fibrous than the yellow fat of the central compartment. The retropulsion maneuver should be performed to aid in herniation through the iatrogenic septal defect. Any excess fat is excised directly with the CO_2 laser by rolling the fat over top of a moistened cotton-tip applicator (see lower eyelid blepharoplasty). No preclamping or electrocautery is required in most instances, but occasionally, an

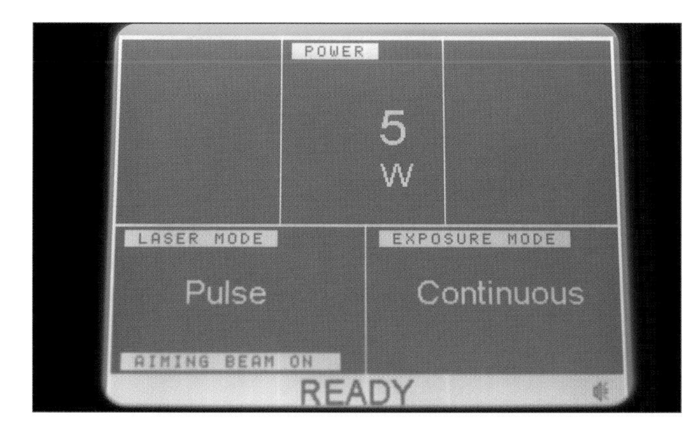

Fig 7-18h Common settings for CO_2 laser–assisted blepharoplasty. Note that these settings may vary depending upon the type and make of laser used. Check recommended settings and manufacturer guidelines for all other laser use.

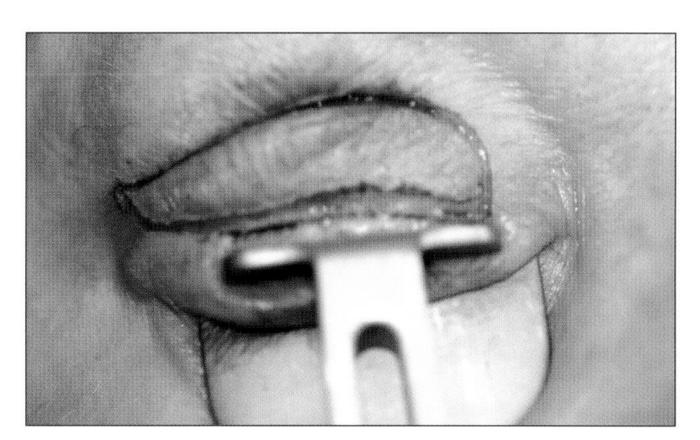

Fig 7-18i CO_2 laser skin incision proceeds uniformly through skin only along planned markings.

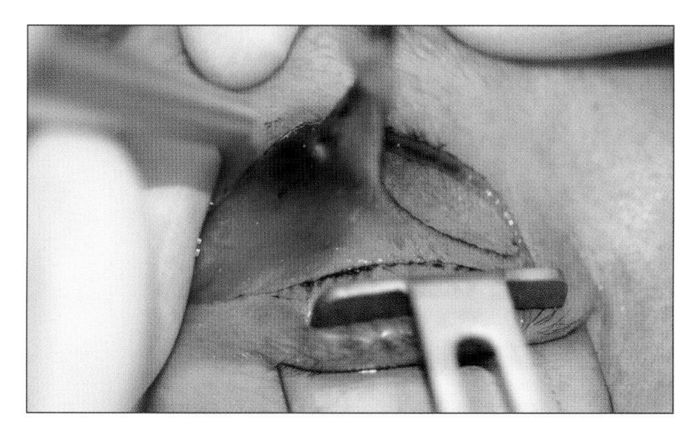

Fig 7-18j CO_2 laser skin excision takes place from lateral to medial in a plane superficial to the orbicularis oculi.

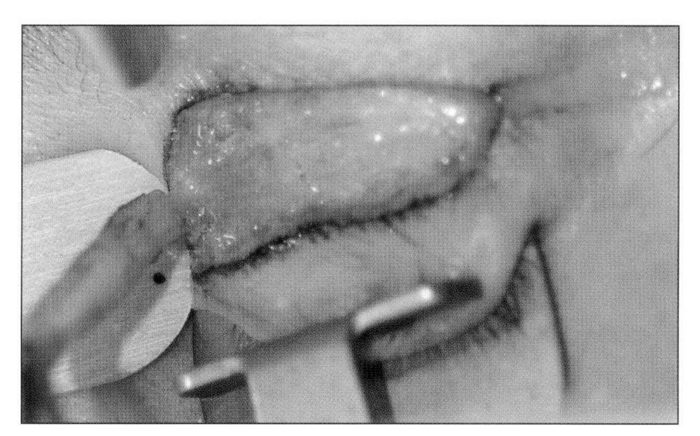

Fig 7-18k A sterile tongue depressor placed inside the medial extent of the incision protects medial and nasal skin from unwanted exposure to the CO_2 laser during final skin excision.

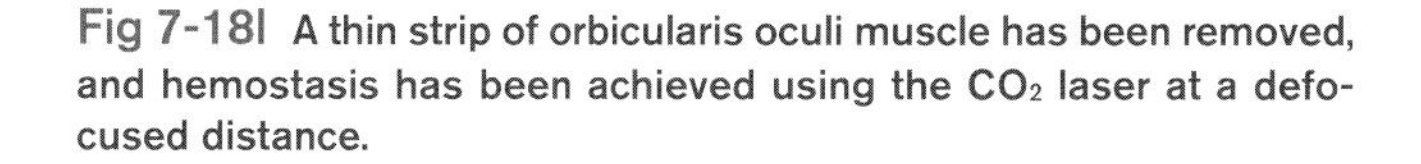

Fig 7-18l A thin strip of orbicularis oculi muscle has been removed, and hemostasis has been achieved using the CO_2 laser at a defocused distance.

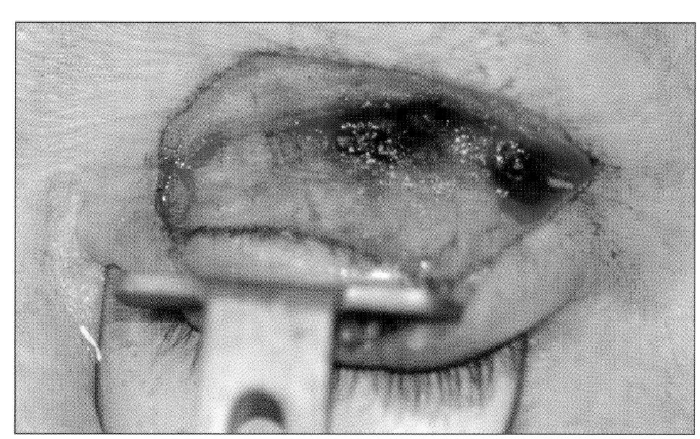

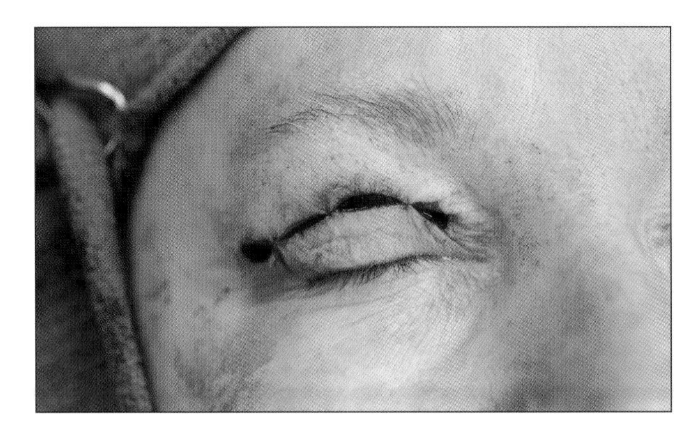

Fig 7-18m Initial closure and wound approximation proceeds with three 6-0 fast gut sutures.

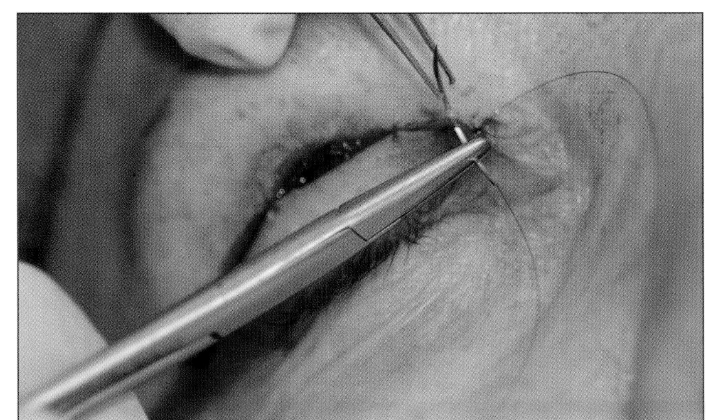

Fig 7-18n Definitive upper eyelid incisional closure proceeds in one layer with a running 6-0 Prolene suture. Care is taken to incorporate skin only into the bites.

additional injection of local anesthesia directly into the medial fat pad may be required. The fat can be gently teased out to help with this step, but it should never be pulled in an attempt to excise or liberate more. Rather, surgeons should only "take what is given to them." Excess manipulation and teasing can lead to the rupture of postseptal blood vessels or direct damage to the superior oblique muscle, which is rarely seen. Once completed, attention is turned to absolute hemostasis using the CO_2 laser at a defocused distance.

Wound closure can be performed with several varied sutures and techniques. The author of this chapter prefers fast gut and polypropylene sutures (Prolene, Ethicon). Initially, the upper and lower limb margins are oriented using three to four 6-0 fast gut standard interrupted sutures (Fig 7-18m), which minimize the chance for medial and lateral dog-ears. Next, a continuously advancing 6-0 Prolene suture is placed from medial to lateral (Fig 7-18n). Tissue bites are carefully taken at regular intervals and at controlled depths, with the needle passing only through skin. It is not desirable to incorporate any underlying muscle in the bite because muscular movement will inadvertently be transmitted more efficiently to the incision line and lead to a greater chance for scarring or dehiscence. Additional tissue trauma is minimized by using a fine 0.5-mm pickup on the subcuticular tissue, only as needed. The wound is thus closed in one layer (skin only) with no need for septal or muscular closure. If medial tissue redundancy or dog-earing persists after closure with the 6-0 Prolene suture, it is easily corrected by removing small Burrow triangles (base down along the longer redundant wound edge), which do not require suturing. Prolene sutures should be used in place of nylon sutures, where possible, because Prolene is the most nonreactive suture available and the easiest to remove. Many surgeons, in-

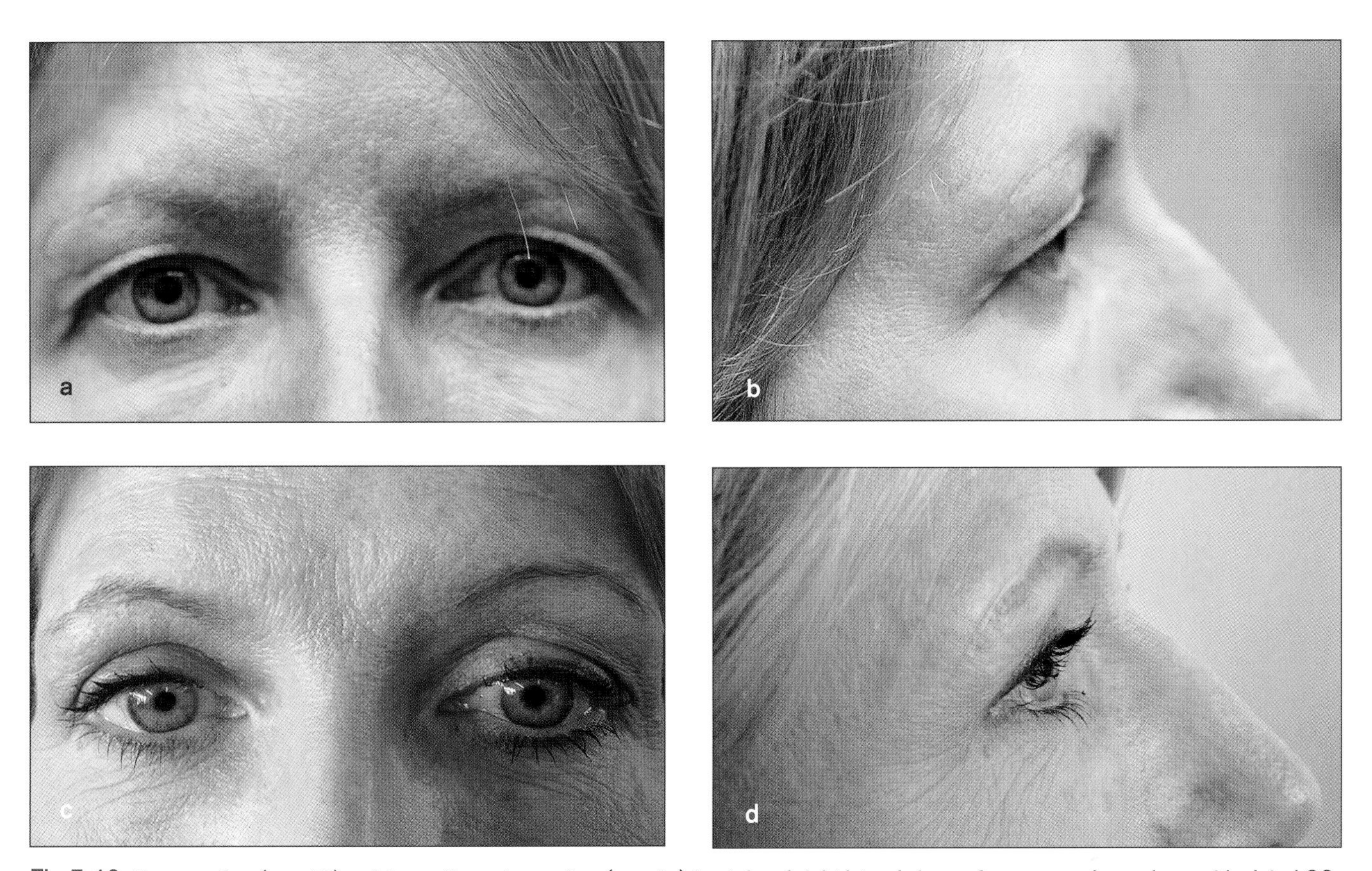

Fig 7-19 Preoperative *(a and b)* and 9-month postoperative *(c and d)* frontal and right lateral views of a woman who underwent isolated CO_2 laser–assisted bilateral upper eyelid blepharoplasty.

cluding the author of this chapter, anecdotally believe it produces the finest scars. Nylon sutures are an acceptable alternative, but nylon is somewhat more reactive and more difficult to remove when placed as a running suture. Resorbable sutures are the most reactive in the skin, producing a redness that is not seen with Prolene sutures. Regardless, many cosmetic oculoplastic surgeons regularly use fast gut sutures for blepharoplasty procedures with excellent results. The author uses the 6-0 fast gut suture sparingly in the upper eyelid. Braided or multifilament sutures are the worst to use for cosmetic blepharoplasty skin incision closure because they leave suture tunnels and skin suture marks. They should be used only as buried sutures, where required.

Following these procedures can lead to successful CO_2 laser–assisted bilateral upper eyelid blepharoplasty (Figs 7-19 to 7-21).

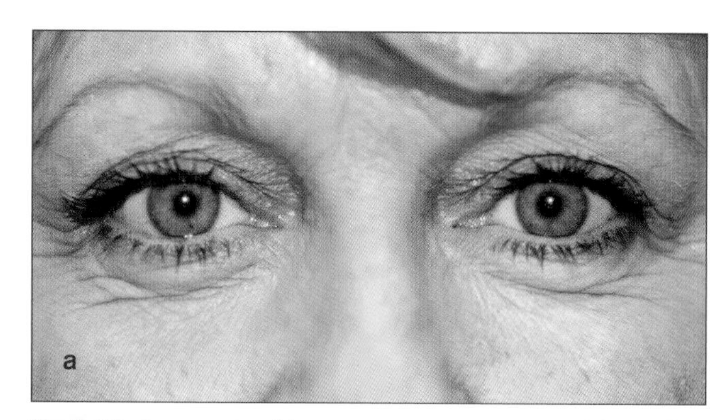

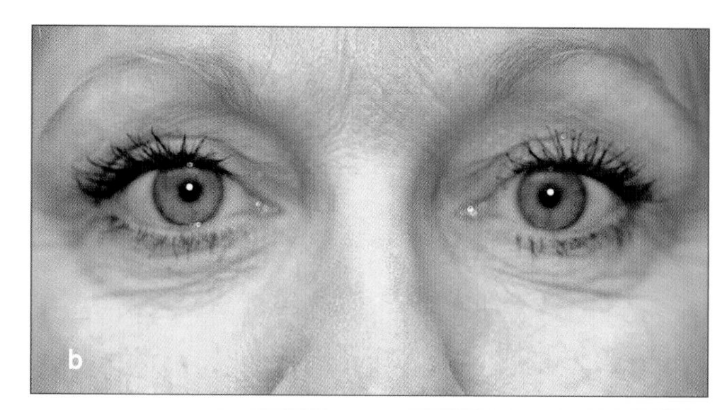

Fig 7-20 Preoperative *(a)* and 5-month postoperative *(b)* frontal views of a woman who underwent CO_2 laser–assisted bilateral upper eyelid blepharoplasty and a minimal incision facelift.

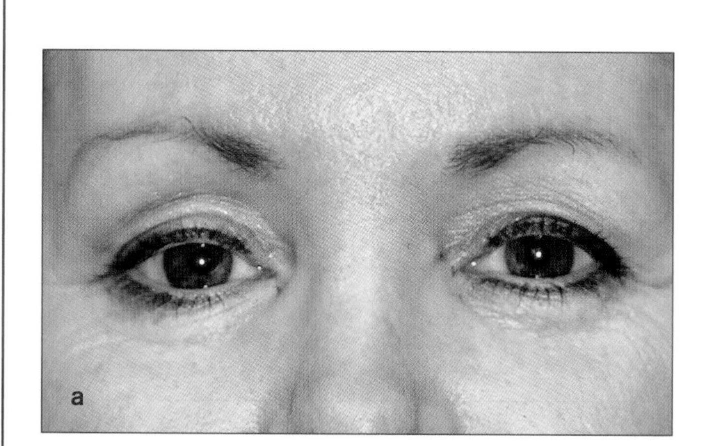

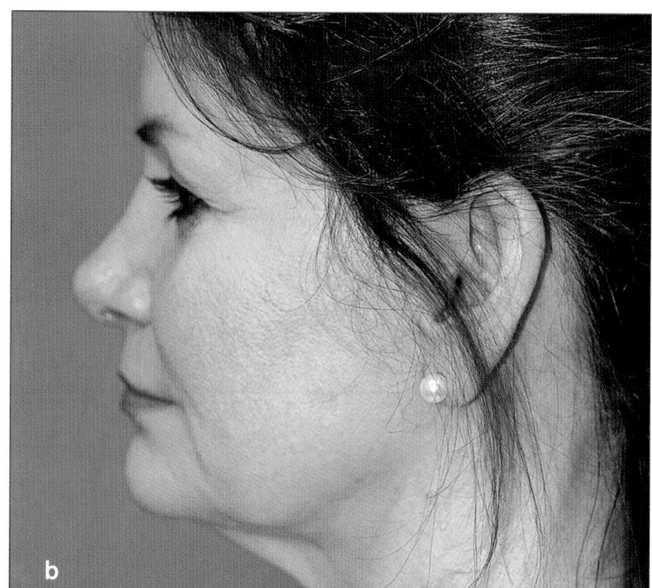

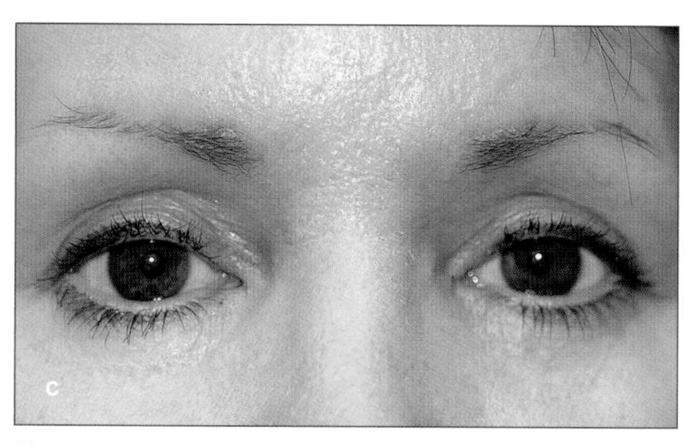

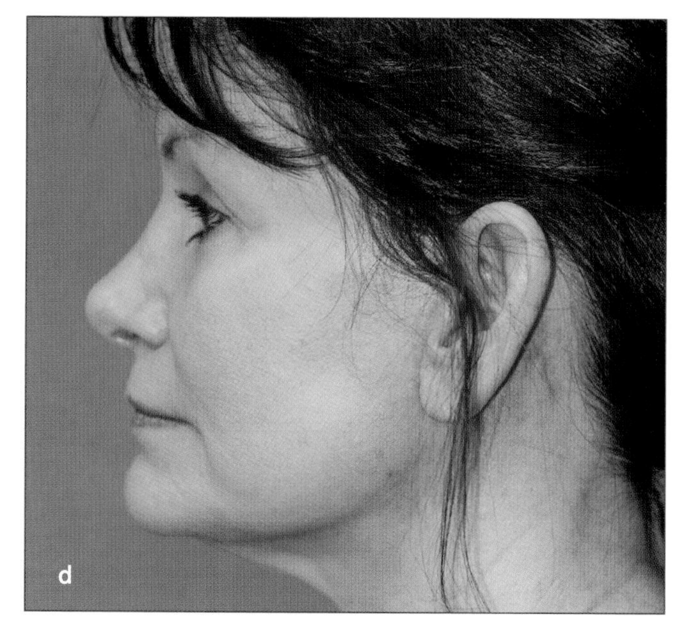

Fig 7-21 Preoperative *(a and b)* and 5-month postoperative *(c and d)* frontal and right lateral views of a woman who underwent CO_2 laser–assisted bilateral upper eyelid blepharoplasty and a minimal incision facelift.

Lower eyelid blepharoplasty: SMF approach

The SMF approach is used less frequently than the transconjunctival approach in both the author's cosmetic blepharoplasty and routine maxillofacial trauma practice. When required, the SMF approach begins in the lateral region of the lower eyelid along the premarked lateral horizontal extension. A sharp incision using a no. 15 scalpel is made through skin down to the level of the orbicularis oculi muscle in this region only. Strabismus scissors are then used to bluntly dissect down to the periosteum over the lateral rim. This periosteum is, as mentioned previously, confluent with the orbital septum and lower tarsal plate. Once down to the periosteal/orbital septal plane, these same scissors are redirected and are sequentially opened so as to dissect and ultimately separate the underlying orbital septum away from the muscle, thereby creating an SMF. The scissors are then repositioned parallel to the skin and are used to carefully cut through the muscle and skin from lateral to medial, in one continuous motion, along the planned subciliary line. By angling the scissors as described, the muscle gets cut at a lower level than the skin, so a portion of the pretarsal muscle structure and functional tone is preserved. This is believed to decrease the postoperative chance of lower eyelid retraction or ectropion. With the use of presterilized cotton-tip applicators, further inferior blunt dissection can proceed medially, inferiorly, and laterally over top of the orbital septum and periosteum, as required. A decision is made at this point to excise, preserve, or reposition the orbital fat. When abundant fat is present in all compartments, some fat must be removed.

The scissors are used to create buttonholes in the orbital septum over top of the postseptal fat pads. Blunt scissor and cotton-tip applicator dissection combined with careful teasing and globe retropulsion readily exposes excess fat arising from within all three compartments (Fig 7-22a). The most obvious fat pad first encountered is the central pad, whereas the most difficult to access is the medial pad. Excess fat from all three compartments is draped over a moistened cotton-tip applicator and then directly excised and simultaneously cauterized using the CO_2 laser. Once the preliminary resection is completed, the surgeon should go back to the lateral compartment to be sure that the proper amount of fat has been removed.

One of the most common complaints following lower lid blepharoplasty is the presence of persistent bulging in the area of the lateral fat compartment. Final fat contouring and hemostasis are achieved using the laser at a defocused distance (Fig 7-22b). The orbital septum is not sutured. The SMF is then redraped superolaterally, and a decision is made at this point to excise, preserve, or reposition the skin and muscle. This is the trickiest part of the procedure. Decisions regarding lateral canthal support and laxity are made first. In almost all cases, lateral canthal support is advantageous. Occasionally, lid tightening or canthoplasty procedures are also necessary. Some of these techniques are outside the scope of this chapter, but the author of this chapter commonly performs a lateral retinacular suspension in a number of SMF patients. It is accomplished by passing a 4-0 clear nylon or Prolene suture through the lateral canthal ligament in a horizontal mattress fashion. It is secured superolaterally to the orbital periosteum (Fig 7-22c). Exact vectors and tension vary from patient to patient. Once complete, the orbicularis SMF is then redraped superolaterally. In some instances, precise skin and muscle tissue trimming can proceed at

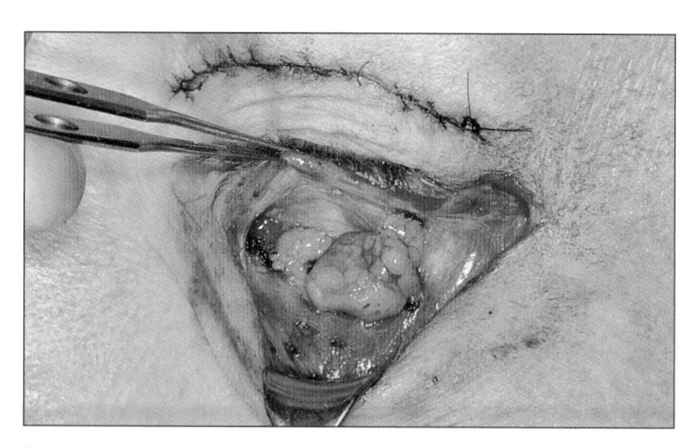

Fig 7-22a SMF approach for lower eyelid blepharoplasty. The orbital septum is being selectively incised to allow for access to the postseptal fat compartments. The medial and central fat pads are visualized.

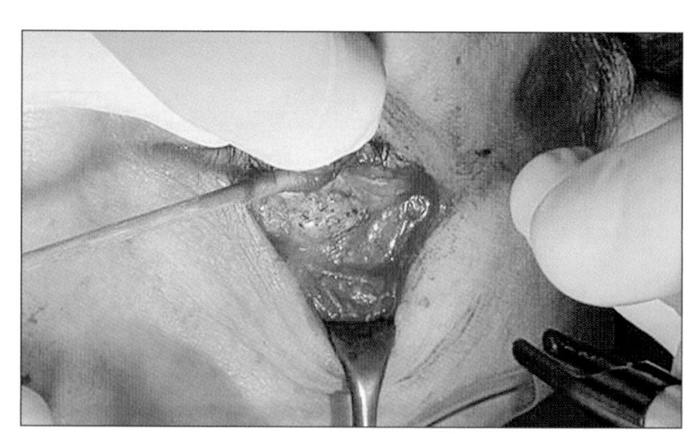

Fig 7-22b SMF approach with final orbital fat contouring and hemostasis using the CO_2 laser at a defocused distance.

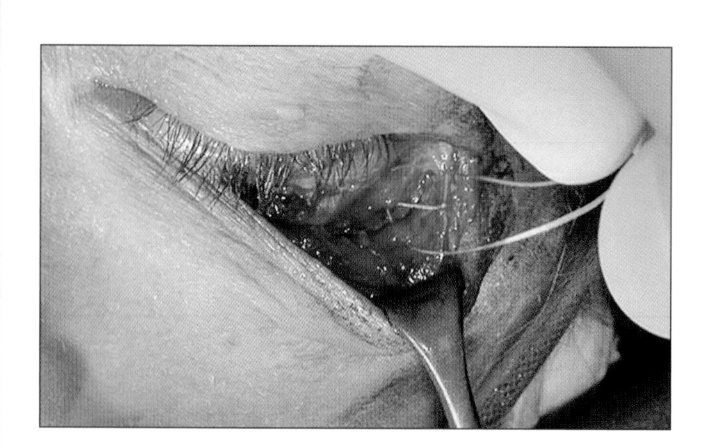

Fig 7-22c Lateral retinacular suspension in an SMF approach. A 4-0 clear nylon suture is passed through the lateral canthal ligament in a horizontal mattress fashion and is secured superolaterally to the orbital periosteum. Vectors and tension are adjusted intraoperatively on a patient-by-patient basis.

this point. This occurs when acceptable orbicularis tone and lower eyelid–to-midface contours exist.

Occasionally, the orbicularis muscle requires further advancement and elevation above and beyond what can be tolerated by the skin. In these instances, the skin must be carefully dissected free of the underlying muscle for a short distance. Care is taken to avoid buttonholing the skin, and once complete, the muscle is then plicated and advanced to the lateral orbital rim periosteum. It is fixated in this position with one to two separate 4-0 Vicryl sutures (Johnson & Johnson). This often reestablishes the lower eyelid–to-midface junction without causing distraction of the lower eyelid away from the globe. This is possible due to the separate but simultaneous lateral retinacular canthopexy procedure. Excess orbicularis muscle is then excised, and the skin flap is repositioned for final tissue trimming with scissors. This step ideally takes place with the patient looking in an upward gaze. Skin closure is accomplished with one to two separate standard interrupted 6-0 Prolene or nylon sutures placed in the lateral canthal region. The remainder of the incision is closed in a running, continuously advancing fashion using the same suture.

Lower eyelid blepharoplasty: TCB and SPT

The TCB approach to the orbit is well known to the oral and maxillofacial surgeon. As is described with orbital trauma, this technique can be performed via either a retroseptal or preseptal approach. The author of this chapter exclusively uses the retroseptal approach and will describe it here because the preseptal version involves incising the orbital septum and so removes most of the advantages that this technique possesses over the SMF technique.

The surgery starts with retraction of the lower eyelid inferiorly using the assistant's thumb and index finger. This facilitates gentle insertion of a small- to medium-sized Desmarres retractor. The globe is then protected and retracted posteriorly with the Jaeger lid plate. Many different versions of these two instruments exist. When using a CO_2 laser, the surgeon should ensure that they are laser-safe with a highly polished surface designed for direct atraumatic contact with the lid or globe and an opposing dull, nonreflective finish designed to prevent laser light scatter. Rubber-coated retractors should not be routinely used in place of the laser-specific ones because melting of the coating can take place.

Placement of the incision 3 to 4 mm below the inferior aspect of the inferior tarsal plate is most common, though the author attempts to place the incision directly over the place where the fat is most accessible. In some patients, this is halfway between the inferior tarsal border and the inferior fornix, while in others, this may be located more posteriorly. The Jaeger plate, Desmarres retractor, and gentle retropulsion together are all used to identify the fat bulge and thus the incision site. When not easily identifiable, it is safer to keep the incision positioned more anteriorly toward the inferior orbital rim rather than continue dissecting posteriorly toward the globe. Using the CO_2 laser, the conjunctival incision is made medially from the lacrimal punctum laterally to the lateral canthal area in one smooth pass (Fig 7-23a). The assistant holding the Desmarres retractor travels laterally along the lid as the laser is advanced. The most common mistake made with the initial TCB incision is failure to incise far enough laterally. Following initial incision, the Jaeger plate and Desmarres retractor are moved slightly to sit in the conjunctival wound, thereby widening it under tension to facilitate deeper dissection. Dissection continues with the laser down through the capsulopalpebral fascia until orbital fat is encountered.

The central compartment is usually encountered first. Further blunt dissection medially and laterally using a presterilized cotton-tip applicator allows for identification of the medial and lateral fat pads (Fig 7-23b). Occasionally, fibrous encapsulations of the fat pads are incised to allow full access to them. Excess fat from each pad is then resected in a controlled fashion by rolling the fat pad out and over top of a moistened cotton-tip applicator. In this way, the CO_2 laser can be used to simultaneously cut and coagulate without fear of damage to underlying structures. Fat removed from each pad is compared to that from the opposing eyelid to ensure subjective symmetry at the end of the case. Instruments are periodically removed, and the external fat pad markings of the preexisting "bags" are evaluated to determine if adequate resection has been accomplished. Final fat ablation and hemostasis are achieved with the laser from a defocused distance.

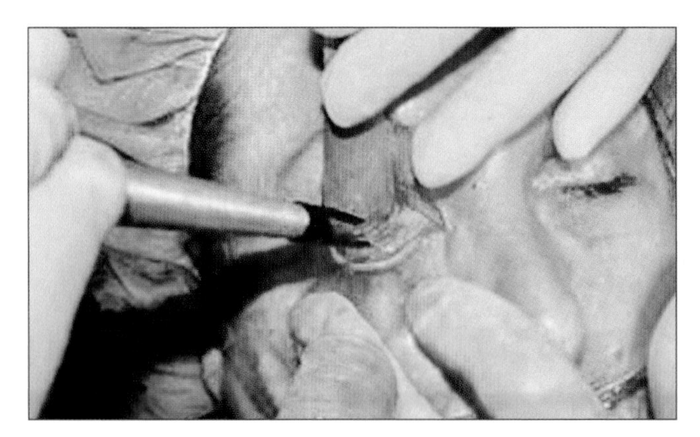

Fig 7-23a Transconjunctival incision being made with CO_2 laser. The Desmarres retractor has been removed to aid with photographic visualization.

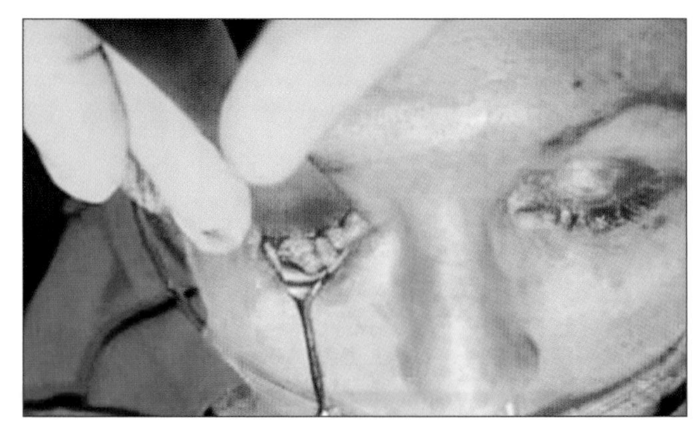

Fig 7-23b Transconjunctival approach for lower eyelid blepharoplasty with exposure of postseptal fat pads.

TCB incisions very rarely require closure with sutures and so are left open to heal by themselves. The next step is to address the excess lower eyelid skin. This chapter focuses on the SPT, but clinicians should be aware that other options, including chemical peeling and fraxel ablative resurfacing, are available.

The SPT involves the removal of a small quantity (usually less than 5 mm) of excess skin from the subciliary region of the lower eyelids. No additional local anesthesia is required when it is completed alongside a TCB. First, the amount of skin to be removed is assessed by pinching the subciliary region from lateral to medial with a pair of cotton pliers or small nontoothed pickups (Fig 7-24). Next, this pinched skin is crimped from lateral to medial with a fine hemostat two to three times, causing a distinct ridge of excess skin to become apparent. The excess crimped skin is then removed with a pair of fine scissors. The underlying blood vessels are cauterized with the CO_2 laser prior to closure with a running 6-0 Prolene or nylon suture.

Following this technique can lead to a successful CO_2 laser–assisted bilateral lower eyelid TCB with or without the SPT (Figs 7-25 and 7-26).

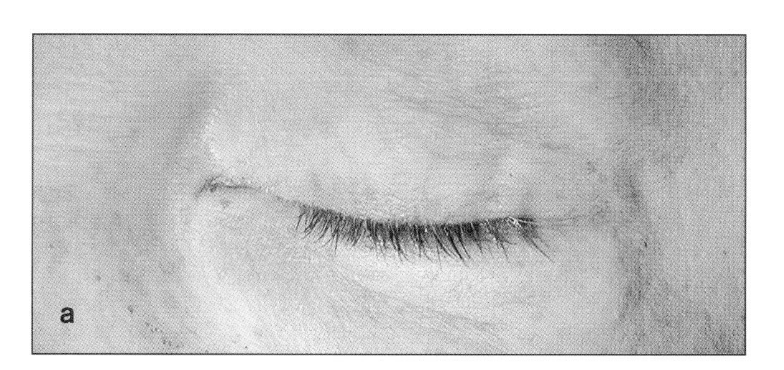

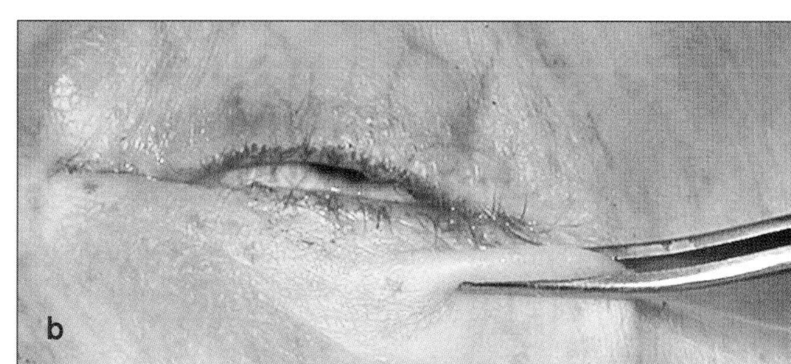

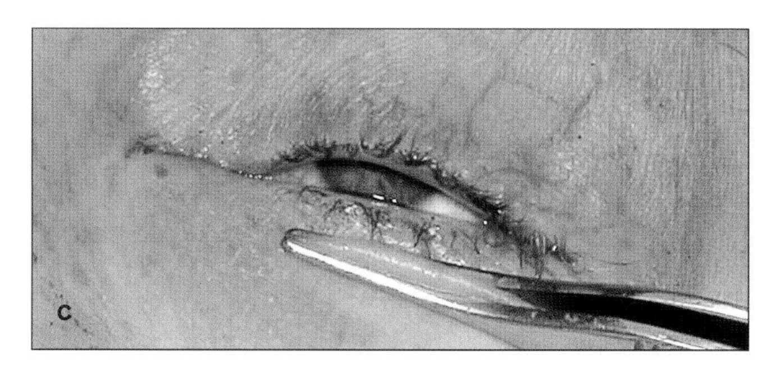

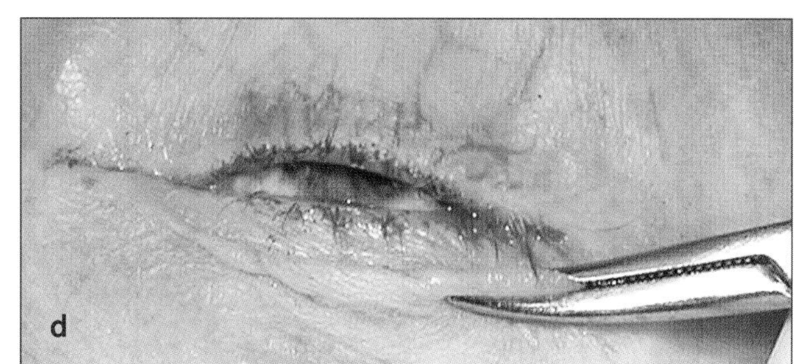

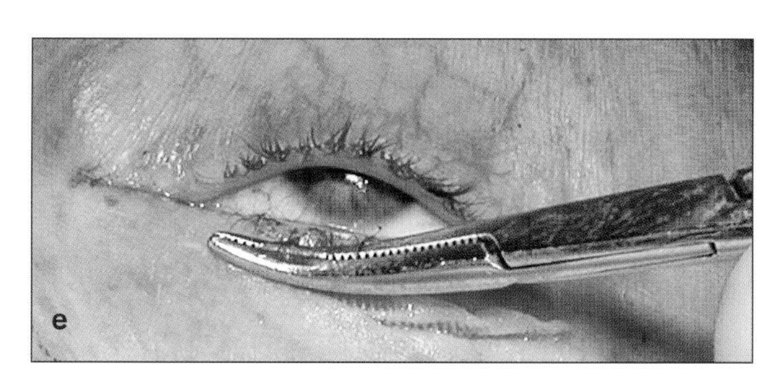

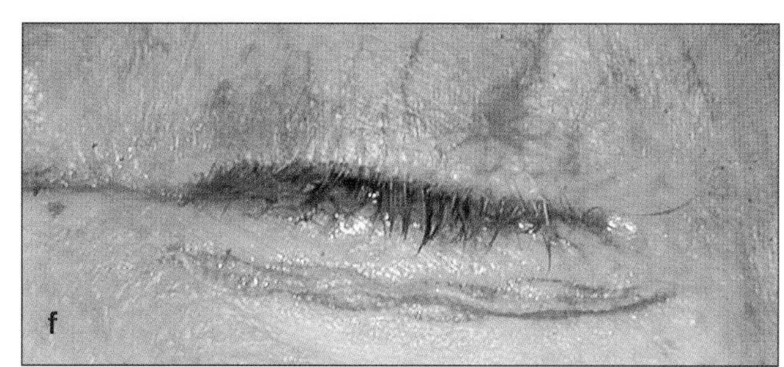

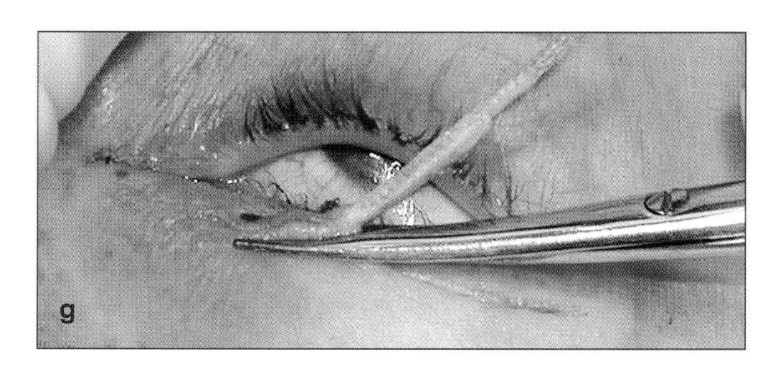

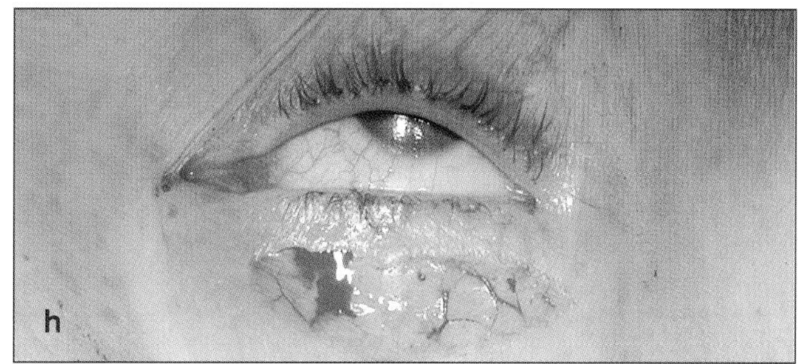

Fig 7-24 SPT for lower eyelid blepharoplasty. *(a)* Preoperative view. *(b and c)* Nontoothed forceps are used to pinch excess lower eyelid skin from lateral to medial. *(d to f)* Following the pinch, skin is further crimped from lateral to medial with a fine hemostat until a distinct ridge of excess skin becomes apparent. *(g)* The excess crimped skin is then removed with a pair of fine scissors. *(h and i)* Hemostasis of blood vessels is achieved with the CO_2 laser prior to closure with a running 6-0 Prolene or nylon suture.

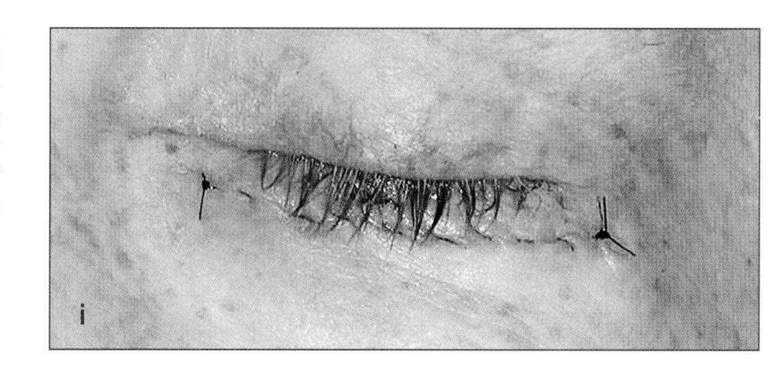

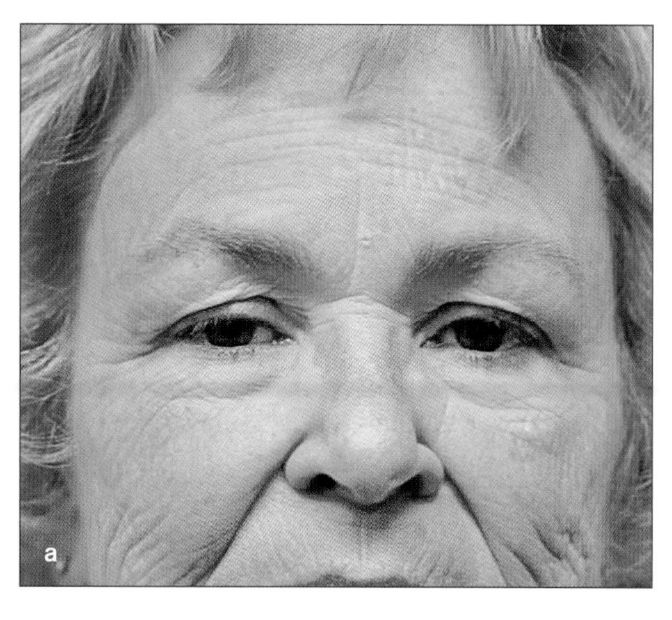

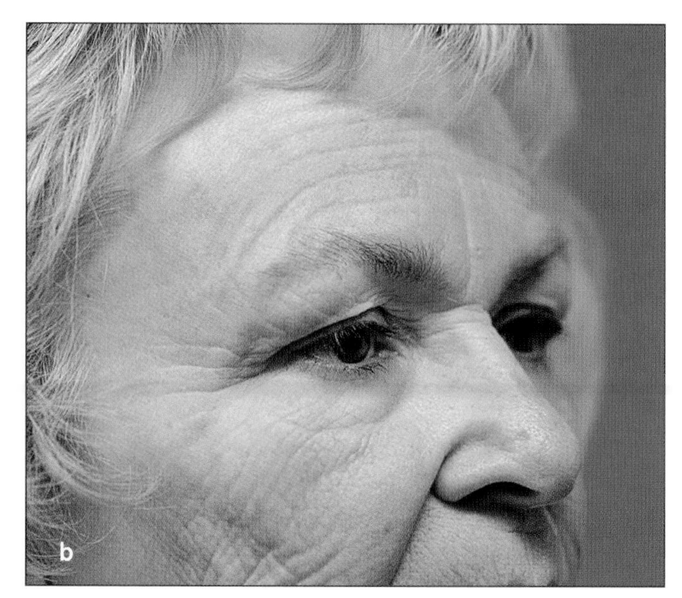

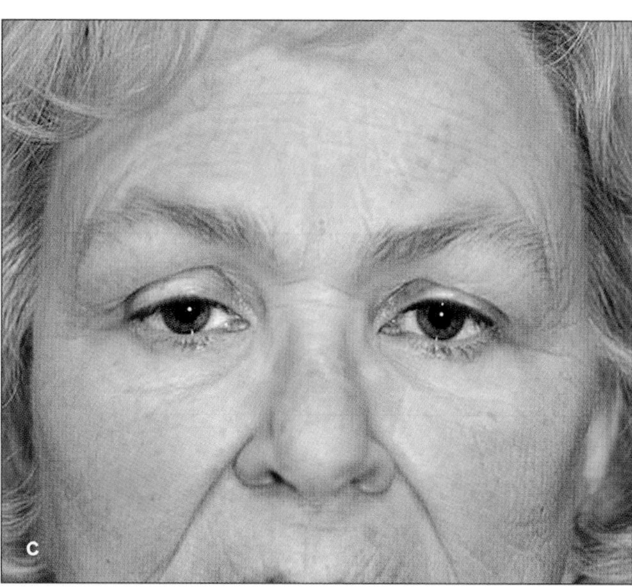

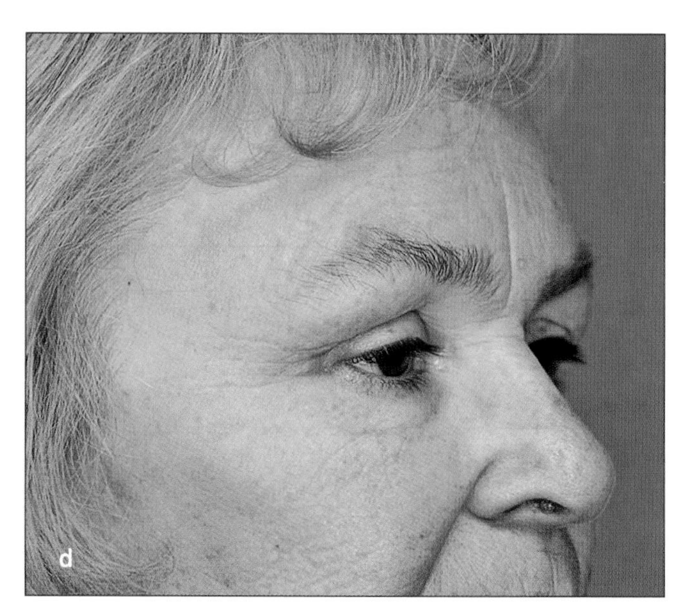

Fig 7-25 Preoperative *(a and b)* and 6-month postoperative *(c and d)* frontal and right three-quarter views of a woman with multiple facial esthetic concerns. The preoperative photographs show presence of bilateral brow ptosis, upper and lower eyelid dermatochalasis, lower eyelid pseudoherniation, generalized advanced facial rhytidosis, cervicofacial tissue laxity, and midface ptosis. Over a two-stage surgical approach, an endoscopic brow lift, bilateral lower TCB/SPT blepharoplasty, and periorbital 20% TCA peel were performed, followed by bilateral CO_2 laser–assisted upper blepharoplasty and formal cervicofacial rhytidectomy. Note persistent postoperative midface ptosis and deep nasolabial folds. The patient declined both a midface lift (recommended simultaneously with the endoscopic brow lift) and postoperative full-face fractional CO_2 resurfacing.

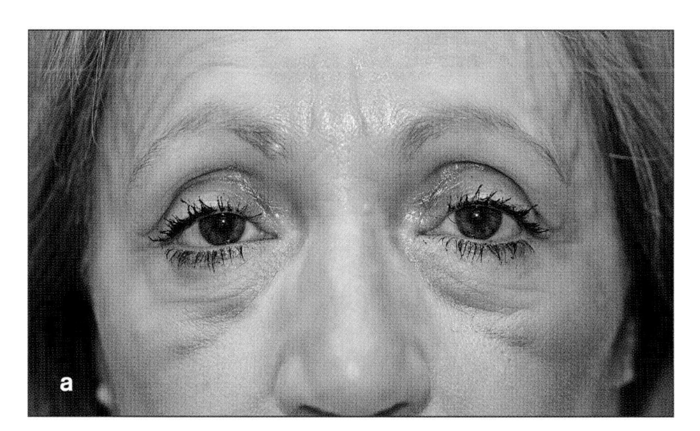

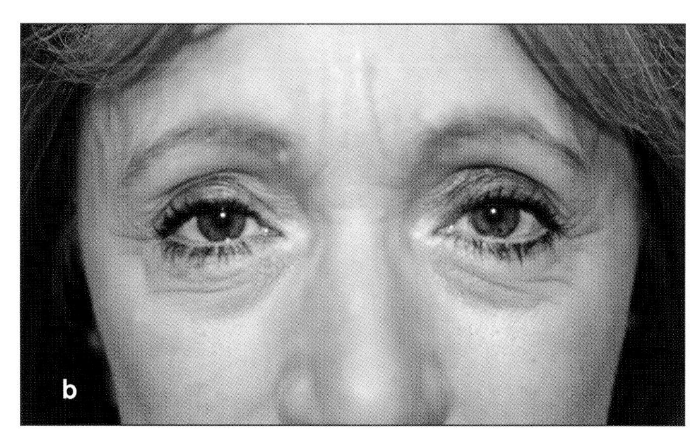

Fig 7-26 Preoperative *(a)* and 6-month postoperative *(b)* frontal views of a woman who underwent CO_2 laser–assisted bilateral lower eyelid TCB and a minimal incision facelift.

Fig 7-27 Immediately following CO_2 laser–assisted bilateral upper eyelid blepharoplasty. The surrounding periorbital skin has been gently cleansed to remove blood and/or debris, and the incision lines have been dressed with an ophthalmic-grade antibiotic ointment.

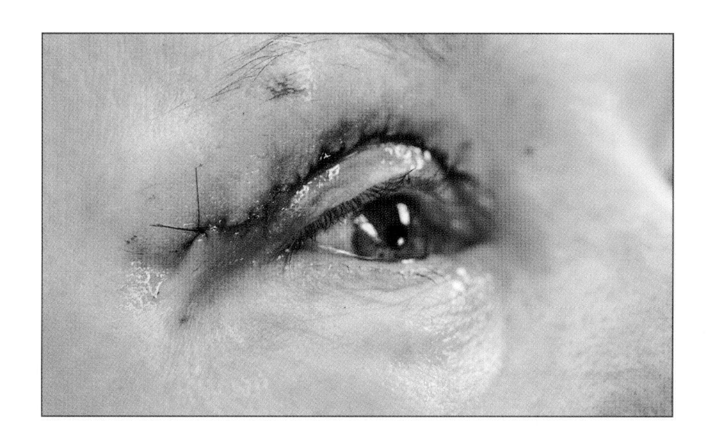

Postoperative Care

The surrounding periorbital skin is gently cleansed to remove blood and debris, and the incision lines are dressed with an ophthalmic-grade antibiotic ointment (Fig 7-27). No bandages are required for upper or lower eyelid blepharoplasty alone, but the eyes should be covered by cold compresses as continuously as possible for the first 24 hours following surgery. Patients are sent home with detailed written instructions along with a prescription for analgesics, antibiotics, and lubricating eye drops. Postoperative pain is an uncommon complaint with isolated blepharoplasty. However, it is not uncommon for patients to experience blurred vision (secondary to ointment) and a burning sensation for 1 to 1.5 hours after surgery. Maximum postoperative edema occurs 48 to 72 hours following surgery, so patients should have their first scheduled follow-up on the second postoperative day. When blepharoplasty incisions are made with a CO_2 laser, sutures are removed 1 week after surgery. Removal at 5 days, as with conventional scalpel incision, is not recommended because a higher rate of wound dehiscence can occur. Additional time is necessary with the CO_2 laser to allow for adequate tissue cohesiveness and strength because it takes longer for the body to remove the thermal-induced eschar created with CO_2 laser incision. Mascara can be applied on the fourth postoperative day, but patients are asked to refrain from the use of eye shadow and contact lenses for 1 week. Bruising and residual edema are highly variable (Figs 7-28 and 7-29), but most patients feel comfortable returning to work or normal activities on the fifth to seventh postoperative day. Strenuous exercise and activity can begin after 2 weeks.

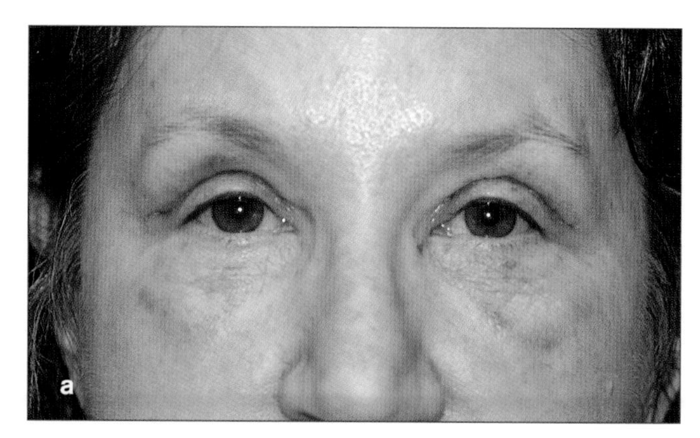

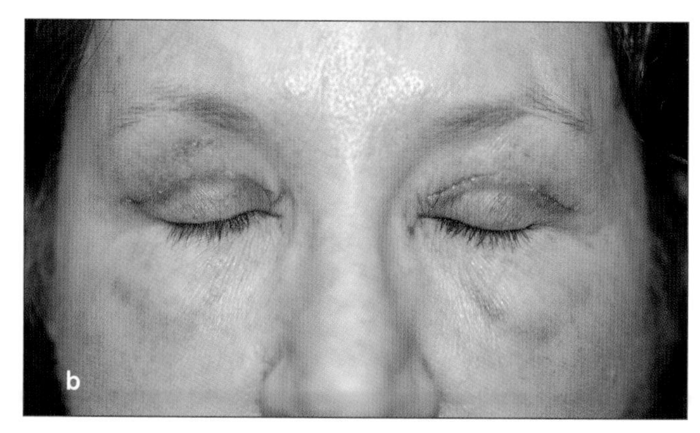

Fig 7-28 One-week postoperative eyes-opened *(a)* and eyes-closed *(b)* frontal views of a woman who underwent isolated CO_2 laser–assisted bilateral upper eyelid blepharoplasty.

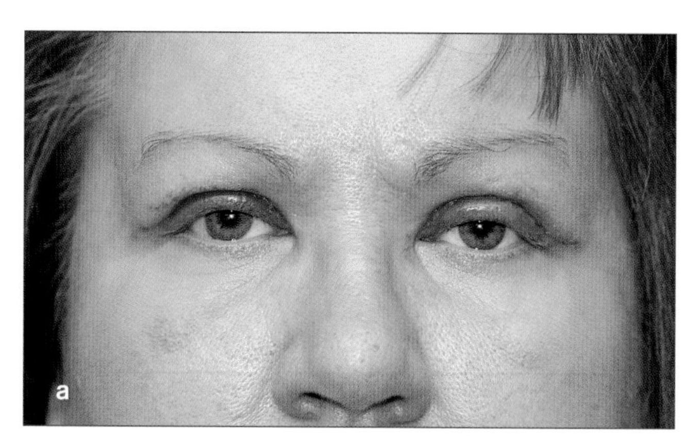

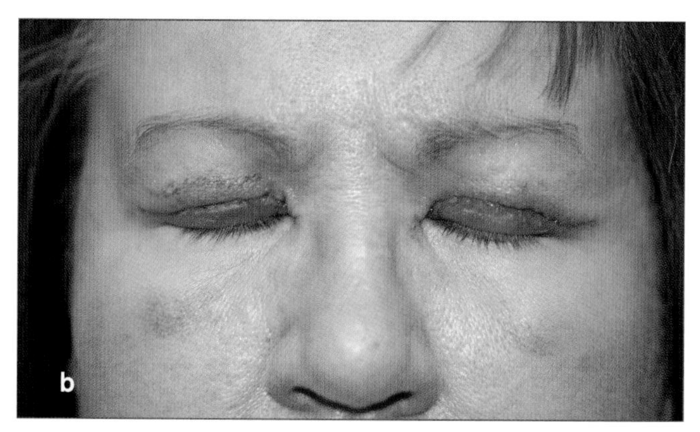

Fig 7-29 One-week postoperative eyes-opened *(a)* and eyes-closed *(b)* frontal views of a woman who underwent isolated CO_2 laser–assisted bilateral upper eyelid blepharoplasty. Bruising and edema are variable when compared to the patient in Fig 7-28.

Complications

Thorough preoperative planning, patient selection, and meticulous technique will most often prevent or at least decrease the risk of complications following blepharoplasty. Serious complications are usually functional in nature and are, fortunately, uncommon.[11] They include persistent dry eye syndrome, persistent epiphora, orbital hematoma, persistent diplopia, and blindness. Blindness secondary to blepharoplasty is extremely rare. Reported cases have been associated more frequently with lower blepharoplasty than with upper blepharoplasty and presumably occur secondary to orbital hematoma. Most reported orbital hematomas take place within the first 24 hours following surgery. They almost always are associated with postseptal procedures; therefore, even seemingly simple techniques such as orbital fat removal must be treated with respect. Orbital hematomas are true emergencies that require immediate medical and surgical attention.[2] Clinicians should suspect such a complication in the presence of severe, throbbing, retrobulbar pain or frank proptosis.

Monocular diplopia is an ominous sign following blepharoplasty and should be investigated. Binocular diploplia persisting longer than 24 to 48 hours is usually caused by extraocular muscle trauma or damage. Fortunately, most diplopias spontaneously resolve. In those that do not, exploration and repair of damaged or transected musculature is indicated after several months of healing. While tearing, or epiphora, and dry eye syndrome may be early common problems following blepharoplasty, they should not persist as long-term nuisances. When present, persistent problems should be evaluated and managed definitively by an ophthalmologist. In the case of dry eye syndrome, the primary surgeon is responsible for ensuring that the affected eye is kept properly lubricated and protected until the patient is assessed by an ophthalmologic colleague.

Minor complications associated with blepharoplasty can be functional and esthetic and are divided temporally into early (less than 2 weeks for resolution) and prolonged (more than 2 weeks) problems. Common early sequelae include tearing; pretarsal/periorbital swelling, bruising, ecchymosis, and/or related lid asymmetries; subconjunctival hemorrhage; chemosis; and eyelid/periorbital paresthesia.[2] Eyelid swelling and periorbital bruising, while expected, can occur to varying degrees between patients. Special attention should be placed on identifying potential "bleeders" preoperatively. Postoperative instructions and home care should likewise be reinforced.

Unwanted esthetic complications can occur despite good esthetic intentions. In the upper eyelid, the surgeon should be aware of the potential for persistent excess skin, scarring, suture marks, lagophthalmos, and blepharoptosis. Blepharoptosis is most often a result of a preexisting upper eyelid ptosis that was present but undiagnosed prior to surgery.[6] It can, however, occur as a result of iatrogenic damage leading to traumatic levator disinsertion. It is repaired only after full healing has occurred. Lagophthalmos following closure in primary blepharoplasty may approach but should rarely exceed 4 mm. Orbicularis oculi anesthesia can lead to unopposed levator contraction and so may be the contributing factor in many cases where careful preoperative markings and skin resection were undertaken. Clinicians using the CO_2 laser should also account for 1 mm of additional lagophthalmos owing to tissue contraction. Eye openings of greater than 5 to 6 mm have the potential to be problematic. Occasionally, primary blepharoplasty patients may retain enough skin elasticity to allow for eventual spontaneous palpebral closure, but this is not a desirable postoperative situation. Scarring and suture marks are very rare problems. Scars at 6 months postoperatively are generally imperceptible in the majority of patients, regardless of the incisional modality. Scar management is case dependent but may include camouflage with makeup, scar revision, laser resurfacing, or, rarely, repeat blepharoplasty. Suture marks are usually due to delayed removal and can be reduced by proper suture selection.

Esthetic and functional complications unique to lower eyelid blepharoplasty include persistent fat, persistent redundant skin, and retraction or ectropion.[11,14] Persistent orbital fat is most often evident in the lateral fat pad. Repeated intraoperative evaluation is required. Required secondary revisions should not proceed for at least 12 weeks to allow for adequate healing time. Skin redundancy in the lower eyelid is a difficult problem to predict. Overresection can lead to lid retraction, ectropion, and esthetics that are worse than preoperative complaints. Patients should be made aware that postoperative adjunctive tightening and resurfacing techniques may help to enhance the skin redundancy. It is also easier to go back and touch up than it is to try to rectify a disaster. Problems with postoperative retraction and increased scleral show can arise secondary to aggressive lower eyelid skin removal. They also often occur with unrecognized preoperative lower eyelid laxity. The likelihood of success with conservative treatment (ie, massage, taping, squinting exercises) depends on the degree of horizontal laxity and is worse with increasing vertical tissue loss. Surgical intervention by way of lid-tightening procedures is used to address horizontal skin laxity, whereas potentially adjunctive skin or palatal grafting can be used to increase lower eyelid vertical height.[2,11,14]

Summary

Elective cosmetic blepharoplasty remains a fundamental procedure of facial rejuvenation. Complex regional anatomy and widely varied esthetic demands pose unique challenges for the facial cosmetic surgeon. Success requires a thorough understanding of the relevant anatomy, proper patient assessment, appropriate procedural selection, and meticulous surgical technique. Current scope and training within the field of oral and maxillofacial surgery makes its practitioners uniquely suited to perform elective cosmetic blepharoplasty. When performed skillfully, these rejuvenation procedures will provide both patient and surgeon with rewarding results with a low risk of complications.

Blepharoplasty Tray

- Blepharoplasty scissors (KLS-Martin)
- Strabismus scissors, curved (Snowden-Pencer)
- Castroviejo caliper (KLS-Martin)
- Scalpel handle, two (KLS-Martin)
- Aspirating syringe, two (KLS-Martin)
- Adson-Brown forceps, two (KLS-Martin)
- No. 9 periosteal elevator (KLS-Martin)
- Towel forceps, four (KLS-Martin)
- Cogswell suction tube (KLS-Martin)
- Mosquito hemostat, four (KLS-Martin)
- Single-prong skin hook (KLS-Martin)
- Senn retractor (Snowden-Pencer)
- Bishop-Harmon forceps (KLS-Martin)
- Bishop-Harmon forceps, no teeth (KLS-Martin)
- Dean scissors (KLS-Martin)
- Fomon scissors (KLS-Martin)
- Castroviejo needle holder, two (Snowden-Pencer)
- Titanium microscissors (Snowden-Pencer)
- Desmarres lid retractors, two (Snowden-Pencer)
- Jaeger lid plate (Oculo-Plastik)
- David Baker lid clamp, small (Oculo-Plastik)
- David Baker lid clamp, large (Oculo-Plastik)
- Desmarres retractor (Oculo-Plastik)
- Iodine cup (Biomet)

References

1. Gentile RD. Upper lid blepharoplasty. Facial Plast Surg Clin North Am 2005;13:511–524.
2. Pastorek N, Bustillo A. Blepharoplasty. In: Azzizadeh B, Murphy MR, Johnson CM (eds). Master Techniques in Facial Rejuvenation. Philadelphia: Saunders, 2007:59–88.
3. Espinoza GM, Holds JB. Evolution of eyelid surgery. Facial Plast Surg Clin North Am 2005;13: 505–510.
4. Dresner SC, Marshak H. Transconjunctival lower blepharoplasty. In: Azzizadeh B, Murphy MR, Johnson CM (eds). Master Techniques in Facial Rejuvenation. Philadelphia: Saunders, 2007:89–98.
5. Most SP, Mobley SR, Larrabee WF Jr. Anatomy of the eyelids. Facial Plast Surg Clin North Am 2005; 13:487–492.
6. Putterman AM. Evaluation of the cosmetic oculoplastic surgery patient. In: Fagien S (ed). Putterman's Cosmetic Oculoplastic Surgery, ed 4. Philadelphia: Saunders, 2008:21–30.
7. Kim DW, Bhakti AM. Upper blepharoplasty in the Asian eyelid. Facial Plast Surg Clin North Am 2005;13:525–532.
8. Niamtu J 3rd. Cosmetic blepharoplasty. Atlas Oral Maxillofac Surg Clin North Am 2004;12:91–130.
9. Harris PA, Mendelson BC. Eyelid and midcheek anatomy. In: Fagien S (ed). Putterman's Cosmetic Oculoplastic Surgery, ed 4. Philadelphia: Saunders, 2008:45–63.
10. Fagien S. Upper blepharoplasty: Volume enhancement via skin approach. Lowering the upper lid crease. In: Fagien S (ed). Putterman's Cosmetic Oculoplastic Surgery, ed 4. Philadelphia: Saunders, 2008:81–103.
11. Lee AS, Thomas JR. Lower lid blepharoplasty and canthal surgery. Facial Plastic Surg Clin North Am 2005;13:541–551.
12. Massry G. Ptosis repair for the cosmetic surgeon. Facial Plast Surg Clin North Am 2005;13:533–539.
13. Putterman AM. Transconjunctival approach to resection of lower eyelid herniated orbital fat. In: Fagien S (ed). Putterman's Cosmetic Oculoplastic Surgery, ed 4. Philadelphia: Saunders, 2008:155–160.
14. Putterman AM. Treatment of lower eyelid dermatochalasis, herniated orbital fat, and hypertrophic orbicularis muscle: Skin-muscle flap approach. In: Fagien S (ed). Putterman's Cosmetic Oculoplastic Surgery, ed 4. Philadelphia: Saunders, 2008:181–185.
15. Niamtu J 3rd. Radiowave surgery versus CO laser for upper blepharoplasty incision: Which modality produces the most aesthetic incision? Dermatol Surg 2008;34:912–921.
16. Baker SS, Muenzler WS, Small RG, Leonard JE. Carbon dioxide laser blepharoplasty. Ophthalmology 1984;91:238–244.

8

Dermal Fillers and Botulinum Toxin Treatment

RAYMOND J. HAIGNEY II, DDS
KING KIM, DMD
JOHN E. GRIFFIN, DMD

There are myriad ways in which moderate to severe wrinkles of the face can be addressed. These include surgical intervention, rhytidectomy (see chapter 2), laser resurfacing (see chapter 9), autogenous fat transfer, and injection with dermal fillers and botulinum toxin. With so many people concerned about economic cost, surgical rejuvenation is being used less than ever in favor of more economical cosmetic procedures, and this chapter focuses on the rapidly growing field of injectable fillers and neurotoxins.

The use of both dermal fillers and neurotoxins to create volume and provide a smooth, youthful facial appearance has been very successful. Static lines of the face—including moderate to deep marionette lines, glabellar lines, crow's feet, and nasolabial folds—and hollow areas of the infraorbital region are best treated with a dermal filler (Fig 8-1). In contrast, dynamic lines caused by hyperkinetic facial musculature are best treated with botulinum toxin (Fig 8-2). Over time, dynamic lines become static lines.

Dermal Fillers

It has been more than 20 years since the first dermal filler gained clearance from the US Food and Drug Administration (FDA), and for the past quarter-century, the gold standard of dermal fillers has been bovine collagen. Due to bovine collagen's potential for allergic reaction, a test spot was initially placed on the arm, and 30 days was allowed to pass to ensure that no reaction took place before it would be injected with impunity into the facial region. Since those pioneering efforts were made, a variety of materials have been added to the cosmetic practitioner's armamentarium.

In general, dermal fillers are indicated for injection into the mid to deep dermis to correct moderate to severe facial wrinkles and folds and soft tissue deficiencies. Some have more limited application, such as restoration of signs of facial fat loss in people with human immunodeficiency virus (HIV), and others are also indicated for use to fill areas of acne scars or other soft tissue deficiencies (Fig 8-3).

Currently, there are more than a dozen FDA-cleared dermal fillers available.[1] These products vary from biologic to synthetic materials and from resorbable to nonresorbable compounds, the majority of which have been developed since 2000. The following section highlights many of the current FDA-cleared dermal fillers.

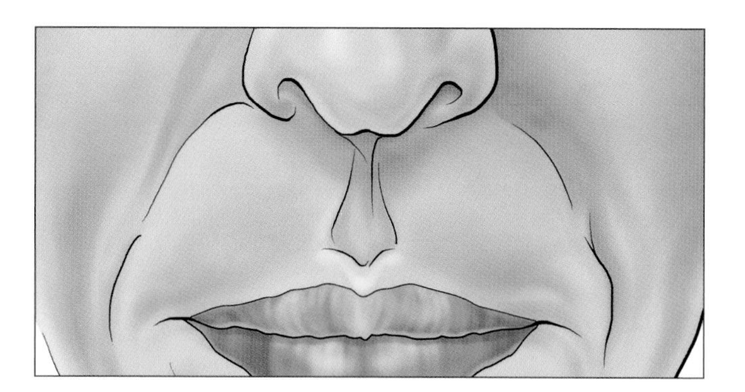

Fig 8-1 Static rhytids of the face. These nasolabial folds are unchanged with muscle movement.

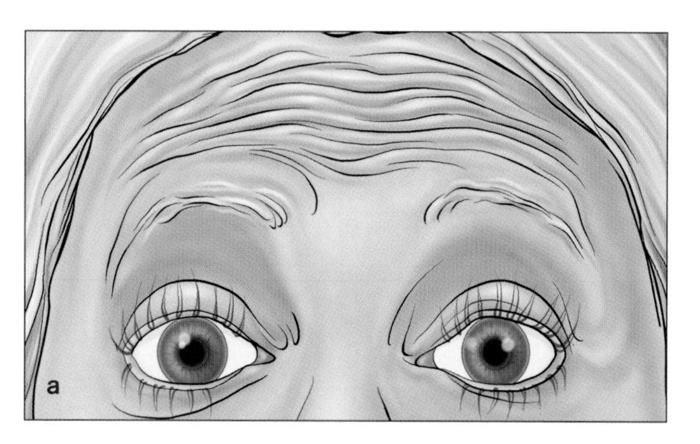

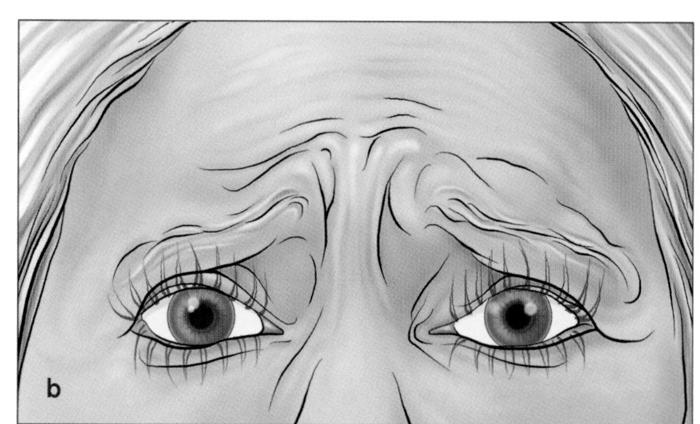

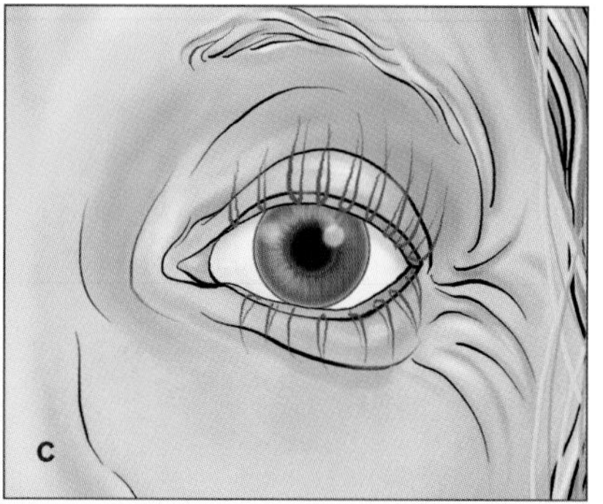

Fig 8-2 Dynamic rhytids of the face. *(a)* Contraction of the frontalis muscle creates lines on the forehead. *(b)* Contraction of corrugator supercilii muscles and procerus muscle produces lines on the glabella. *(c)* Activity of the orbicularis oculi from smiling leads to crow's feet lines in the periorbital region.

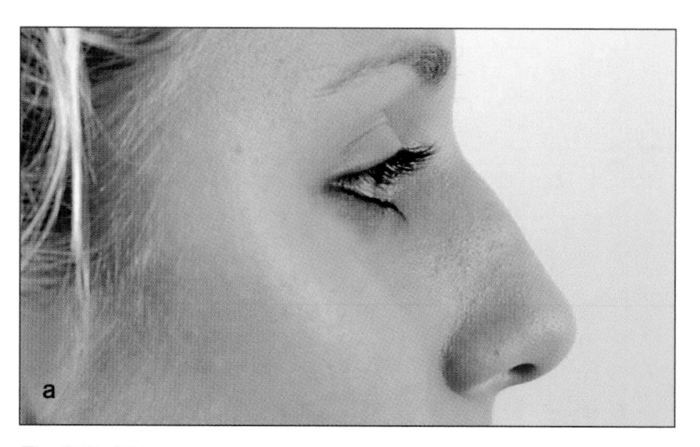

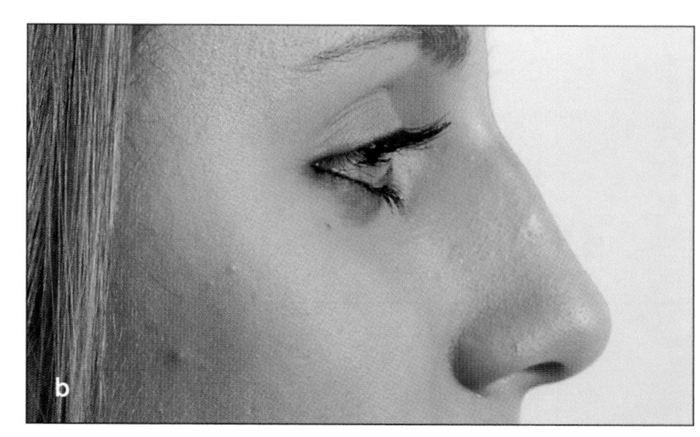

Fig 8-3 *(a)* Pretreatment profile of a woman with a prominent dorsal hump. *(b)* Posttreatment profile following dermal filler injection to smooth the dorsal hump.

Types of dermal fillers

Natural collagen (nonresorbable)

Evolence porcine collagen dermal filler (Colbar Lifesciences) can be used for the correction of moderate to severe deep facial wrinkles and folds, such as the nasolabial folds. It is composed of a biodegradable type 1 fibrillar porcine collagen that is cross-linked using D-ribose and suspended in phosphate buffered saline. Evolence is available at a concentration of 35 mg/mL. Various antigenic portions of the collagen molecule have been removed.[1]

Cosmoderm (Allergan) and Cosmosplast (Allergan) are human-based (H-B) collagen implants. Cosmoderm is injected into the superficial papillary dermis for correction of soft tissue contour deficiencies, such as wrinkles and acne scars. It is derived from highly purified fibroblast cell culture and is dispersed in phosphate buffered physiologic saline containing 0.3% lidocaine.[1] Cosmoplast H-B collagen is also used for the correction of soft tissue contour deficiencies, but it is injected into the mid to deep dermis.[1] Cosmoplast H-B collagen is derived from highly purified fibroblast cell culture that is cross-linked with glutaraldehyde and dispersed in phosphate buffered physiologic saline containing 0.3% lidocaine.

Zyderm (Allergan) and Zyplast (Allergan) are bovine collagen implants. Zyderm is composed of highly purified bovine dermal collagen dispersed in phosphate buffered physiologic saline containing 0.3% lidocaine and is indicated for the correction of contour deformities of the dermis in areas that are not weight bearing.[1] Zyplast is composed of highly purified bovine dermal collagen that is lightly cross-linked with glutaraldehyde and dispersed in a phosphate buffered physiologic saline containing 0.3% lidocaine.[1] It is indicated for the correction of contour deformities of soft tissue.

Natural resorbable dermal fillers

Hylaform (Genzyme Bioscience), Hylaform Plus (Genzyme Bioscience), and Captique (Genzyme Bioscience) are indicated for injection into the mid to deep dermis for correction of moderate to severe facial wrinkles and folds, such as nasolabial folds. All three fillers are clear, colorless gels composed of cross-linked hyaluronic acid derived from rooster combs and gram-positive bacteria.[1] They are injectable, sterile, nonpyrogenic, and viscoelastic.[1]

Restylane (Medicis Aesthetics) and Perlane (Medicis Aesthetics) are suspensions of hyaluronic acid generated by streptococcal bacteria.[1] Restylane is indicated for mid to deep dermal implantation for the correction of moderate to severe facial wrinkles and folds, such as nasolabial folds. Perlane is indicated for implantation from the deep dermis to the superficial subcutis for the correction of moderate to severe facial folds and wrinkles, such as nasolabial folds.

The Juvederm gel implants (Allergan)—Juvederm Ultra and Juvederm Ultra Plus—are injectable gels indicated for injection into the mid to deep dermis for correction of moderate to severe facial wrinkles and folds, such as nasolabial folds. The hyaluronic acid in Juvederm is produced by *Streptococcus equi* bacteria and suspended in a physiologic buffer.[1]

Sculptra (Aventis Pharmaceuticals) is intended for restoration and/or correction of the signs of facial fat loss (lipoatrophy) in people with HIV or receiving treatment for HIV. It is an injectable poly-L-lactic acid implant in the form of a lyophilized cake.[1]

Synthetic dermal fillers

Nonresorbable

The only nonresorbable dermal filler that has received FDA clearance is Artefill (Artes Medical). It is used for the correction of nasolabial folds. Artefill is an implant composed of nonresorbable polymethylmethacrylate microspheres that are 30 to 50 μm in diameter and are suspended in a water-based carrier gel composed of 92.6% buffered isotonic water, 3.5% bovine collagen, 2.7% phosphate buffer, 0.9% sodium chloride, and 0.3% lidocaine.[1]

Resorbable

Radiesse (Bioform Medical) is a hydroxyapatite product that is used for subdermal implantation for the correction of moderate to severe facial wrinkles and folds, such as nasolabial folds.[1]

Injection techniques

There are essentially four techniques employed in delivering dermal filler: *(1)* the serial injection, *(2)* the threading push, *(3)* the thread pullback, and *(4)* the fan techniques. Practitioners may find it beneficial to use a combination of all four techniques to create volume, depending on the location of the injection.

Serial injection

In the serial injection technique, small advancing injections are placed along the area of concern. With this technique, even the novice injector should be able to achieve precise, predictable results.

Threading push

In the threading push technique, the needle first is injected into the dermal plane with the bevel up. Then, the contents are slowly and gently delivered as the needle is advanced along the desired path. This technique is thought to minimize bruising and swelling.

Thread pullback

In the thread pullback technique, the needle is introduced into the dermal plane with the bevel up. It is positioned along the entire planned distance for delivering the filler. The practitioner then slowly injects the filler as the needle is withdrawn. The advantage of this technique is that the needle creates a plane or a space to inject into, which allows for a smooth, even distribution of the product.

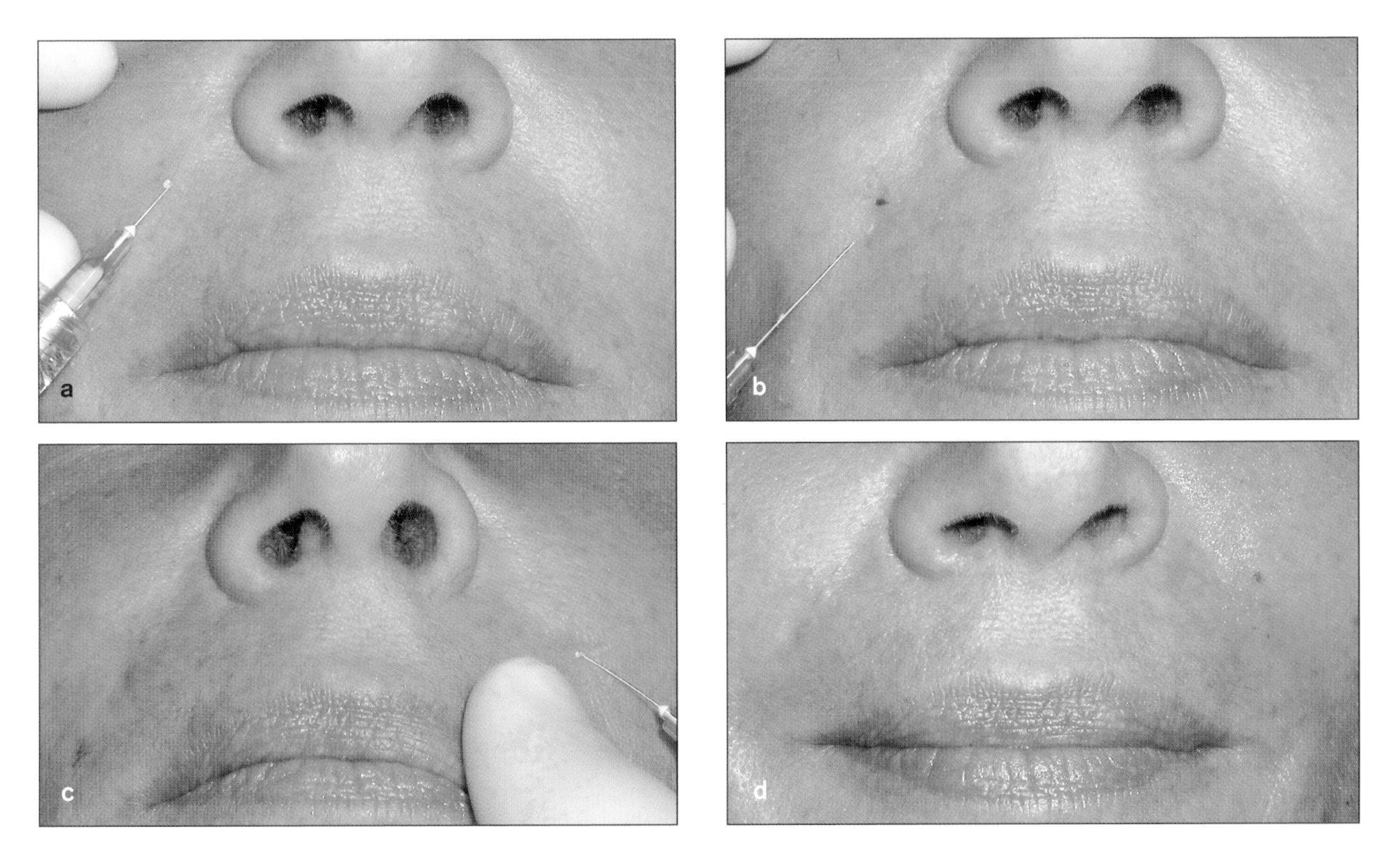

Fig 8-4 *(a to d)* **Dermal filler used in the nasolabial folds.**

Fan injection

In the fan technique, the needle is introduced, and material is injected without removing the needle as it approaches the entry point. Rather, a new direction is taken again and again in the shape of a fan. This technique is beneficial because it saves the patient from having multiple injection points at the skin surface. Therefore, adequate volume of product can be deposited in a wide area with a single skin prick.

Anatomical considerations

Nasolabial region

Care must be exercised in the region of the nasolabial fold to allow the filler to enter only the side of the cutaneous lip and not the area lateral to the fold, which would create the unintended consequence of making the fold more acute than obtuse. The goal of using dermal filler in this area is not to completely efface the fold, which would appear unnatural, but to create a smooth transition from cheek to lip (Fig 8-4).

Lips

When injecting the lips, the practitioner first asks several questions to help determine the desired final outcome:

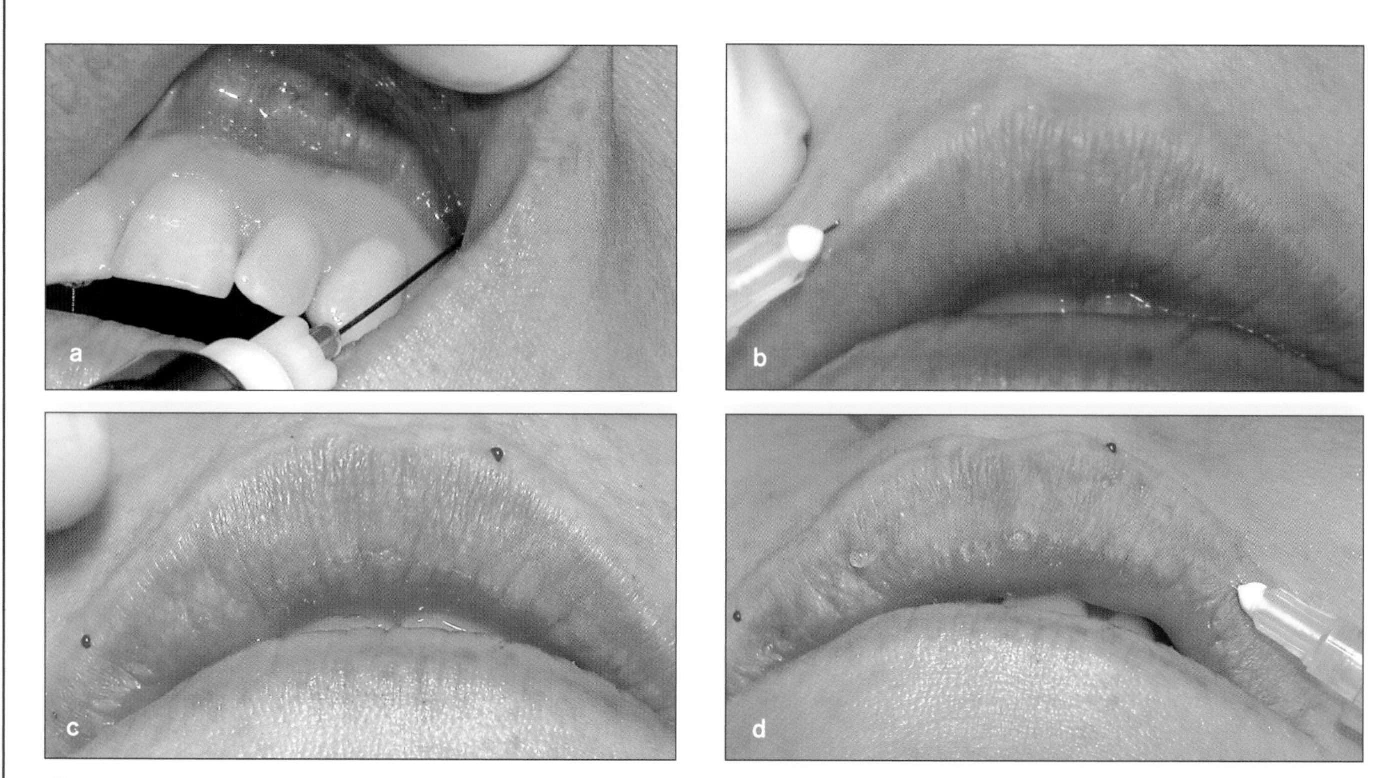

Fig 8-5 *(a)* Local anesthesia (2% lidocaine and 1:100,000 epinephrine concentration) is administered to provide patient comfort prior to injecting the dermal fillers. Intraoral injections keep from masking the areas that need to be treated. *(b to d)* Serial injection technique of dermal filler on an upper lip.

- What needs to be accentuated, the white roll or the vermilion border?
- Does the Cupid's bow need more definition?
- Does the wet line need to be addressed?
- Is the patient concerned about the amount of mucosal or pink portion of the lip that is showing?

There are several possible injection sites in the lips. Beginning at one of the oral commissures, the tissue filler product can be injected in sequential fashion following the vermilion border to the opposite oral commissure. The result may look awkward at first, but patients should be aware that over 2 to 3 weeks the vermilion will be augmented and will slowly begin to take on a more natural appearance.

Injections can also be made in the general area of the mucosal portion of the lips to add overall volume. When injecting the filler, gentle bimanual palpation is essential for good placement and even distribution of the product. Massaging the area is reserved for the end of treatment. After that, no further injections should be made that day. Ideally, the final outcome will leave the upper lip approximately 80% the size of the lower lip, and the lower lip in a position slightly anterior to the upper lip (Figs 8-5 and 8-6).

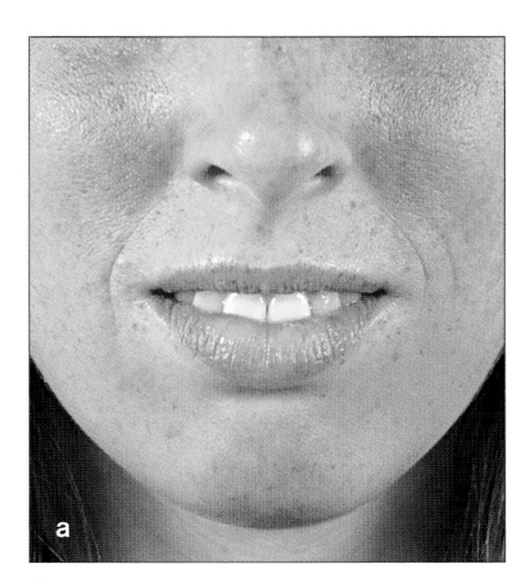

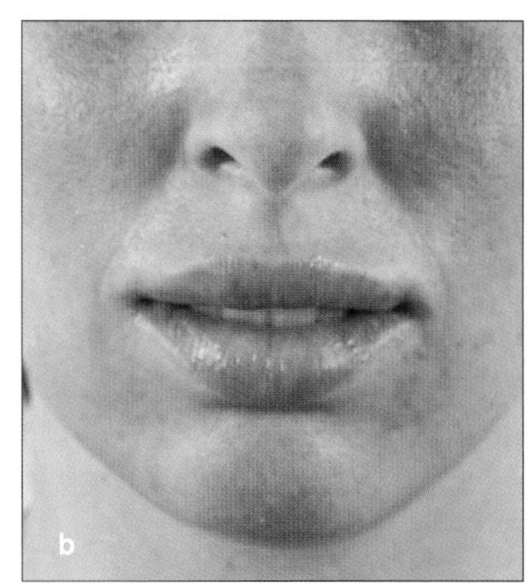

Fig 8-6 *(a)* Pretreatment view of a woman with a thin upper lip. *(b)* Posttreatment view of a woman following upper lip injection with Juvederm Ultra Plus.

Postoperative care

Patients are informed that redness, minor swelling, and potential bruising may occur at the injection site. They are advised to avoid alcohol, vigorous exercise, the use of medicated skin care products, and sunbathing for 24 hours following the procedure to minimize the potential for bruising, swelling, and skin irritation. Ice may be applied, and makeup may be used immediately following the injection. Patients are scheduled for a follow-up visit within the first week to assess the final outcome and make any necessary adjustments.

Complications

The most common side effects associated with dermal fillers are swelling, redness, pain, bruising, and tenderness at the injection site, which typically resolve within 7 days. Serious but rare side effects include delayed-onset infections, recurrence of herpetic eruptions, and superficial necrosis at the site of the injection. Dermal fillers should be used with caution in patients recently treated with anticoagulants or platelet inhibitors to avoid bleeding and bruising, and their use is contraindicated in patients known to have a hypersensitivity to the filler material, a history of severe allergy or anaphylaxis, or bleeding disorders. Furthermore, the safety of dermal fillers for use during pregnancy and breastfeeding or in patients under 18 years of age has not been established.

Botulinum Toxin A

Clostridium botulinum is a gram-positive, spore-forming anaerobe that produces seven serologically distinct strains of neurotoxin, labeled A to G. Currently, there are two botulinum toxin type A preparations cleared by the FDA for cosmetic use: Botox Cosmetic (Allergan) and Dysport (Medicis). In this chapter, all references are to Botox.

Botulinum serotype A produces temporary chemical denervation by blocking the presynaptic release of acetylcholine (Ach) at the neuromuscular junction. It achieves this by cleaving synaptosome-associated protein of 25,000 daltons (SNAP-25), a presynaptic membrane protein necessary for the fusion of Ach-containing vesicles. This cleavage, therefore, inhibits the release of Ach into the neuromuscular junction. The paralysis typically takes 24 to 48 hours to become fully effective, which reflects the time needed for cellular metabolism of the toxin. In some cases, several days to 1 week may pass before the local paralysis is complete. The localized effects of standard botulinum toxin injections last for approximately 90 days but may last as long as 6 months.[2–4]

The recovery time corresponds to the hypothesized mechanism of recovery that occurs in two phases. First, new axonal sprouting allows limited Ach release. Second, new SNAP-25 production, the major pathway of recovery, results in a resumption of Ach release across the neuromuscular junction. In patients who receive repeated, long-term botulinum toxin treatment, localized denervation muscle atrophy can be expected. Anecdotal reports also suggest that in patients who start botulinum toxin treatment at a young age and receive frequent injections, a hypothesized "permanent retraining" of the muscles of facial expression may be seen, which ultimately may result in the patients no longer needing to use botulinum toxin.

Botulinum toxin reconstitution

Botulinum toxin A is precipitated, purified, filtered, and processed into a fine, vacuum-dried powder. Each standard vial of Botox contains 100 units of botulinum toxin A, 0.9 mg of sodium chloride, and 0.5 mg of human albumin,[5] and it must be stored at or below -5°C prior to its final reconstitution to prevent degradation. Its rehydration presents one controllable variable in the effectiveness and duration of treatments. The manufacturer recommends that the botulinum toxin be reconstituted with 2.5 mL of preservative-free saline, which yields 4 units of botulinum toxin per 0.1 mL.[5] Furthermore, they recommend that the 100-unit vial be used completely on the same day that it is reconstituted.

In general, most cosmetic practitioners have not followed these recommendations for years and, in some cases, to good effect. For example, mixing the botulinum toxin with bacteriostatic saline instead of preservative-free saline results in significantly less discomfort to the patient upon injection, and in the authors' experience, it allows the reconstituted botulinum toxin to be stored for several weeks without an appreciable decrease in efficacy. Furthermore, practitioners differ in how much saline they use to reconstitute botulinum toxin, which commonly varies from 1 to 4 mL. The authors of this chapter use 2.0 to 2.5 mL of bacteriostatic saline, yielding 4 to 5 units of botulinum toxin per 0.1 mL, because it has yielded more predictable outcomes and decreased the number of "touch-up" appointments than those achieved with the manufacturer recommendations. Unfortunately, our communities are filled with individuals who expect cosmetic perfection immediately and at the least cost possible.[6–8]

Regardless of the amount of saline used for botulinum toxin reconstitution, the saline should be added slowly and gently into the bottle to minimize the potential for premature degradation of the purified protein. The plunger is controlled so the botulinum toxin is reconstituted with as few bubbles as possible. The bottle is then gently rolled, not shaken. Finally, the cap is removed, and the botulinum toxin solution is drawn up into 1-mL tuberculin syringes connected as one piece to a 0.5-inch, 30-gauge needle. By removing the cap and drawing up the solution in this fashion, the needles stay sharper, and less solution is left behind in the vial.

Complications

Botox has a high safety profile, as indicated by the rare occurrence of irreversible medical complications over the past 25 years. It is reassuring that any potential adverse reaction may be short-lived, localized, and reversible, given the short-term, localized effects of botulinum toxin injections.[9–12]

Botulinum toxin works most effectively at the local site of injection; however, there is the potential for it to spread to areas that may not have been the intended muscular target. When this happens, it may result in a poor cosmetic outcome, such as the loss of proper facial expression or, more concerning, upper eyelid ptosis. Minute quantities of botulinum toxin may also enter the circulatory system, eliciting a regional or systemic reaction. The potential for systemic botulinum exposure has raised the question of antibody development and potential long-term, immune-mediated complications. The development of antibodies to botulinum toxin may be related to a patient's exposure to it in high doses.[13,14]

Contraindications

Botox is contraindicated in patients with a known hypersensitivity or allergy to botulinum toxin A or human albumin and in those who have a neuromuscular disorder, such as multiple sclerosis, Eaton-Lambert syndrome, or myasthenia gravis. In addition, aminoglycoside antibiotics interfere with neuromuscular transmission and increase the effects of botulinum type A. Patients taking this class of medication should avoid using botulinum toxin treatments or delay treatment until the completion of the antibiotic regimen.[2]

Botulinum toxin treatment is contraindicated during pregnancy and during breastfeeding. Many women have unknowingly been pregnant when injected with botulinum toxin and have experienced no associated complications. Nevertheless, the FDA classifies Botox as a category C drug, reflecting that its safety profile during pregnancy has not been studied. Also, the concentration of botulinum toxin in human breast milk and its effect on a nursing infant are not known.[15]

Consent

A proper informed consent is obtained from the patient prior to cosmetic treatments. Botulinum toxin A has been cleared for moderate to severe lines associated with the glabellar region. The consent form should state that its injection in other areas of the face and neck are considered off-label uses. The practitioner can then explain to the patient that botulinum toxin has been used safely in these other areas for years and performs remarkably well, but that the manufacturer does not wish to undergo the extensive and financially expensive process required to gain FDA clearance for these other regions of the face and neck that are only inches away.

Both common and rare side effects and risks are discussed with the patient. These include swelling at the injection site and local bruising, which may be exacerbated by aspirin or nonsteroidal anti-inflammatory medications. Headaches during the first few days following injection are not uncommon. Flulike symptoms and allergic reactions, though rare, are possible. Unintended migration may cause untoward esthetic outcomes. Finally, it may behoove practitioners to explain that there is great variability among individuals and the amount of botulinum toxin that may be needed. They are advised to make it clear to patients that touch-up injections, if desired, are the financial responsibility of the patient.

Patient selection

Botox is FDA cleared for the treatment of moderate to severe glabellar lines in patients aged 18 to 65 years. It also is commonly used for off-label uses as well, such as the temporary reduction of other fine lines and wrinkles of the face and neck. Nevertheless, botulinum toxin is not the proverbial hammer for every nail. To identify those patients who are good candidates for this procedure, clinicians need a clear understanding of both the underlying causes of their patients' facial aging and the inherent strengths and limitations of botulinum toxin treatment.

Patients who will receive the most satisfactory results are those with good skin elasticity and those with fine lines accentuated by facial animation. Botulinum toxin is effective in effacing the rhytids caused by hyperfunctional muscles of facial expression. It is not effective, however, in treating rhytids associated with poor skin elasticity or those associated with gravitational rhytidosis, such as the deep rhytids from jowling. Individual wrinkles can be evaluated by a spread test, in which the lines should easily disappear when gentle pressure is applied to spread apart the wrinkle.

Commonly treated regions

The three areas most commonly treated with botulinum toxin injections are the glabella, the forehead, and the lateral periorbital region (Figs 8-7 and 8-8).

Glabellar region

The glabellar region is usually treated with a series of five injections. The central injection, located between and slightly below the medial eyebrows, weakens the procerus muscle that causes the horizontal rhytids in this area. The corrugator muscle is injected bilaterally, which effaces the "angry 11s"—the angry-looking vertical lines between the brows. The total amount of botulinum toxin used in this area, as in all areas, varies greatly, depending on the patient's and the provider's preferences. The authors of this chapter typically use a total of 20 to 25 units in this area.

Fig 8-7 Markings for botulinum toxin injections in the glabellar region (1), forehead (2), and periorbital region (3).

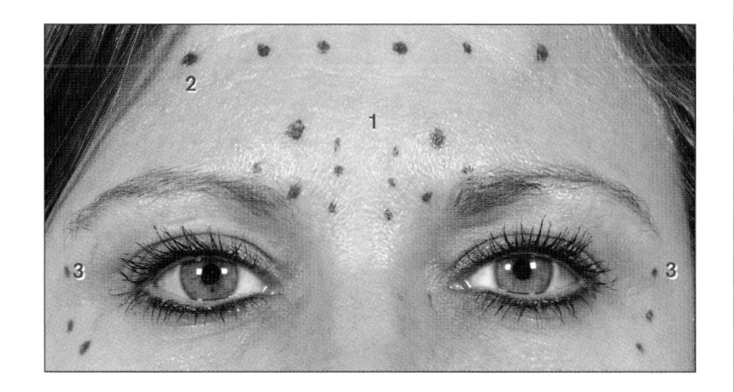

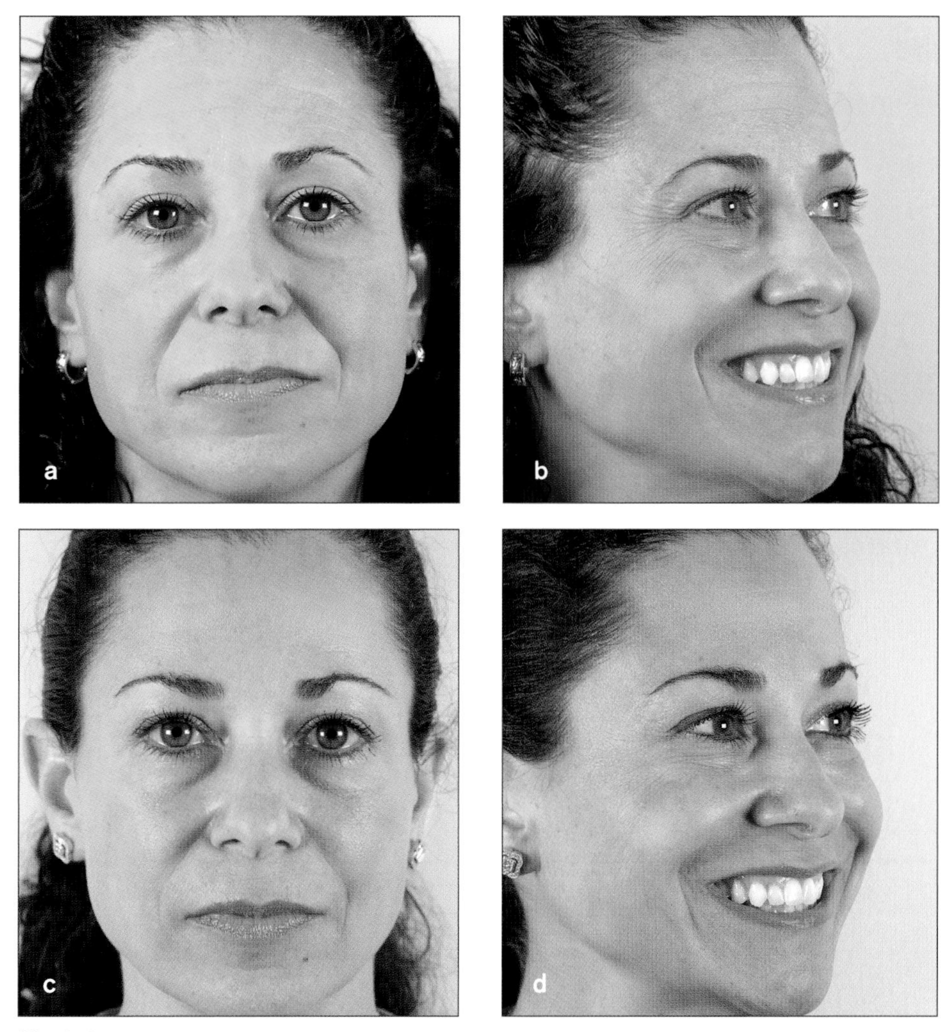

Fig 8-8 *(a and b)* Pretreatment frontal and three-quarter views. Notice marked rhytids on the forehead and periorbital regions. *(c and d)* Frontal and three-quarter views following botulinum toxin A injections.

Forehead

The forehead is treated with a series of 4 to 8 injections for a total of 16 to 32 units of botulinum toxin. Care must be exercised in this area to prevent penetration so deep that no movement of the eyebrows is achieved or, worse yet, that brow ptosis or upper eyelid ptosis occurs. Patients do not return if they develop brow ptosis and feel heaviness in the upper eyelid. It is essential to determine whether patients have proper brow position before treatment. If they do not, let them know that the rhytids just superior to the brow cannot be effaced without causing the "frozen forehead look" and a sensation of heaviness in the upper eyelids.

Periorbital region

In the lateral periorbital region, where crow's feet occur, patients typically receive 2 to 4 injections, for a total of 10 to 20 units of botulinum toxin, to achieve gentle elevation of the tail of the brow and smoothing of the rhytids that radiate laterally from the lateral canthal region. In this area of the face, the authors of this chapter use two approaches that differ from the techniques used in other parts of the face: *(1)* An ice cube is rubbed on the skin prior to injection to shrink the well-vascularized vessels in this area, and *(2)* injections are made in a subcutaneous plane. These two modifications help to avoid bruising of the area.

Other areas

Though less frequently treated, the so-called bunny lines may also benefit from botulinum toxin injections. Bunny lines are caused by hyperkinetic nasalis contracture and can usually be smoothed with 2 to 3 injections of 2 units of botulinum toxin A into the muscle. Other areas that have gained wide acceptance and popularity for botulinum toxin treatment outside of the traditional upper third of the face are the vertical rhytids of the perioral area, the platysmal banding of the anterior neck, the marionette lines just lateral to the commissure of the lips (caused by the risorius muscle), and the dimpled chin (caused by the mentalis muscle).

Summary

It is imperative that the practitioner who uses botulinum toxin and injectable tissue fillers have a good knowledge of the musculature and an understanding of the science behind these products. Clinicians need to explain to patients that botulinum toxin injections will limit facial expression and that their primary effect is in treating dynamic rhytids. Injectable fillers, on the other hand, are more suited for camouflaging static rhytids. Botulinum toxin provides the best results when injected into the muscle, whereas tissue fillers are injected superficial to the muscle, in either a subdermal or intradermal plane. Because of the rapidly growing popularity of cosmetic procedures and facial rejuvenation, many practitioners have become clinical providers of injectable dermal fillers and botulinum toxin. Oral and maxillofacial surgeons have a unique advantage in their understanding of the face and are easily poised to become leaders in patient satisfaction.

References

1. Food and Drug Administration. Center for Devices and Radiological Health Office of Device Evaluation. General and Plastic Surgery Devices. Panel Public Advisory. Committee Meeting. November 18, 2008.
2. Vartanian AJ, Dayan SH. Facial rejuvenation using botulinum toxin A: Review and updates. Facial Plast Surg 2004;20:11–19.
3. Singh BR. Molecular basis of the unique endopeptidase activity of neurotoxin. In: Brin MF, Hallett M, Jankovic J (eds). Scientific and Therapeutic Aspects of Botulinum Toxin. Philadelphia, PA: Lippincott Williams & Wilkins, 2002:75–88.
4. Montecucco C, Schiavo G. Tetanus and botulinum neurotoxins: A new group of zinc proteases. Trends Biochem Sci 1993;18:324–327.
5. Botox [package insert]. Irvine, CA: Allergan, 2002.
6. Klein AW. Dilution and storage of botulinum toxin. Dermatol Surg 1998;24:1179–1180.
7. Huang W, Foster JA, Rogachefsky AS. Pharmacology of botulinum toxin. J Am Acad Dermatol 2000;43:249–259.
8. Alam M, Dover JS, Arndt KA. Pain associated with injection of botulinum toxin A exotoxin reconstituted using isotonic sodium chloride with and without preservative: A double-blind, randomized controlled trial. Arch Dermatol 2002;138:510–514.
9. Blitzer A, Binder WJ, Boyd JB, Carruthers A. Management of Facial Lines and Wrinkles. Philadelphia: Lippincott Williams & Wilkins, 2000.
10. Carruthers JA, Kiene K, Carruthers J. Botulinum A exotoxin use in clinical dermatology. J Am Acad Dermatol 1996;34:788–797.
11. Matarasso SL. Complications of botulinum A exotoxin for hyperfunctional lines. Dermatol Surg 1998;24:1249–1254.
12. Blitzer A, Binder WJ. Current practices in the use of botulinum toxin A in the management of facial lines and wrinkles. Facial Plast Surg Clin North Am 2001;9:395–404.
13. Lange DJ, Rubin M, Greene PE, et al. Distant effects of locally injected botulinum toxin: A double-blind study of single fiber EMG changes. Muscle Nerve 1991;14:672–675.
14. Goschel H, Wohlfarth K, Frevert J, Dengler R, Bigalke H. Botulinum toxin therapy: Neutralizing and nonneutralizing antibodies—Therapeutic consequences. Exp Neurol 1997;147:96–102.
15. Jankovic N, Brin MF. Therapeutic uses of botulinum toxin. N Engl J Med 1991;324:1186–1194.

9

FACIAL SKIN REJUVENATION

KING KIM, DMD
ALEXANDRA DOWNEY

Several options can be considered for rejuvenating the skin of the aging face. Popular nonsurgical modalities include ablative laser therapy (carbon dioxide [CO_2] and erbium-doped yttrium aluminum garnet [Er:YAG]), nonablative laser therapy (neodymium-doped yttrium aluminum garnet [Nd:YAG]), radiofrequency resurfacing, dermabrasion, and chemical peels (superficial, medium, and deep). This chapter focuses on the following facial skin rejuvenation procedures: fractional CO_2 laser therapy, Er:YAG laser therapy, and chemical peels. The use of a prescription home skin care regimen is also discussed.

Preoperative Evaluation for Laser Therapy

The patient desiring skin rejuvenation often presents with facial and/or neck rhytidosis, photodamaged skin, dyschromia, acne scars, or skin laxity. Discussion should ensue regarding laser and chemical modalities of treatment in those patients wanting minimal recovery time, skin tightening, and harmonious, even skin texture and coloration. It should be kept in mind that lasers thermally ablate the skin and that the primary goal of facial laser resurfacing is to replace the epidermis with healthy cells and the dermis with new collagen and elastin fibers (Fig 9-1). It has been shown that an average of 90 days after laser skin resurfacing, mild wrinkles are virtually effaced, and moderate to severe wrinkles improve by one class (severe becomes moderate, moderate becomes mild). Improvements after laser skin resurfacing can also be seen up to 18 months posttreatment as the dermal collagen continues to remodel.[1]

Patients desiring laser therapy should be assessed for the amount of skin pathosis in the form of scarring and dyspigmentation, the ability of the skin to tan or burn (Table 9-1), and the overall degree of wrinkling and photodamage (Table 9-2). Patients with Fitzpatrick skin types I and II have a decreased likelihood of developing pigment changes following laser resurfacing but may be more apt to develop postoperative erythema than do patients with skin types V and VI.[1] Patients with Glogau skin types I and II may be more amenable to less aggressive laser techniques than those with skin types III and IV, who likely require more invasive measures than laser therapy alone to achieve a desirable outcome.

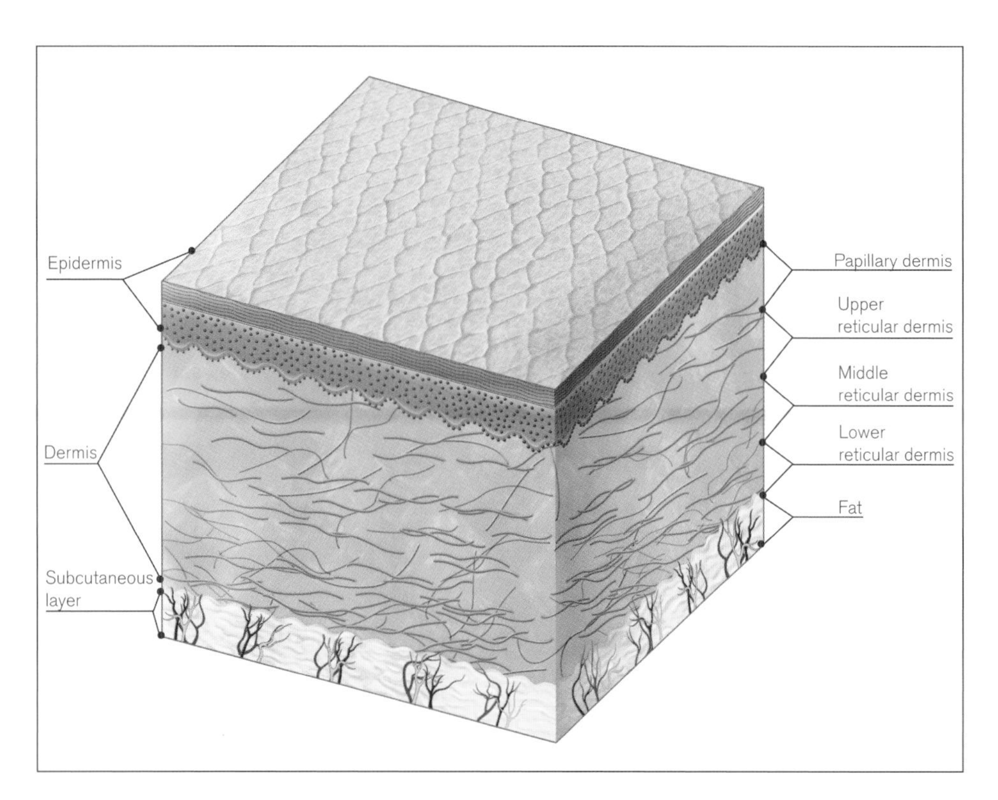

Fig 9-1 Cross section of skin layers.

Table 9-1 Fitzpatrick classification according to the ability of skin to tan or burn

Ability	I (Very fair)	II (Fair)	III (Light olive)	IV (Olive)	V (Dark brown)	VI (Very dark)
Burn	Always	Always	Sometimes	Rarely	Never	Never
Tan	Never	With difficulty	Gradually	Easily	Very easily	Always

Table 9-2 Glogau classification skin according to photodamage

Characteristic	I (Early)	II (Moderate)	III (Advanced)	IV (Severe)
Age	20s and 30s	30s and 40s	50s and 60s	60s and 70s
Wrinkles	Few	Dynamic lines	Static lines	Profound
Keratoses	None	Early	Actinic	Actinic
Makeup use	Rare	Sometimes	Always	Heavy
Acne scarring	Minimal	Mild	Moderate	Severe
Discoloration		Early lentigines	Skin dyschromia	Yellow to gray skin color
Other			Telangiectasia	History of skin cancer

Contraindications for using laser therapy include patients who possess one or more of the following: inflammatory skin conditions, such as psoriasis; history of developing keloids; active bacterial, fungal, or viral infection; severe smoking habit; and history of isotretinoin use. Smokers should be alerted to the risk of retarding wound healing because of diminished tissue oxygenation with subsequent risk of infection, scarring, and dyspigmentation.[2] Those patients who have used isotretinoin within a year of laser treatment may have an increased risk of scarring; it has been witnessed in those receiving chemical peels and dermabrasion.[3] It is recommended that patients who undergo laser resurfacing have a 1- to 2-year isotretinoin-free period to decrease the risk of scar formation.[1]

All patients undergoing facial laser rejuvenation should undergo prophylaxis against a herpes simplex virus outbreak and bacterial infection. Laser resurfacing may trigger a viral outbreak in the laser-treated areas, resulting in increased pain, recovery time, and likelihood of scarring. Options for viral prophylaxis include acyclovir 400 mg by mouth, 3 times a day; valacyclovir 500 mg by mouth, 2 times a day; and famciclovir 250 mg by mouth, 2 times a day.[1] Famciclovir has been shown to have the most bioavailability.[2,4] These antiviral medications should be implemented 48 hours prior to the procedure and then continued for 10 days postoperatively. In addition, prophylaxis against bacterial infections of the laser-treated, sloughed skin should also be exercised. Options here are cephalexin 500 mg by mouth, 4 times a day, or in penicillin-allergic patients, azithromycin 250 mg a day with a 500-mg loading dose.[1,5] The bacterial prophylaxis should be started 1 day prior to surgery and continued for 5 days postoperatively.

Those patients who are darker skinned and fit in the Fitzpatrick IV, V, or VI categories may be at risk of developing postinflammatory hyperpigmentation following laser resurfacing. Bleaching agents such as 4% hydroquinone, kojic acid, and azelaic acid can be used from 1 to 3 months prior to the procedure to minimize this risk. To further minimize the risk of postinflammatory hyperpigmentation, patients should avoid suntanning for several weeks prior to the procedure.

Various skin-conditioning products can be used in conjunction with laser resurfacing to provide a higher comfort level and better results. The use of tretinoin 6 weeks prior to chemical peels and dermabrasion improves recovery time and reepithelialization of the epidermal layer.[1] It has also been shown to reverse epidermal changes of damaged skin.[6–8] In addition, α-hydroxy acids (AHAs), due to their effects of decreasing corneocyte cohesion and increasing the quality of collagen and elastic fibers, can be used as an additional adjunct.[2] Topical local anesthetic cream, either with 4% lidocaine or eutectic mixture of local anesthetic (EMLA) cream (AstraZeneca), should also be prescribed prior to the procedure. Patients are instructed to apply the cream in the areas being treated 1 hour prior to laser resurfacing.

Fractional CO_2 Laser Therapy

The fractional CO_2 laser has the benefits of the traditional continuous wave and superpulse CO_2 laser with the added characteristic of being less invasive to the skin, which results in a diminished healing time (Fig 9-2). Although less invasive than the traditional continuous wave CO_2 laser, the fractional CO_2 laser is still effective in contracting dermal collagen fibers and enabling the formation of new, healthy collagen.

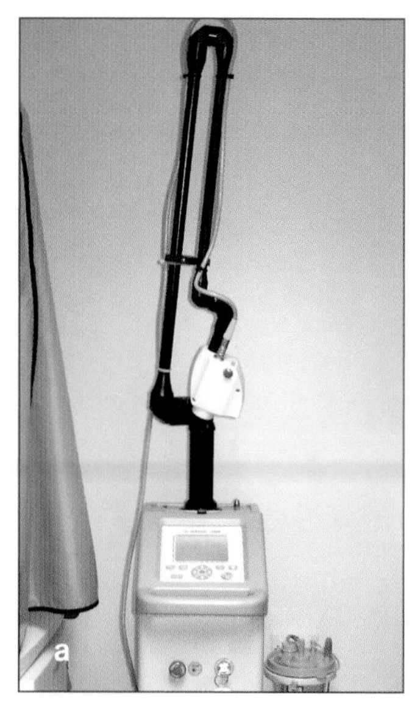

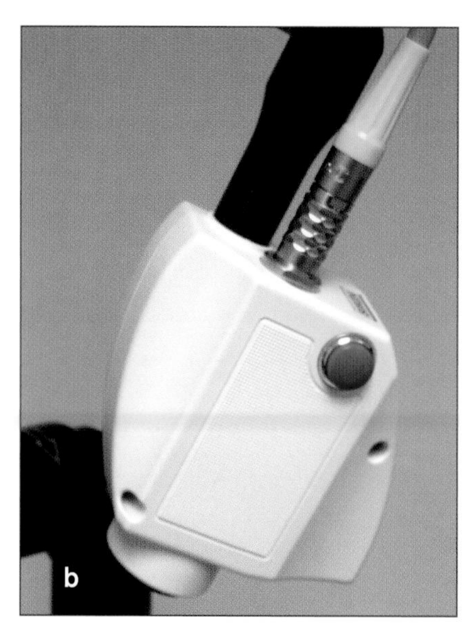

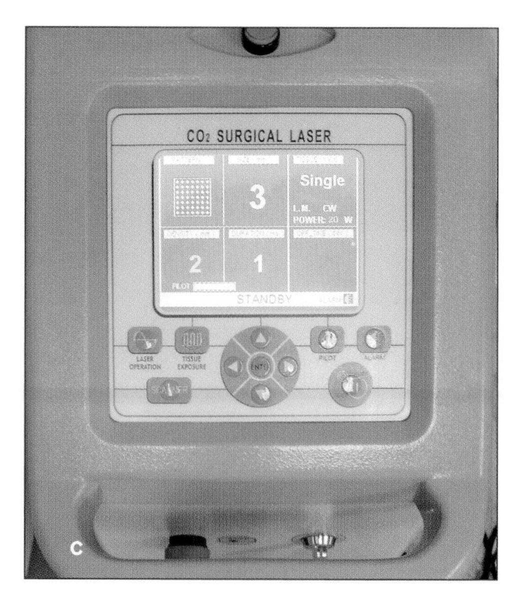

Fig 9-2 *(a)* **Fractional CO_2 laser unit (Sandstone Medical).** *(b)* **Articulated-arm delivery system.** *(c)* **Laser unit control panel.**

The remodeling of thermally damaged tissues via reepithelialization and new collagen formation is the process that creates improved, younger-looking skin.

The continuous wave CO_2 laser wavelength (10,600 nm) is absorbed by water, penetrates down to the papillary dermis, ablates 50 to 150 µm of tissue, and has an epidermal thermal relaxation time of 1 millisecond.[2,9] The diameter of the thermal damage created by each laser pulse, known as the *spot size*, is usually from 2 to 3 mm. The downfall, however, is that the CO_2 laser causes up to 100 µm of thermal damage, which can result in prolonged wound healing, scarring, and dyspigmentation[10–12] (Fig 9-3a). Because of these side effects, fractional CO_2 laser systems have been developed to minimize thermal damage by decreasing pulse duration while keeping tissue vaporization effective.

The fractional CO_2 laser essentially heats the cellular fluids to the point of vaporization, somewhere from 400°C to 600°C . Cellular rupture occurs, creating fragmented tissue debris. This laser essentially ablates small columns of epidermal and dermal tissue in evenly spaced points over a fraction of the skin surface, and it is considered the less invasive means to resurface the face compared with the traditional high-energy CO_2 laser ablative system.[13] The fractional CO_2 laser ablates only a "fraction" of the total skin area. It delivers pinpoint spots that penetrate approximately 600 µm into subdermal tissue (Fig 9-3b). The spot sizes are only 150 µm across, as opposed to the 2- to 3-mm spot sizes of the traditional continuous wave CO_2 laser. Although the laser penetrates deeper, it does so in such a small area that the actual surface damage is decreased, resulting in less erythema to the skin clinically. A laser-treated area with a 150-µm spot size heals more quickly than one with a 3-mm spot size. In addition, there is healthy, undamaged tissue between the spots that helps the thermally damaged skin to heal faster. To illustrate the difference, imag-

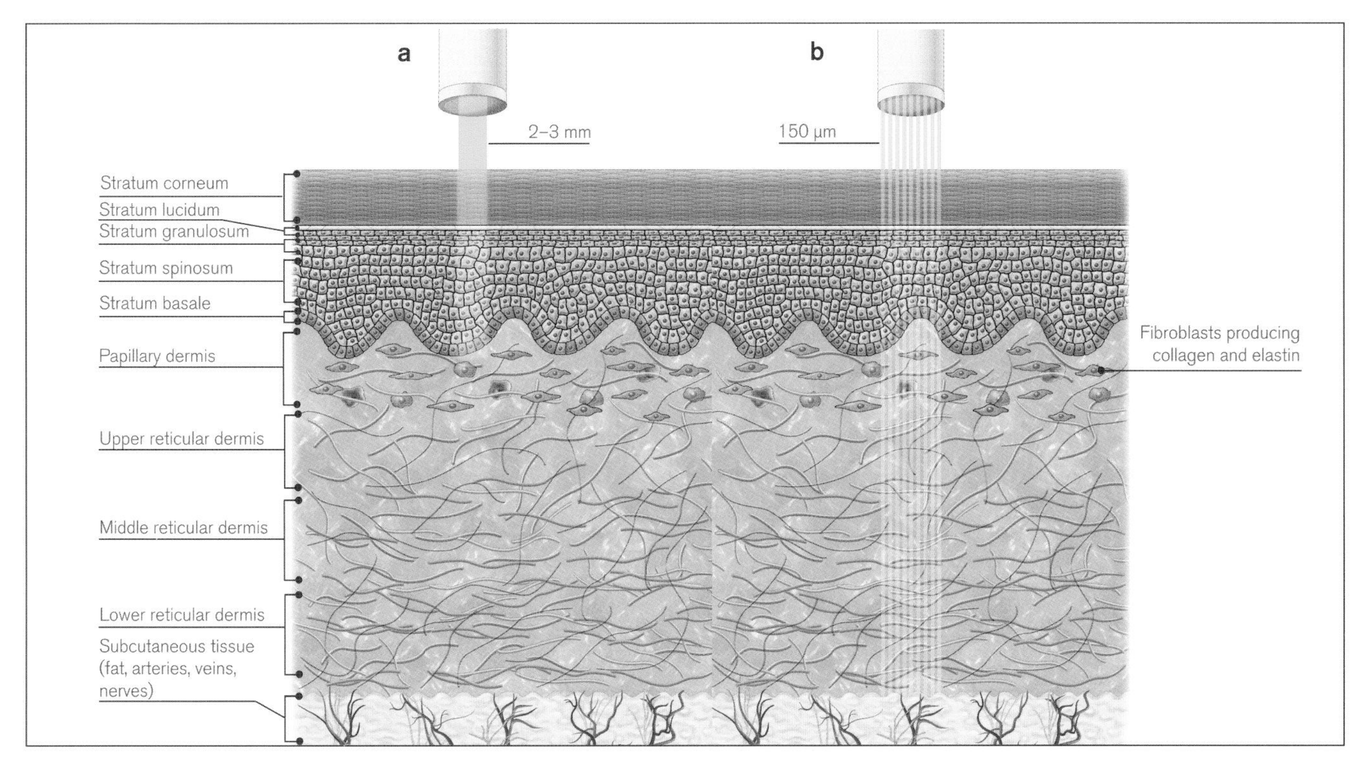

Fig 9-3 **Cross section of skin.** ***(a)*** **Spot size (2 to 3 mm) and penetration depth of thermal damage (100 µm) from a continuous wave CO_2 laser.** ***(b)*** **Spot size (150 µm) and penetration depth of vaporization (600 µm) from a fractional CO_2 laser.**

ine penetrating tissue with a spinal needle compared with a tissue biopsy punch. The spinal needle penetrates deeper but has a much smaller diameter, causing less tissue trauma and requiring less healing time.

The use of a fractional CO_2 laser at a 10,600-nm wavelength has been proven to be effective for resurfacing epidermal and dermal tissue and treating facial rhytids, hyperpigmentation, abnormal texture, and skin laxity, while proving to be safer than the traditional CO_2 laser ablative system.[14] In addition, positive results following CO_2 laser resurfacing have proven successful even after long-term follow-up.[15,16] The primary reason the fractional CO_2 laser promotes quicker wound healing and patient recovery is that there is less residual thermal damage to the skin. As the epidermal and dermal layers are vaporized by the laser, inflammatory cells migrate to the wound to induce angiogenesis, reepithelialization, and dermal remodeling. Prolonged erythema and delayed wound healing can occur as a result of excessive inflammation of the wound. An abundance of nonviable tissue created by peripheral thermal damage will act as an obstacle to optimal tissue recovery.[17] Therefore, it is crucial that adjacent tissue damage to the skin be minimized to promote faster wound healing. This is the primary means by which the fractional CO_2 laser is considered less invasive and results in quicker recovery.

Laser safety

The safe operation of laser equipment is an important element in the treatment process. It is crucial that safe practices be implemented to avoid unnecessary injuries to the surgeon and patient. Laser safety goggles should be worn by the surgeon as well as any assistants while the laser is being used. It has been shown that direct penetration or reflection of the laser to the eye can injure the anterior chamber and cornea.[2,18] Bulky laser safety goggles may interfere with treatment of the patient; therefore, small moistened gauze pads should be placed gently over the patient's eyes while the eyes are shut.

Another important safety measure is to prevent airborne particles ejected from the patient's vaporized tissue from being inhaled. Infectious viral DNA particles have been shown to be present in the laser plume.[2] High-flow suction held within 2 to 3 cm of the treated areas can be used to help evacuate the airborne debris. The use of masks by all persons in the treatment room is another way to minimize exposure to infectious organisms.

Laser settings

Settings for the fractional CO_2 laser for full-face laser resurfacing include power level (depth of penetration for each pulse), density (distance between spots), and pulse duration (length of time each pulse penetrates the skin). Power level can be adjusted according to the extent of the pathology. Deeper rhytids, dyschromia, and sun-damaged skin will likely be treated with a higher power level. It is recommended that the power level be lowered around the eyes, neck, and nose. The higher the density, the farther apart are the spot sizes. Densities range from 0.2 mm to 2.0 mm. A setting of 0.2 mm is equal to 90% coverage of the treated skin, whereas 2.0 mm is equal to 13% coverage of the treated skin. The pulse duration setting can be adjusted according to skin type. Thicker skin types may be more suited for a pulse duration of 3.0 milliseconds and thinner types for a pulse duration of 2.0 milliseconds. Ideal settings include a power level of 22 to 23 W, a density of 1.0 mm, and a duration of 2 milliseconds. The practitioner becomes more adept at determining which settings work best after performing multiple treatments.

Technique

The patient is instructed to apply EMLA cream (a good mixture includes 2.5% lidocaine and 2.5% prilocaine) on the areas planned for resurfacing 1 hour prior to the procedure. This will likely be done at home, prior to arriving at the office. No additional anesthetic is required as the fractional CO_2 laser is a bloodless and relatively painless procedure. Once in the office, the patient is positioned comfortably in the chair, semisupine at approximately a 45-degree angle.

With this laser system, a cooling apparatus in the form of a cold air blower is helpful. This allows the patient to be more comfortable during the procedure while the cool air is applied over the treated areas during the treatment itself. The cold air

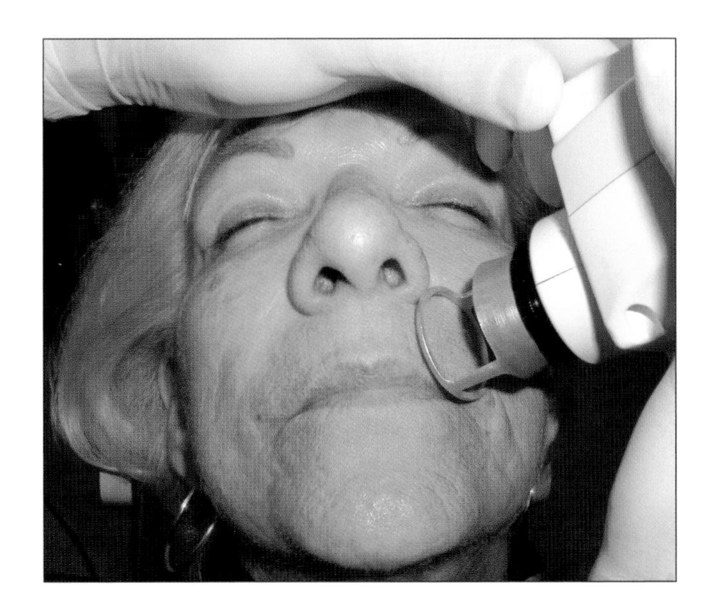

Fig 9-4 Focusing the pattern generator around the lips.

blower should have different power levels to adjust the intensity of the air according to patient comfort.

The computer pattern generator (CPG) is set from the laser console and is useful in that the computer places each laser spot within the chosen pattern. The CPG creates a safer, more precise, and more uniform result. It should be set on the larger pattern for more open areas such as the forehead, cheeks, and neck. For more refined areas requiring laser passes—such as areas surrounding the eyes, lips, and nose—the smaller pattern can be selected (Fig 9-4).

The laser scanner is placed against the skin, and the resurfacing procedure commences according to the pattern created by the CPG. It is important to overlap each successive pattern 1 to 2 mm to assure uniform treatment. Resurfacing of the face can proceed in any desired order but should cover the upper face (forehead), midface (cheeks, periorbit area, and nose), and lower face (perioral area, chin, and neck) (Figs 9-5a to 9-5f). The first pass vaporizes the epidermis, causing contraction of the skin and leaving a pink color indicative of penetration into the upper papillary dermis (Fig 9-5g). Subsequent passes of the fractional CO_2 laser leaves a proteinaceous, eschar residue that should be removed immediately to prevent adjacent thermal damage. Additional passes may cause the treated areas to yellow, which indicates that the laser has penetrated the upper reticular dermis. No bleeding should be observed with the fractional CO_2 laser because the laser itself closes off small blood vessels.[2] Bleeding during the procedure indicates entry into the midpapillary dermis. The fractional CO_2 laser creates a nice blend between the treated and nontreated areas, so it is not necessary to feather the junction between the treated and nontreated areas as with the Er:YAG laser. Regions of the face and neck that have significant skin pathosis can be treated with two passes, but more than two passes is not recommended because of the increased possibility of eschar formation, residual thermal damage, and scarring.

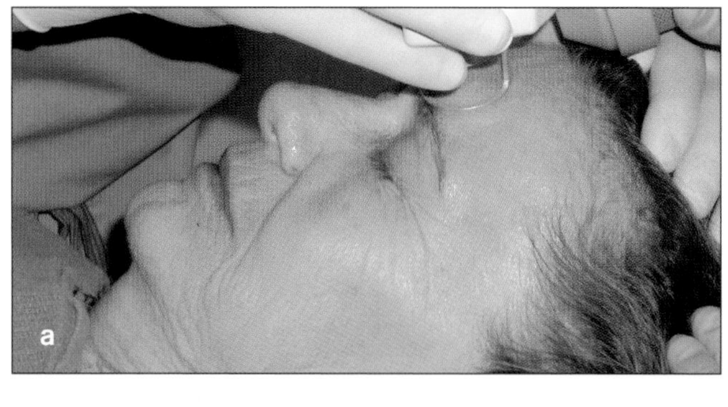

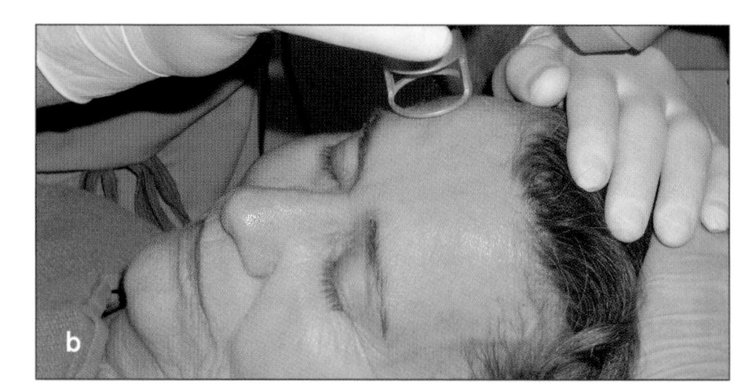

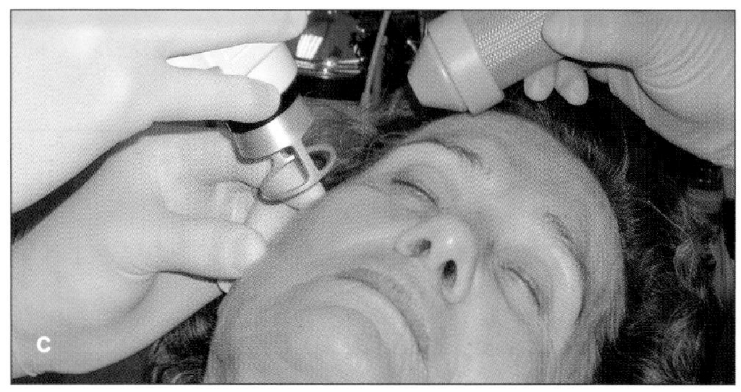

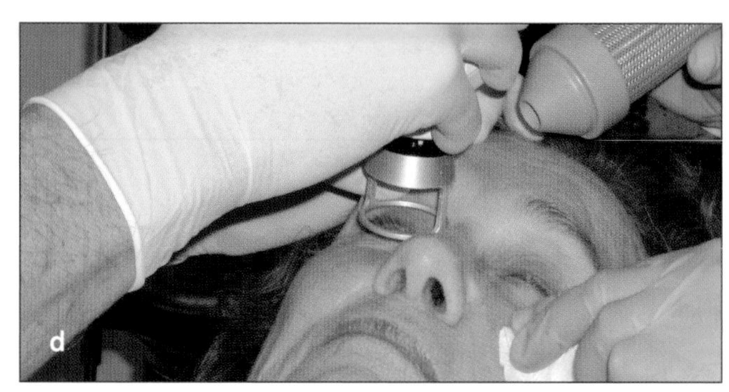

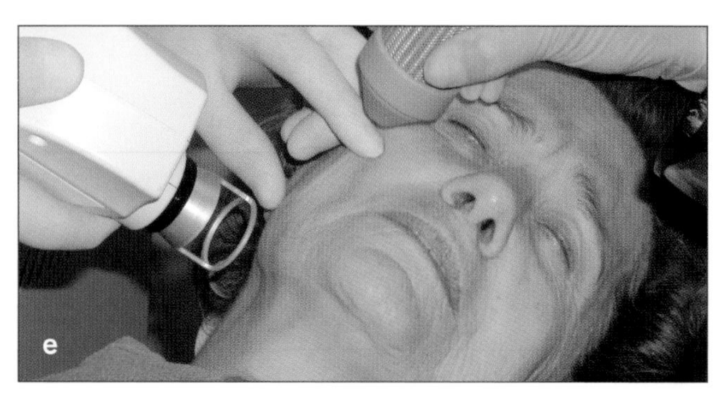

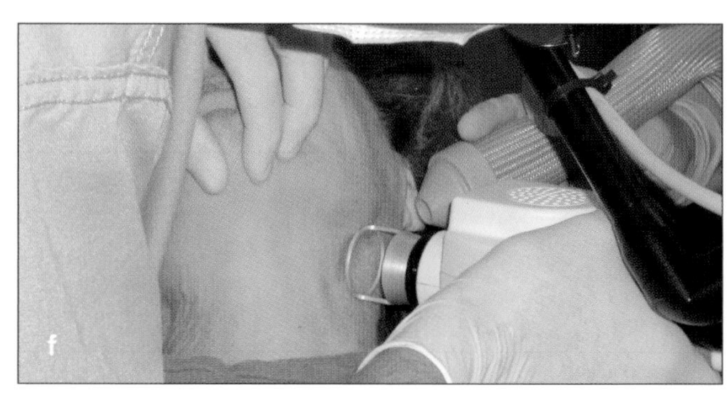

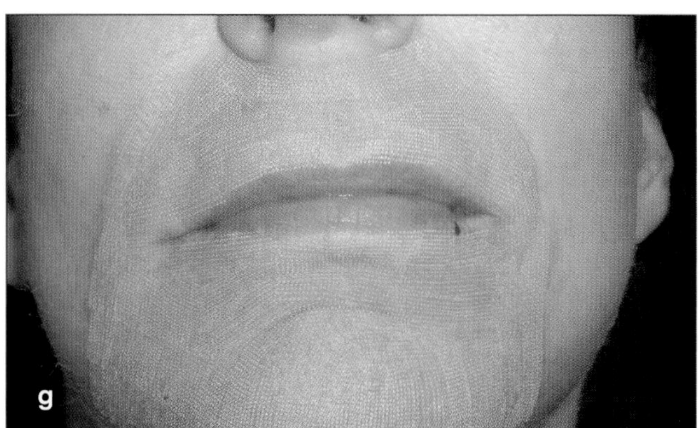

Fig 9-5 *(a and b)* Treatment of upper face. *(c and d)* Treatment of midface. *(e and f)* Treatment of lower face. *(g)* After the first pass, skin treated by the fractional CO_2 laser is pink.

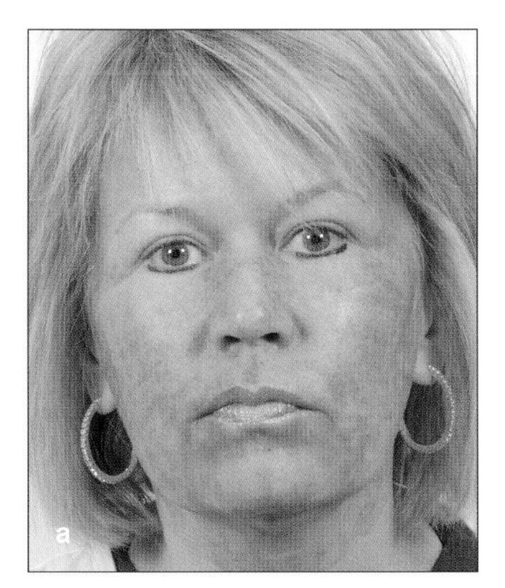

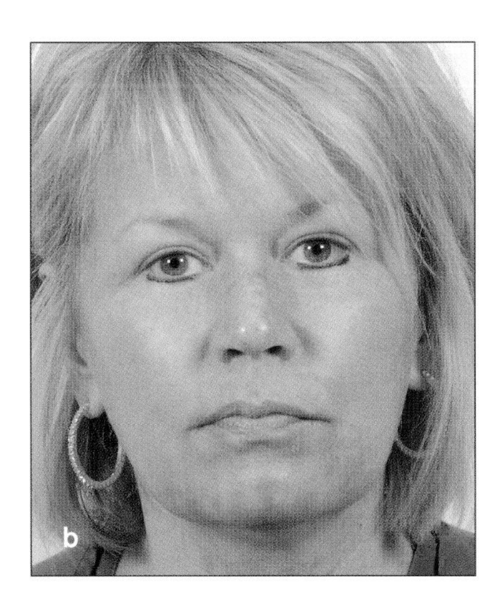

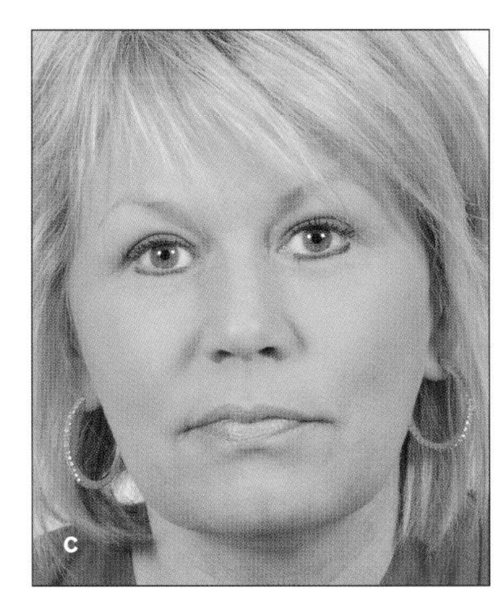

Fig 9-6 **Results of treatment with fractional CO_2 laser 24 hours *(a)*, 4 days *(b)*, and 7 days *(c)* postoperatively.**

After completion of the laser resurfacing procedure, the patient can immediately be dismissed. Patients are instructed to apply ointment on the face for the next 2 weeks to keep the treated areas moist. In addition, the prophylactic antimicrobial medications should be taken. Reepithelialization of the epidermis takes only about 7 days with the fractional CO_2 laser—one of the benefits of using this method (Fig 9-6).

Er:YAG Laser Therapy

The Er:YAG laser is primarily used in skin rejuvenation only for the treatment of fine rhytids and mild to moderate photoaging of the skin (Glogau classes I and II) and is also the preferred treatment modality for patients with darker skin.[19] This laser has a 13-times greater affinity for water than does the CO_2 laser. Because the skin is 70% water, skin ablation with the Er:YAG is ideal. The Er:YAG laser has a wavelength of 2,940 nm, ablation depth of 10 to 80 µm, residual thermal damage of 0 to 50 µm, and reepithelialization in 4 to 10 days.[2] Spot sizes should be 4 to 6 mm. This laser essentially ablates the stratum corneum of the epidermis (Fig 9-7). Because the Er:YAG laser has a higher affinity for water than does the CO_2 laser, it causes a much finer level of tissue ablation and produces less thermal injury to the tissues. As a result, there is a low incidence of scarring, fibrosis, prolonged erythema, and pigmentary changes, and the treated areas are able to reepithelialize quickly, which corresponds to rapid patient recovery.[2] Because this laser acts superficially, less dermal collagen remodeling occurs than with the deeper penetrating CO_2 laser. Thus, it has been shown that the Er:YAG laser is more effective for fine lines and superficial facial scarring whereas the CO_2 laser is better suited to treat more accentuated rhytids, scars, and photodamaged skin.[19,20]

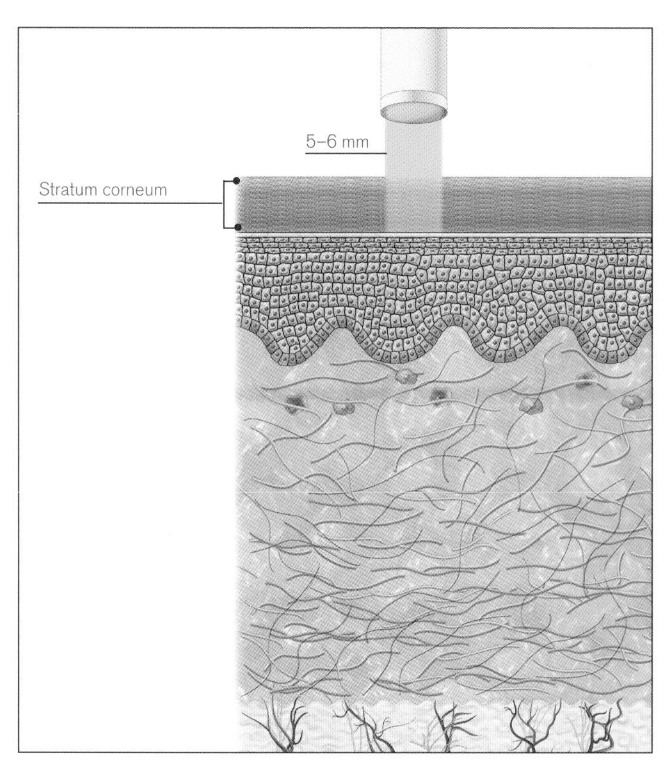

Fig 9-7 **Cross section of skin depicting spot size (5 to 6 mm) and ablation penetration depth (10 to 80 μm) of an Er:YAG laser.**

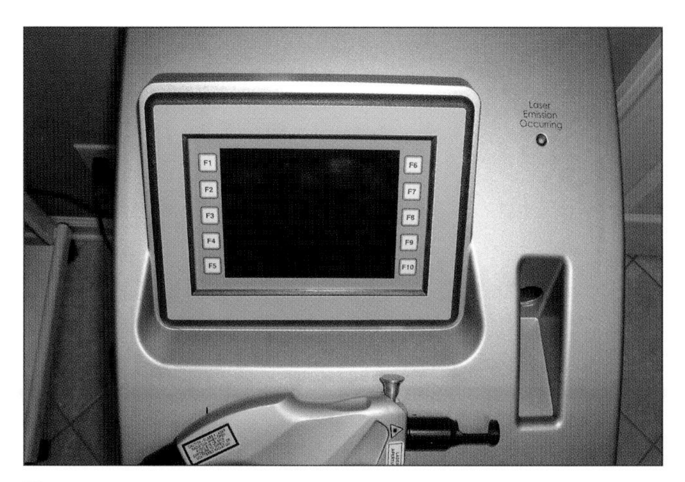

Fig 9-8 **Er:YAG laser unit.**

Laser settings

The Er:YAG laser can be set at a power level of 200, 400, or 600 mJ (Fig 9-8). The amount of power used is subjective and based primarily on the treatment goal. For rhytids and dyschromia, the 600-mJ setting is ideal. For removal of acne scarring, a 400-mJ power level may be enough. If the neck is to be treated, the 200-mJ setting is optimal because of the thinner skin. The operator should get a feel for what setting works best for each scenario.

Operating at 5 to 10 Hz is optimal for facial skin rejuvenation. Approximately 4 μm of tissue is vaporized per J/cm^2 of energy used.[21] The settings can be adjusted according to the amount of tissue vaporization the surgeon desires. A fluence of 5 J/cm^2 will ablate the epidermis with four passes, whereas a fluence of 8 to 12 J/cm^2 will ablate the epidermis in two passes.[1,22] The pulse duration used depends on the amount of thermal coagulation and skin shrinkage that is desired.[1] Optimal pulse duration for full-face laser resurfacing in most circumstances is 0.3 milliseconds. Shorter pulse durations are more ideal for treating finer rhytids and minimal photodamage.

Technique

Patients are asked to apply the EMLA cream 1 hour prior to their arrival, as stated previously. Patients are placed in a comfortable reclined position for the procedure. An exfoliating cleanser is applied to the face to condition the skin prior to treatment,

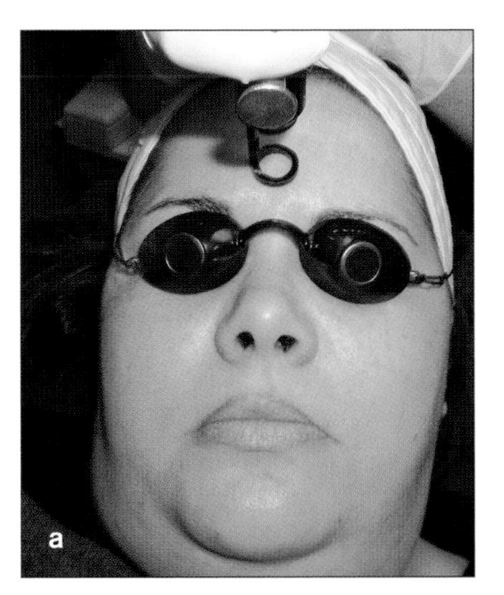
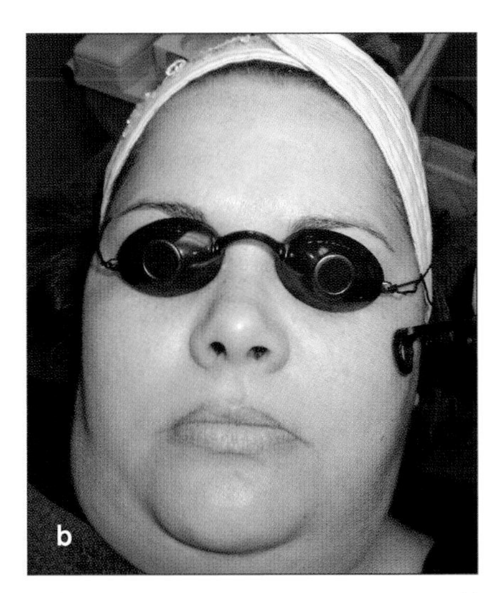
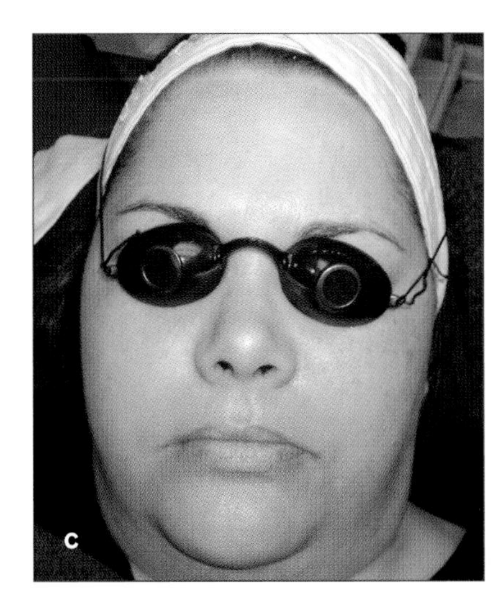

Fig 9-9 *(a)* Er:YAG laser treatment of upper face. *(b)* Er:YAG laser treatment of midface. *(c)* Pink hue of Er:YAG laser–treated skin.

and an isopropyl alcohol scrub is then used to prepare the skin. The alcohol is wiped off cleanly with a water sponge. The water residue needs to be completely removed prior to laser treatment. If water is left on the skin, the laser will have no penetration effect because water is the chromophore for this laser. If the laser targets water on the skin, a brown mark will appear, indicating the need to wipe the face dry.

The laser scanner is placed against the planned treatment areas, and the pulses are administered. The Er:YAG laser produces a loud, sharp popping sound with each pulse, which indicates that tissue is being ejected from the body. The pulses should be spaced out with about 10% to 20% overlap. The laser scanner is then continuously passed over the entire face (Figs 9-9a and 9-9b). Unlike the CO_2 laser, proteinaceous debris is not encountered with the Er:YAG laser, as the laser ablates the debris with each pass. To blend the treated and nontreated areas, the laser should be feathered out into the nontreated areas with a lower fluence, which helps lower the contrast between the two areas.

The number of passes performed is at the surgeon's discretion. With each pass, the laser penetrates deeper into the skin, and upon entering the deep papillary dermis, bleeding may be encountered. Penetration into the papillary dermis with the Er:YAG laser is marked by a smooth, glistening appearance, whereas entry into the reticular dermis demonstrates an irregular surface with the emergence of sebaceous glands.[1] Additional passes are performed on the treated areas until the patient's pathosis is removed or until bleeding is visualized. The removal of photodamaged skin and rhytids can be appreciated, and the surgeon can make the decision to end treatment. It is important to avoid being so aggressive with the laser as to cause scarring or permanent pigmentary changes.

After the completion of laser treatment, the skin should have a uniformly pink hue (Fig 9-9c). It is important at this point to apply cold packs over the treated areas to counteract the accumulated heat from the laser. Patients are instructed to keep cold compresses on the treated areas while at home. The laser-treated skin tends to exfoliate over the next 3 to 7 days. Moisturizers are discouraged because they will likely impede the exfoliation process. Patients are also discouraged from tampering with the laser-treated areas, which may promote scarification. Enzyme exfoliants are gentle removers of peeling skin and encourage quicker exfoliation. The red discoloration of skin often dissipates after exfoliation; however, the time required for this varies among individuals. Makeup can be worn the day after laser resurfacing with the Er:YAG laser.

Chemical Peels

A chemical peel is the application of an acid to the skin. It is a controlled exfoliation procedure used to reduce the appearance of fine lines and wrinkles, scars, and hyperpigmentation. The type and concentration of the acid determines the depth of the burn. The superficial peels are AHAs, which are used to improve fine lines and wrinkles. Medium-depth peels are trichloroacetic acids (TCAs), which are designed to help improve scarring, blemishes, wrinkles, and texture. Deep chemical peels are carbolic acid (phenol), which is used only on the face because it can cause scarring on other areas of the body, especially the neck. The peel can be applied to the whole face or to a specific area, such as the upper lip. Caution should be taken when the chemical solution is applied around the eyes. Each peel is designed to fit each patient's needs. Peels can be used in conjunction with surgical procedures, but they are not a substitute.[23] The application technique is similar for all three types of chemical peels:

Step 1: The skin is completely cleansed to remove oils and impurities. An exfoliating cleanser, such as the Nu-Derm Foaming Gel Cleanser (Obagi), is recommended, so the peel can penetrate deeper (Fig 9-10a).

Step 2: The peel is applied evenly with a cotton-tipped applicator or facial brush, with extra care around the eye area. Patients are to keep their eyes closed at all times (Fig 9-10b).

Step 3: At this time, the patient may need a fan to help cool the burning sensation (Fig 9-10c).

Step 4: The peel is neutralized until the burning sensation subsides. The neutralizing solution should be ready because the skin's reaction determines how long the peel stays on the skin. The patient may still feel a tingle after neutralization, which is normal (Fig 9-10d).

Step 5: After neutralization, the skin is cleaned with a gentle cleanser (Nu-Derm Gentle Cleanser, Obagi) (Fig 9-10e).

Step 6: Moisturizer and sunscreen are applied. If a phenol peel was performed, petroleum jelly is applied instead (Fig 9-10f).

Step 7: The patient is given postprocedural instructions.

Superficial peels

Very light

AHA products are the most common type of peel. Common AHAs are glycolic, lactic, and fruit acids (Fig 9-11). These peels typically penetrate only into the stratum corneum of the epidermis (Fig 9-12). Glycolic acid is typically used for oily skin types and is the most aggressive of the AHAs. Lactic acid is typically used for dry, sensitive skin types.

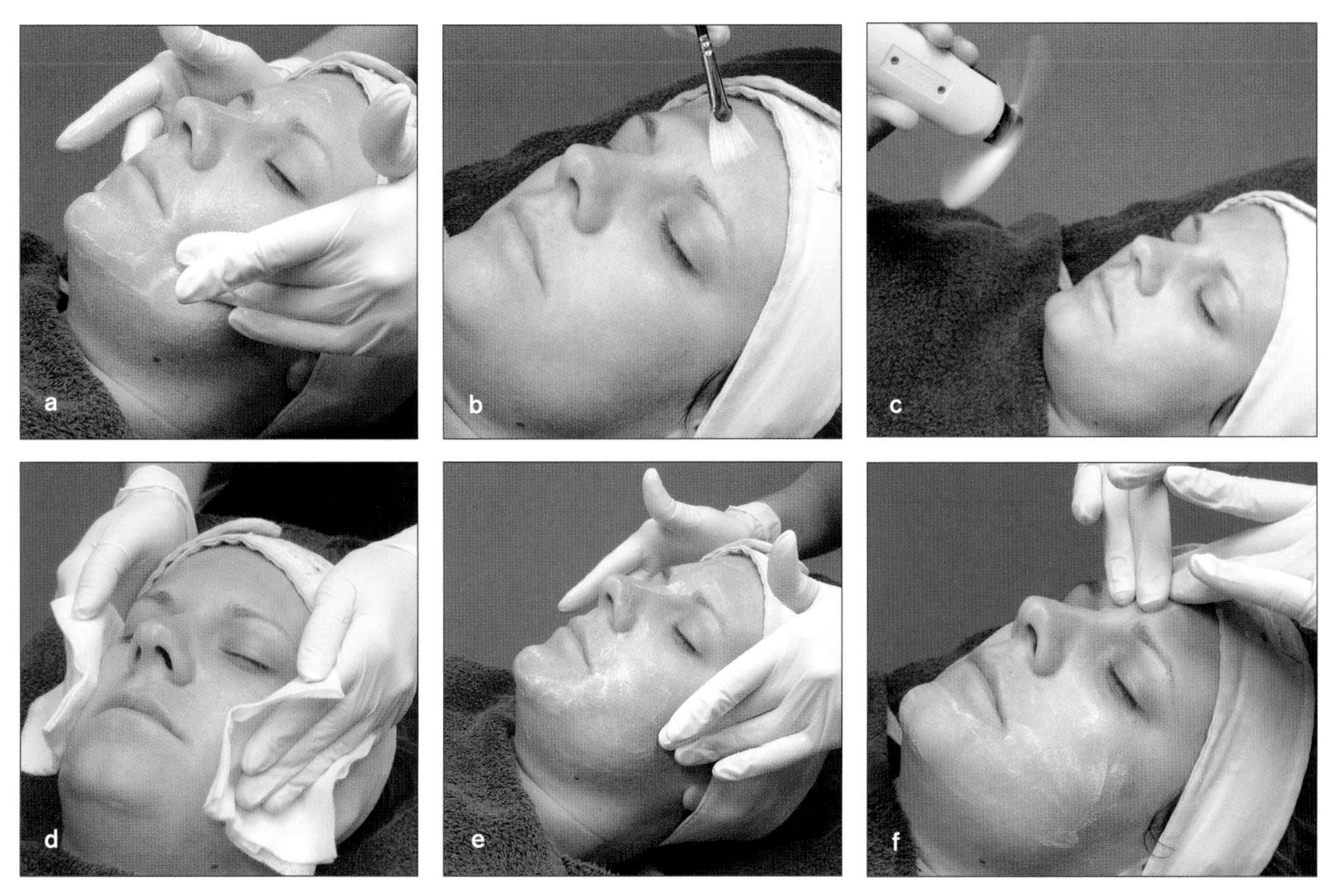

Fig 9-10 *(a)* Application of exfoliating cleanser. *(b)* The chemical peel is applied with a facial brush. *(c)* A fan is used to cool the patient's skin during the treatment. *(d)* The chemical peel is neutralized. *(e)* A gentle cleanser is used to clean the skin. *(f)* Application of moisturizer and sunscreen.

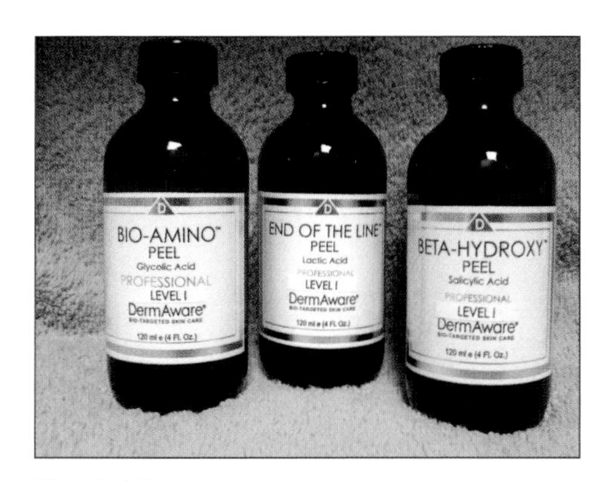

Fig 9-11 Superficial, very light peels: glycolic acid, lactic acid, and salicylic acid.

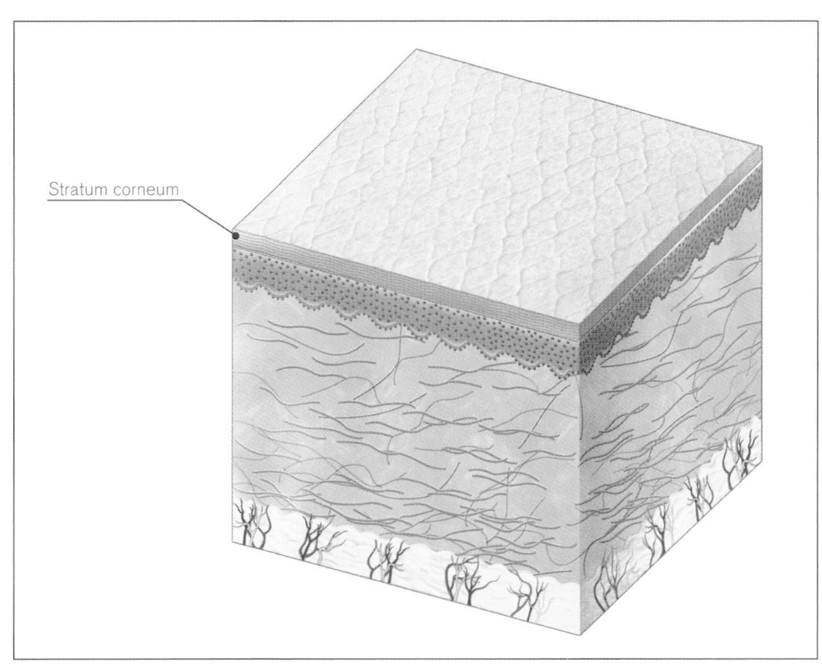

Fig 9-12 Cross section of skin showing the penetration of a superficial, very light chemical peel *(yellow)* into the stratum corneum.

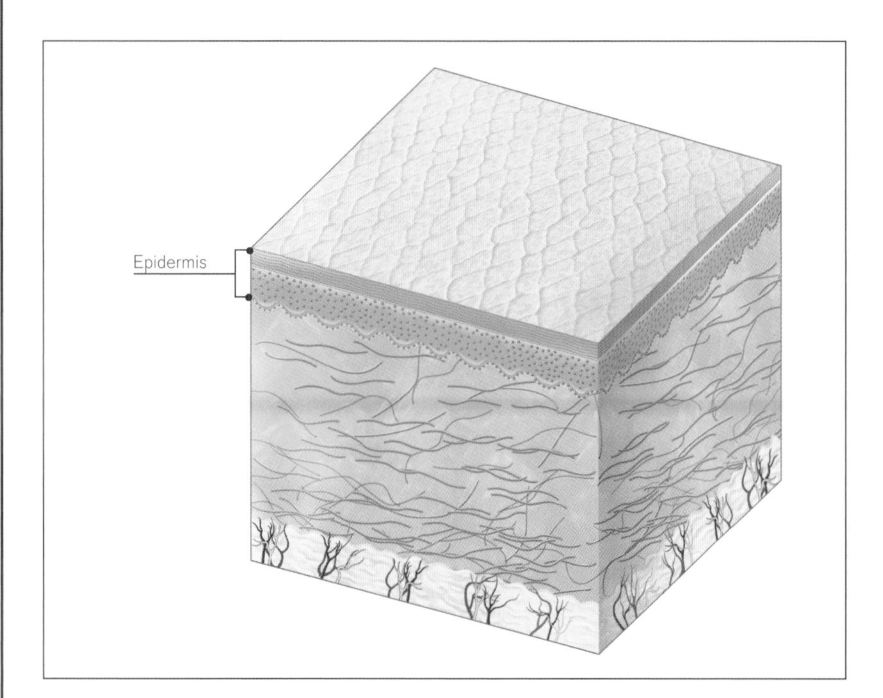

Fig 9-13 Cross section of skin showing the penetration of a superficial light chemical peel *(yellow)* through the entire epidermis.

Another type of commonly used peel is salicylic acid, which is a β-hydroxy acid (BHA). Salicylic acid is recommended for skin types prone to acne. The AHA and BHA peels help smooth and brighten skin and are commonly used by patients who cannot afford the downtime associated with the deeper TCA and phenol peels. These very light peels help to smooth rough, dry skin and improve the texture of sun-damaged skin. Several treatments may be needed to achieve the desired results. These peels also help to condition the skin for more aggressive procedures such as TCA and phenol peels, laser resurfacing, and surgical procedures.

AHA is the main ingredient in most exfoliating cleansers. Some desired results may be accomplished by using these cleansers alone and not in conjunction with a chemical peel. Patients using tretinoin need to be careful while receiving chemical peels because their skin is more sensitive. The very light peels work by removing the stratum corneum layer of the skin, which increases cellular turnover. A glycolic peel will have a stronger effect in a patient using tretinoin than in a patient who is not using tretinoin. Signs of redness, flaking, and peeling may be present for about 5 days. These peels sometimes go by the name of "lunchtime peels" because patients often return to normal activities immediately following the procedure. Patients are instructed to use a gentle cleanser and sunscreen for the next few days to allow their skin to recover.

Light

Light peels penetrate more deeply than the very light peels and are useful for patients with mild photodamage (Glogau I and II), acne, and pigmentary dyschromias.[24] Examples of these peels include 70% glycolic acid and 20% to 30% TCA. These peels produce a superficial wound to a depth of the entire epidermis and sometimes into the papillary dermis (Fig 9-13).

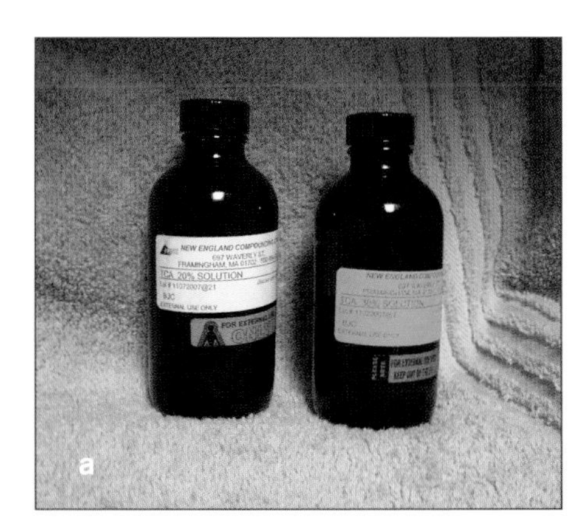

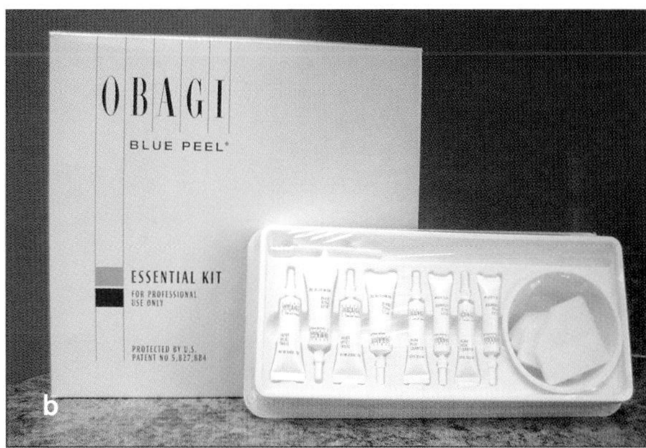

Fig 9-14 *(a and b)* Superficial light TCA peels including the Blue Peel (Obagi).

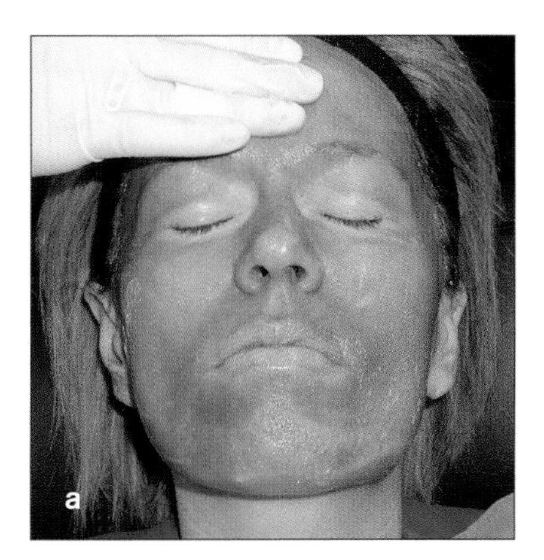

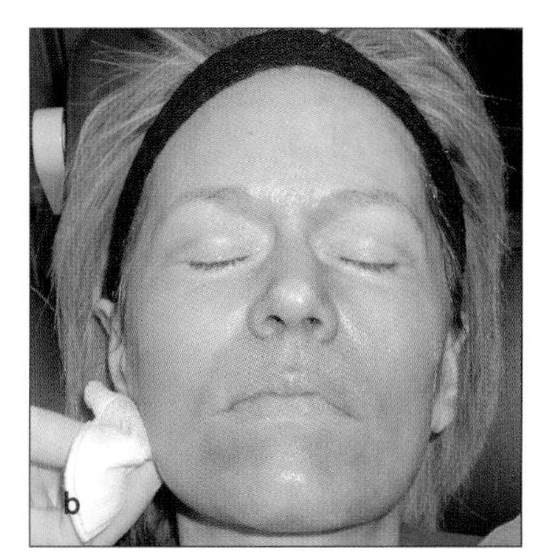

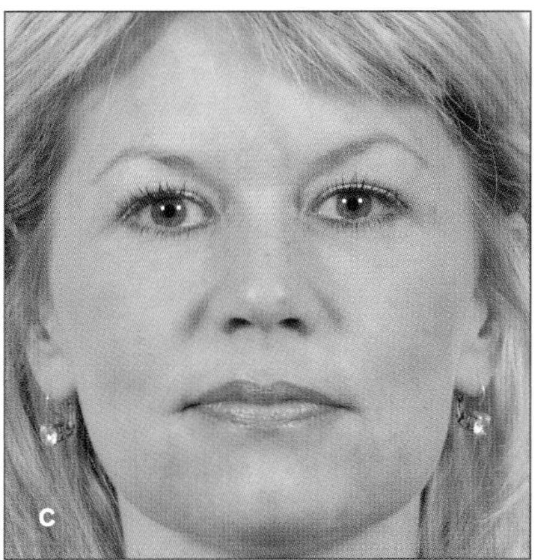

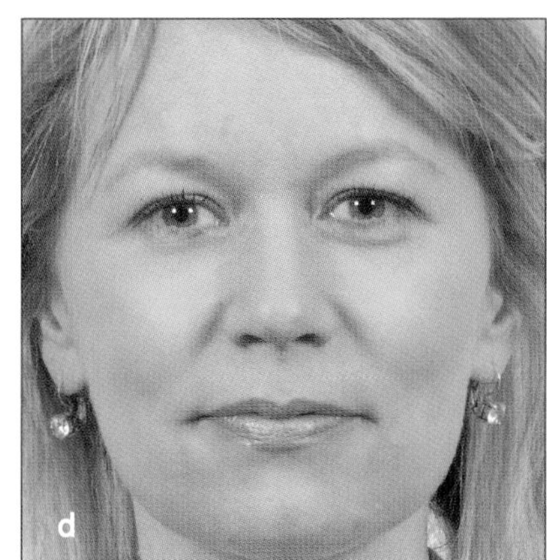

Fig 9-15 *(a)* Application of the Obagi Blue Peel. The Blue Peel is essentially a TCA peel with an added blue dye to distinguish between treated and untreated areas.[24] *(b)* Once treatment is finished, the peel is neutralized and wiped away. *(c)* Pretreatment view. *(d)* Results 8 weeks posttreatment.

TCA is commonly used to correct fine lines and wrinkles, superficial blemishes, pigmentation problems, and scarring (Figs 9-14 and 9-15) and can be used on any part of the body. It is recommended that the skin be pre- and postconditioned with a prescription skin care system (eg, Nu-Derm, Obagi) to achieve the best results. This helps the TCA penetrate deeper and more evenly. The patient's skin type determines the strength of the peel. Thick, sun-damaged skin is better able to handle a strong peel than can thin, fragile skin.

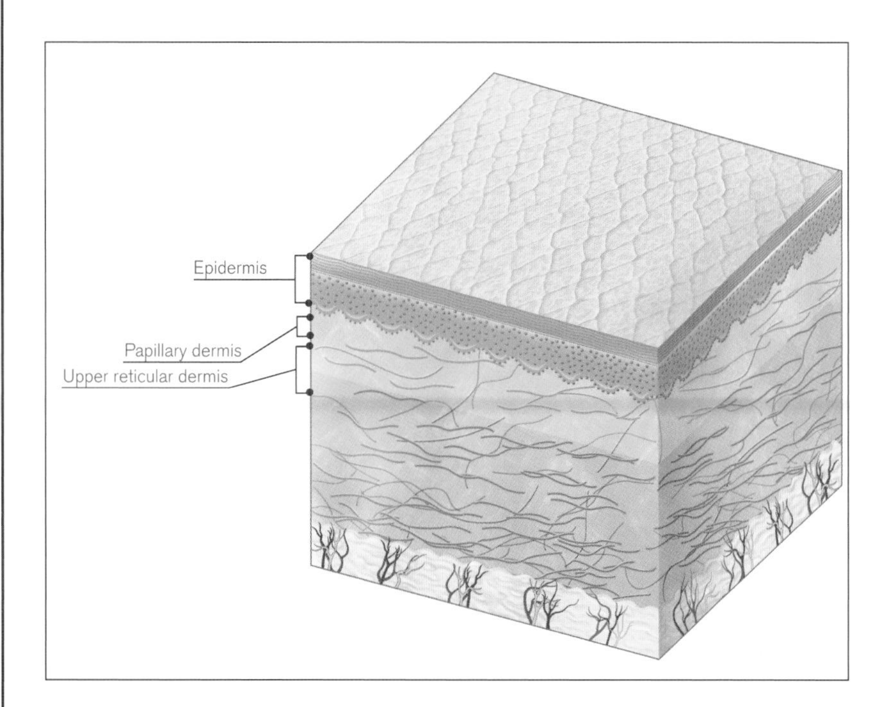

Fig 9-16 Cross section of skin showing effect of a medium-depth chemical peel *(yellow)* down to the upper reticular dermis.

The TCA peel can be deep or superficial depending on the concentration. It burns away the surface skin, allowing new skin to replace it. Anesthesia is typically not recommended because the peel acts as an anesthetic. The treated area may form a crust or scab, and peeling may last from 7 to 10 days. The superficial layers of skin will become stiff and eventually crack and start to peel off. Swelling may also be present for a day or two. The strength of the peel determines the recovery time. Stronger solutions remove more tissue, resulting in a longer recovery time. Recovery can be very similar to that seen with use of a CO_2 laser. Patients must be warned that picking at peeling skin may result in scarring. An enzyme mask, versus a scrub, is recommended to remove the flaking skin because scrubs sometimes irritate healing skin and cause more harm than good. Sun protection is key after a TCA peel. These peels may be repeated every 3 to 6 months for optimal results.

Medium-depth peels

This category of peels includes 88% phenol, 30% to 40% TCA, and a mixture of 70% glycolic acid and 30% to 35% TCA. These peels produce a wound down to the upper reticular dermis (Fig 9-16).

Phenol peels are very potent peel formulations and pose the greatest risks compared with AHA and TCA peels. They are recommended for the face only and are used for coarse facial wrinkles, blotchy or damaged skin, and precancerous growths. Scarring may result if the peel is applied to the neck or any other part of the body. The results of a phenol peel are dramatic and long lasting, because there is a marked increase in collagen production and expansion of the papillary dermis up to 3 months after treatment. Permanent skin lightening and lines of demarcation may occur. This peel is not recommended for patients with dark skin.

Moreover, patients with cardiac, liver, or kidney abnormalities should not receive an 88% phenol peel because phenol is cardiotoxic, hepatotoxic, and nephrotoxic.[23] Individuals for whom this type of peel is planned should have an electrocardiogram and blood work completed prior to the procedure, including complete blood count, serum electrolyte tests, and liver function tests.

Cotton-tipped applicators provide good control of the TCA solution and can be rolled and brushed over the skin to ensure an even, gentle distribution of the peel on the forehead, cheeks, and lips (Fig 9-17a). Use of a semi-wet cotton-tip applicator is recommended on eyelids. Caution should be exercised around the eyelid skin to ensure that no excess solution drips into the eyes (Figs 9-17b).

Once the solution is evenly applied, a white frost will appear on the skin within 30 seconds, indicating the completion of the physiologic reaction of the TCA peel[25] (Fig 9-17c). Three levels of frost may be observed: *(1)* the first level is marked by erythema with white frost streaks, *(2)* the second level is white frost with a halo of erythema, and *(3)* the third level is white frost with no erythema. The third level of frost indicates penetration into the reticular dermis and should be reserved for those patients with thicker, sun-damaged skin.[23] Around thin areas of skin, such as the eyelids, the second level of frost is more desirable.

Ideally, medium-depth peels should be performed with either oral or intravenous sedation to help patients overcome the initial painful part of the procedure. The medium-depth TCA peel is a painful procedure, and patients who do not receive anesthesia may describe discomfort and a very intense burning sensation. However, this initial discomfort settles after the frost has peaked (3 to 4 minutes). If the patient is awake, a light fan can cool the treated areas (Fig 9-17d). Once the peel is completed, application of cold compresses provides relief (Figs 9-17e and 9-17f).

Medium-depth peels may take 1 to 2, hours depending on the area of the face that is being treated, and it is recommended that someone drive the patient home after this procedure. The recovery may be slow and could take several months (Fig 9-17g). Following the peel, the patient's face may become very swollen, even causing the eyes to temporarily swell shut in some cases. It may be a good idea for patients to have someone care for them for a few days until they recover. After the procedure, sun protection must always be used. New skin should begin forming 7 to 10 days after the treatment. It may take up to 2 weeks before the patient can apply makeup and return to normal activities. Following the treatment, the skin should have a dramatic improvement with fewer wrinkles and blemishes (Figs 9-17h and 9-17i).

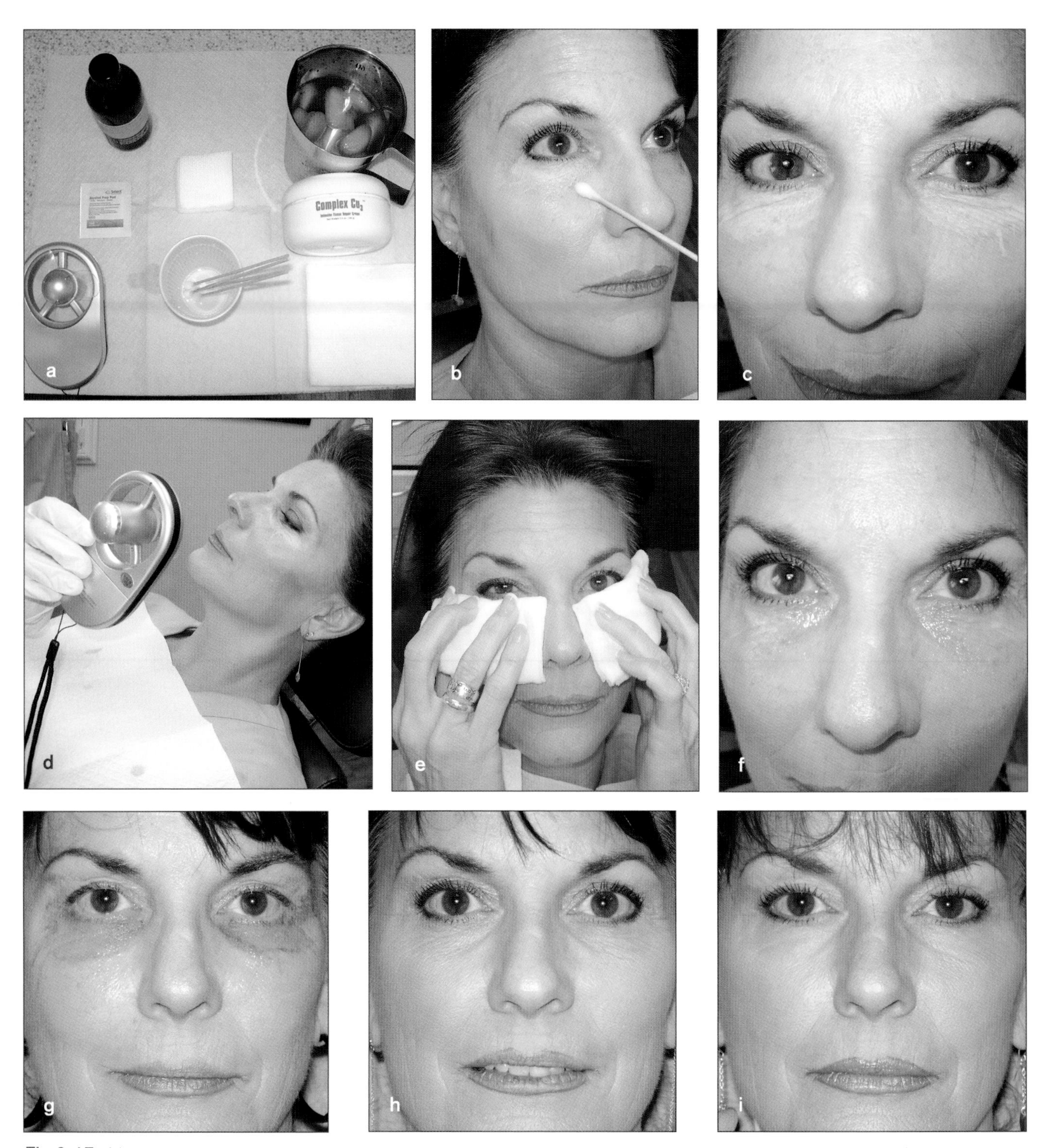

Fig 9-17 *(a)* Treatment setup for a medium-depth peel includes a 30% TCA peel solution (New England Compounding CTR), ice water, alcohol swab, gauze pads, copper peptide cream (Complex Cu3, PhotoMedex), portable fan, and cotton-tip applicators. *(b)* Application of TCA to lower eyelid. *(c)* White frost observed with a halo of erythema (second level), which is desirable for a 30% TCA peel. *(d)* Use of a fan provides cooling comfort to the patient during the treatment. *(e)* After the procedure, application of cold compresses provides relief from the burn of the chemical peel. *(f)* Lower eyelid appearance 20 minutes posttreatment following application of copper peptide cream. *(g)* Lower eyelids 4 days posttreatment. The skin appears reddened, but the patient exhibited no pain. *(h)* View of patient prior to having TCA peel to lower eyelids. *(i)* View of patient 2 weeks posttreatement.

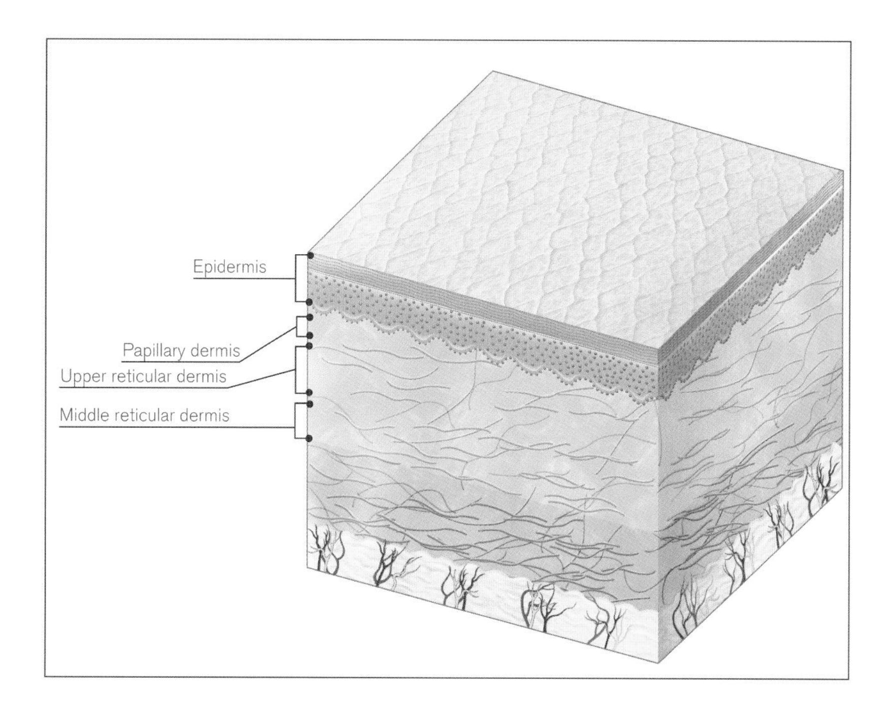

Fig 9-18 Cross section of skin showing the penetration of a deep chemical peel *(yellow)* to the middle reticular dermis.

Deep chemical peels

Deep chemical peels are seldom used because of the amount and depth of tissue destruction that is induced and the potential for postoperative scarring and pigment changes. These peels are reserved only for individuals with extremely photodamaged skin (Glogau IV). Examples of the deep peels include 50% or greater TCA and Baker-Gordon phenol peel, containing 88% phenol, 2 mL of tap water, septisol, and croton oil.[23] Deep peels penetrate to the middle reticular dermis (Fig 9-18). The increased collagen turnover during recovery rejuvenates the skin at a deeper level because of the greater amount of pathosis.

Selecting the right peel

Patients often have difficulty choosing which peel is right for them. As a physician, it is important to recognize a patient's commitment to the procedure. Sometimes, it is better to start patients with the superficial peels and slowly work them up to the more aggressive peels. Light superficial peels are most likely to give patients the best result because they gradually exfoliate the skin and result in less downtime and fewer complications than the medium-depth peels. If the patient is not looking for a dramatic change, then the very light superficial peels are probably the best choice. Refer to Table 9-3 to compare the chemical peels, and select the best peel to suit the patient.

Table 9-3 Treatment applications

	AHA	Salicylic acid	TCA		Phenol
			Low concentration (35%)	High concentration (>50%)	
Target area					
Fine lines	2	1	1	3	4
Acne	4	4	1	1	4
Acne scars	1	1	2	3	4
Deep wrinkles	1	1	1	3	4
Age spots	2	2	3	4	4
Effects (months)	1 to 3	1 to 3	3 to 6	> 12	> 12
Risks	Low	Low	Medium	High	High (including cardiac risks)
Recovery time	Short	Short	Generally short	Long	Long

1—little improvement; 2—some improvement; 3—moderate improvement; 4—good improvement

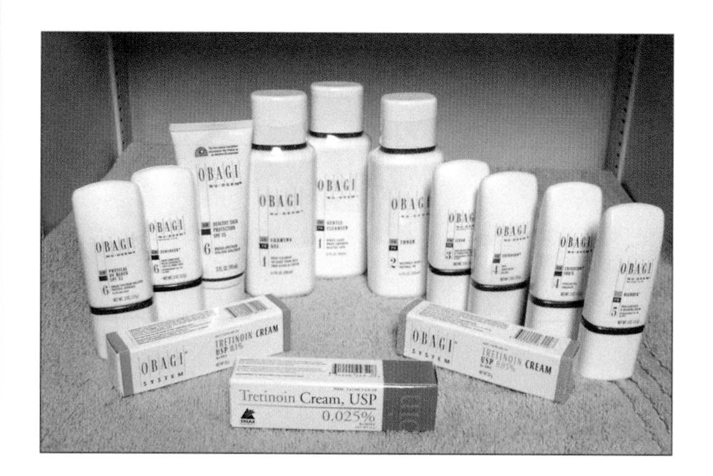

Fig 9-19 Obagi Nu-Derm system for skin care.

Prescription Skin Care

These skin care systems are designed to correct and prevent the signs of aging and can promote normal cellular turnover to exfoliate old skin and replace it with new skin. In addition, some products can stimulate fibroblasts to increase collagen production and reduce melanocyte production, thereby improving the skin's evenness and clarity. Although there are several prescription skin care systems available, the authors of this chapter use Obagi products, and this section will outline the Nu-Derm system (Fig 9-19).

Mechanism of action

Intracellular action

The Nu-Derm system promotes intracellular transcription of keratinocytes that triggers normal cellular production. Tretinoin (0.05% to 0.1%) increases the rates of cell production in the dermis and of keratinocyte turnover. As a result, the epidermis thickens, and the stratum corneum contracts. The stimulation reduces collagen breakdown and slows the natural thinning of the dermis. This system also contains products with 4% hydroquinone—twice the amount of that found in over-the-counter products. As an effective inhibitor of melanogenesis, hydroquinone lightens freckles, age spots, melasma, and postinflammatory hyperpigmentation.

Extracellular action

The key ingredients that facilitate extracellular repair are phytic acid, glycolic acid, lactic acid, antioxidants, and sunscreens. Phytic acid is a plant-derived, non-AHA product that acts as a gentle exfoliant. Glycolic acid, the most common type of AHA, is extracted from sugarcane and works well on oily skin types. Lactic acid is an AHA that is derived from milk and used primarily as a moisturizer on dry, dehydrated skin. Phytic, glycolic, and lactic acids work together to aid in exfoliation; to create a smooth, compact stratum corneum; and to enhance the ability of other skin care products to penetrate the skin.

Product regimen

The products of the Nu-Derm system are designed to work together for superior results and include Foaming Gel Cleanser, Toner, Clear, Exfoderm, Blender, and sunscreens. Products must be used at recommended times (morning, evening, or both) and applied in the correct amounts. Once patients begin the Nu-Derm system, it is important that they stay committed to the daily regimen to see the best results. Particularly when photodamage is being treated, time and possibly some mild skin irritation may be necessary before significant improvement is reported.

The Foaming Gel Cleanser removes dirt, oil, and impurities from the skin. It is recommended for normal to oily skin types and is used mainly for skin types that need exfoliation. The Gentle Cleanser is recommended for normal to dry skin types and is ideal for fragile, sensitive, and menopausal skin. It is recommended for use immediately before and after invasive procedures to condition the skin and reduce irritation.

The Toner balances the pH in the skin and prepares it for the application of active ingredients. It is very important that the toner not contain alcohol, which prevents active products from penetrating the skin.

The Clear product contains 4% hydroquinone and is used to correct upper epidermis hyperpigmentation. The recommended application amount is determined by the condition of the skin and varies from 0.5 g (no excess hyperpigmentation) to 1.0 g (primary patient concern is hyperpigmentation).

Exfoderm has an active ingredient of 3% phytic acid to gently exfoliate the stratum corneum and is recommended for patients with normal to dry skin. The stronger and more aggressive Exfoderm Forte has active ingredients of 6% glycolic acid and 4% lactic acid and is suitable for normal to oily skin. Application amount varies from 0.5 g (minimal exfoliation) to 1.0 g (exfoliation is primary concern). These products are recommended to condition the skin prior to chemical peels, laser treatments, and surgical procedures.

A nighttime application of 0.5 g of the Blender contains 4% hydroquinone and should always be paired with tretinoin cream in order to target lower dermal hyperpigmentation. The tretinoin cream comes in concentrations of 0.025%, 0.05%, and 0.1%. Unless sensitivity is an issue, patients should start with 0.05% tretinoin until their skin has been conditioned enough for the 0.1% concentration. Patients with thick, oily skin may be able to handle 0.1% tretinoin cream from the beginning of treatment.

Using daily sun protection is required while using the Nu-Derm system, because failure to do so can reverse the effects of the system. Patients can participate in normal outdoor activities while using the active products, but they may experience increased sensitivity to sun and heat. When exposed to the sun, patients should reapply sun protection every few hours. The recommended sunscreens are the Healthy Skin Protection, Sunfader, and Physical UV Block. Healthy Skin Protection is recommended for daily use. It has a sun protection factor (SPF) of 35 and contains 9% micronized zinc oxide and 7.5% octinoxate for both physical and chemical protection from ultraviolet (UV) A and B rays. Sunfader contains 4% hydroquinone, has an SPF of 15, and provides chemical UV protection. It is recommended for extra sun protection for patients concerned about hyperpigmentation. The Physical UV Block has an SPF of 32 and is recommended for application immediately following invasive procedures and for patients exposed to direct sunlight. It contains 18.5% micronized zinc oxide that provides physical protection from both UV A and B rays.

Treatment phases

Weeks 1 to 6

Signs of premature aging and acne flares should be corrected as dead cells are replaced with new ones. While the skin is adapting to the skin care system, common side effects are itching, redness, and dryness. However, by week 6, a more even, toned appearance should be apparent.

Weeks 7 to 12

Healthy new cells continue to form and the production of melanin slows and becomes more evenly distributed. Collagen production is stimulated, which creates a noticeable tightness to the skin. By week 12, the skin should be smoother and clearer.

Weeks 13 to 18

New skin cell formation and collagen production continues. Tighter skin and a clearer complexion should be noticeable by week 18, and the skin should look and feel younger, brighter, and healthier.

Maintenance

Patients are recommended to stay on the prescription skin care system for 18 to 24 weeks (Figs 9-20 to 9-23). Once the goal is achieved, maintenance begins. Patients should continue to use the Cleanser, Toner, and sunscreen daily and the other products less frequently throughout the week. How often patients need to use the active products—Clear, Exfoderm or Exfoderm Forte, and Blender in combination with tretinoin—must be determined according to individual need. The skin is monitored closely for a few weeks after the maintenance program starts to make sure symptoms do not return. Typically, patients stay on a maintenance program for 4 to 5 months and then return to the full regimen for 6 weeks.

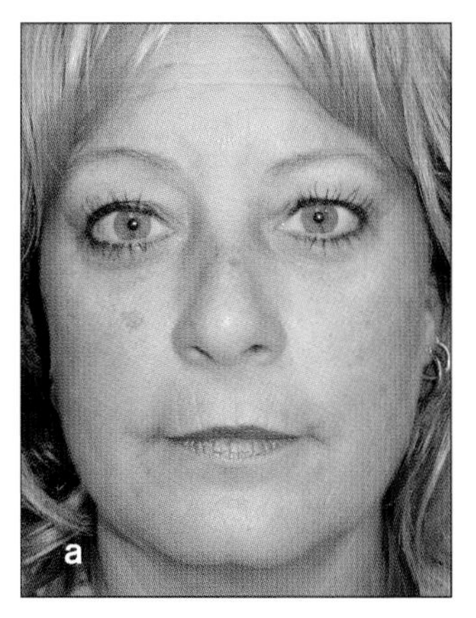
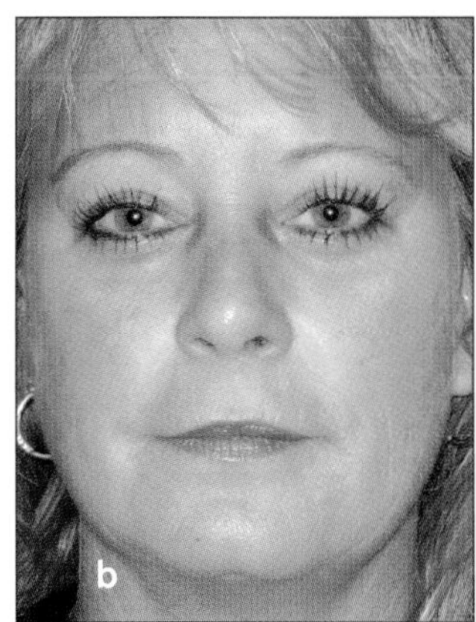

Fig 9-20 *(a)* View of patient prior to treatment. *(b)* Clinical results following 18 weeks of Obagi Nu-Derm treatment.

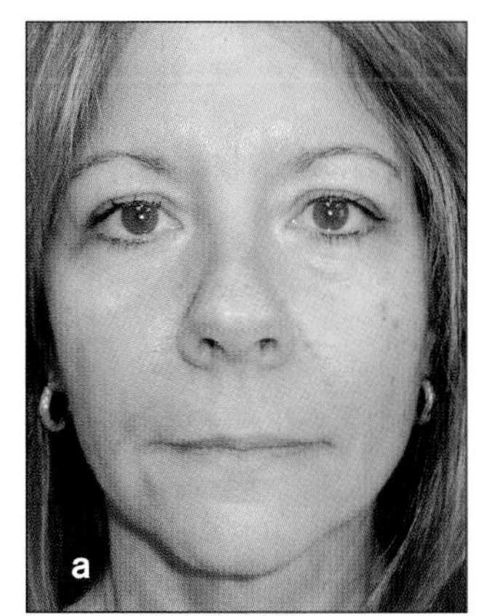
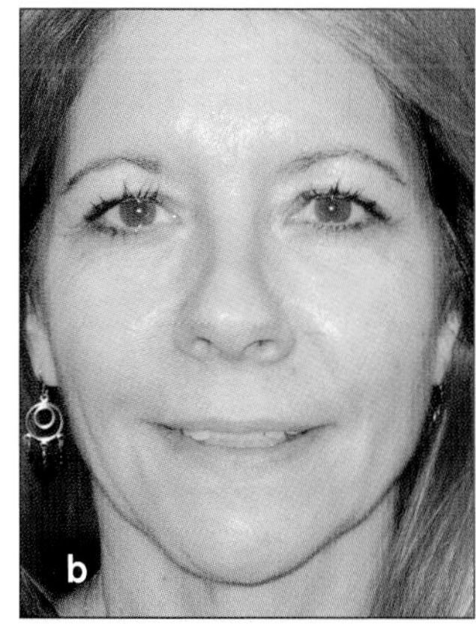

Fig 9-21 *(a)* View of patient prior to treatment. *(b)* Clinical results following 18 weeks of Obagi Nu-Derm treatment.

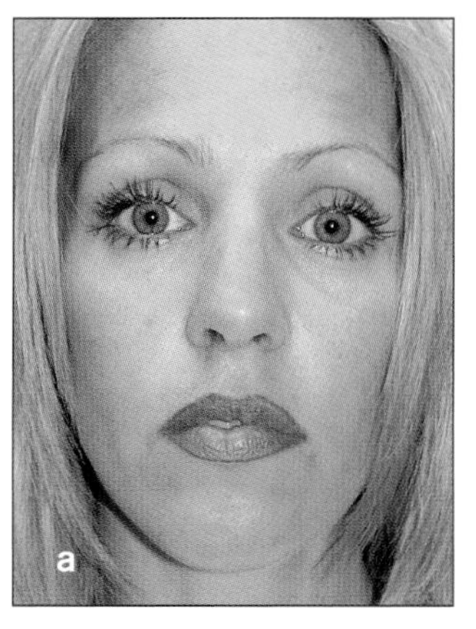
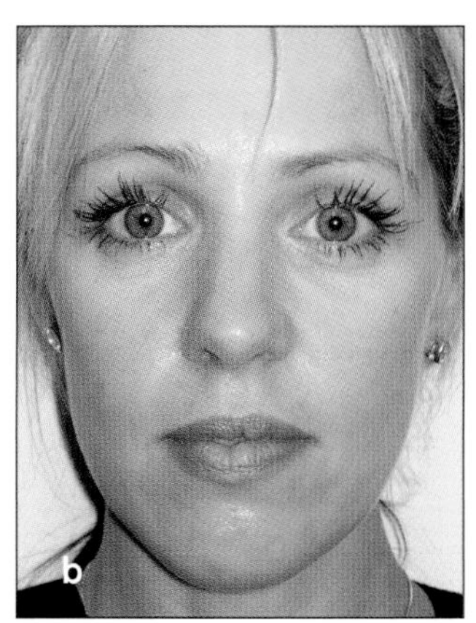

Fig 9-22 *(a)* View of patient prior to treatment. *(b)* Clinical results following 18 weeks of Obagi Nu-Derm treatment.

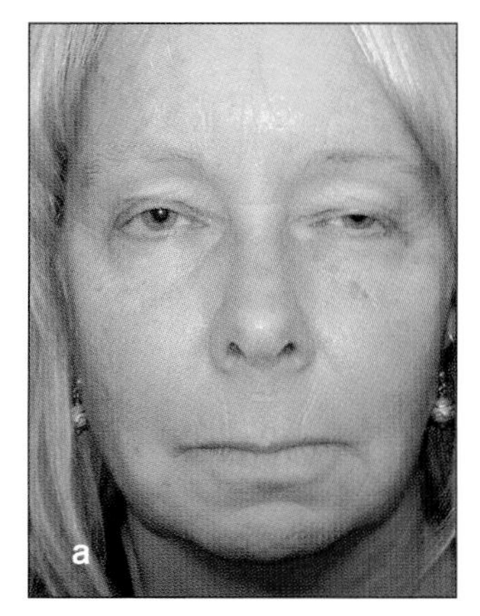
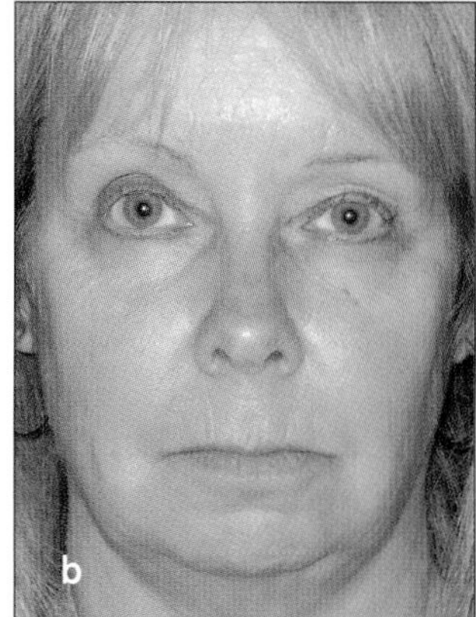

Fig 9-23 *(a)* View of patient prior to treatment. *(b)* Clinical results following 18 weeks of Obagi Nu-Derm treatment.

Complications

Complications associated with skin rejuvenation procedures can be avoided by judicious use of antibacterial, antiviral, and antifungal medications as well as by exercising caution during the procedures. Intraoperative complications, such as misplacing a peeling solution in an undesired area (eg, eyes) or using the incorrect peeling medication, can occur. If a drop of peeling agent were inadvertently placed in the eyes, saline and bicarbonate should be readily available to dilute the substance.

Delayed wound healing may occur after a chemical peel or laser resurfacing, which should alert the practitioner to a possible bacterial, viral, or fungal infection. Failure to quickly intervene in these cases may lead to pigmentary changes and scarring.[25,26] Patients who exhibit delayed wound healing should be treated with moistened dressings, antibiotics, and corticosteroids, when appropriate. Corticosteroids can be used in cases of noninfected contact dermatitis.[26] *Streptococcus* and *Staphylococcus* species can often harbor in ointment-soaked occlusive dressings and subsequently infect wounds. Prevention of infection can be implemented by utilizing 0.25% acetic acid–soaked sponges on the wounds, and by removing all ointment at the dressing changes.[26]

Prevention of herpetic outbreaks following laser treatment or chemical peels is performed with antiviral prophylaxis, as mentioned earlier in this chapter. It is important to continue the antiviral medication for the full 10 days following the procedure because viral replication will continue until the skin reepithelializes. In most instances, reepithelialization takes 7 to 10 days following a CO_2 laser resurfacing or a medium-depth chemical peel.[26] If a viral outbreak ensues, early intervention with antiviral therapy should be performed to prevent scarring of the skin.[25]

Summary

Facial skin rejuvenation procedures are popular and their results can be very gratifying for both practitioner and patient, if done correctly. Patient selection is paramount, and treatment planning must draw on a detailed discussion with the patient over treatment goals and desired appearance. This chapter illustrates a variety of rejuvenation techniques. Chemical peels have the benefit of a much lower startup cost than laser resurfacing procedures, which require an initial investment into the laser unit. Chemical peels and lasers are both effective means of achieving desirable esthetic outcomes, and both techniques require getting used to. Over time, the surgeon will develop a preference and a personalized system to optimize efficiency and results.

References

1. Airan LE, Hruza G. Current lasers in skin resurfacing. Facial Plast Surg Clin North Am 2005;13: 127–139.
2. Price CR, Carniol PJ, Glaser DA. Skin resurfacing with the erbium:YAG laser. Facial Plast Surg Clin North Am 2001;9:291–302.
3. Rubenstein R, Roenigk HH Jr, Stegman SJ, Hanke CW. Atypical keloids after dermabrasion of patients taking isotretinoin. J Am Acad Dermatol 1986;15: 280–285.
4. Physicians' Desk Reference, ed 54. Montvale, NJ: Medical Economics, 2000.
5. Lowe NJ, Lask G, Griffin ME. Laser skin resurfacing: Pre- and posttreatment guidelines. Dermatol Surg 1995;21:1017–1019.
6. Popp C, Kligman AM, Stoudemayer TJ. Pretreatment of photoaged forearm skin with topical tretinoin accelerates healing of full-thickness wounds. Br J Dermatol 1995;132:46–53.
7. Griffiths CE, Russman AN, Majmudar G, Singer RS, Hamilton TA, Voorhees JJ. Restoration of collagen formation in photodamaged human skin by tretinoin (retinoic acid). N Engl J Med 1993;329: 530–535.
8. Weinstein GD, Nigra TP, Pochi PE, et al. Topical tretinoin for treatment of photodamaged skin. Arch Dermatol 1991;127:659–665.
9. Ross EV, Naseef GS, McKinlay JR, et al. Comparison of carbon dioxide laser, erbium:YAG laser, dermabrasion, and dermatome: A study of thermal damage, wound contraction, and wound healing in a live pig model: Implications for skin resurfacing. J Am Acad Dermatol 2000;42:92–105.
10. Fitzpatrick RE, Tope WD, Goldman MP, Satur NM. Pulsed carbon dioxide laser, trichloroacetic acid, Baker-Gordon phenol, and dermabrasion: A comparative clinical and histologic study of cutaneous resurfacing in a porcine model. Arch Dermatol 1996;132:469–471.
11. Rubach BW, Schoenrock LD. Histologic and clinical evaluation of facial resurfacing using a carbon dioxide laser with the computer pattern generator. Arch Otolaryngol Head Neck Surg 1997;123: 929–934.
12. Yang CC, Chai CY. Animal study of skin resurfacing using the ultrapulse carbon dioxide laser. Ann Plast Surg 1995;35:154–158.
13. Alexiades-Armenakas MR, Dover JS, Arndt KA. The spectrum of laser skin resurfacing: Nonablative, fractional, and ablative laser resurfacing. J Am Acad Dermatol 2008;58:719–737.
14. Rahman Z, MacFalls H, Jiang K. Fractional deep dermal ablation induces tissue tightening. Lasers Surg Med 2009;41:78–86.
15. Ward PD, Baker SR. Long-term results of carbon dioxide laser resurfacing of the face. Arch Facial Plast Surg 2008;10:238–243.
16. Fitzpatrick RE, Goldman MP, Satur NM, Tope WD. Pulsed carbon dioxide laser resurfacing of photoaged facial skin. Arch Dermatol 1996;4:395–402.
17. Goldman MP. CO2 laser resurfacing of the face and neck. Facial Plast Surg Clin North Am 2001;9:283–290.
18. Ries WR, Clymer MA, Reinisch L. Laser safety features of eyeshields. Lasers Surg Med 1996;18: 309–315.
19. Papadavid E, Katsambas A. Laser for facial rejuvenation: A review. Int J Dermatol 2003;42: 480–487.
20. Alster TS, Lupton JR. Erbium:YAG cutaneous laser resurfacing. Dermatol Clin 2001;19:453–466.
21. Kaufmann R, Hibst R. Pulsed erbium:YAG laser ablation in cutaneous surgery. Lasers Surg Med 1996;19:324–330

22. Ziering CL. Cutaneous laser resurfacing with the erbium:YAG laser and the char-free carbon dioxide laser: A clinical comparison of 100 patients. Int J Aesth Restor Surg 1997;5:29–37.
23. If you're considering chemical peel. American Society of Plastic Surgeons. http://www.plasticsurgery.org/patients_and_consumers/procedures/cosmetic_procedures/chemical_peel.html. Accessed May 25, 2009.
24. The Obagi Blue Peel System. Obagi Medical Products. http://www.obagi.com/article/forphysicians/ourproducts/obagibluepeelsystem/obagibluepeelsystem.html. Accessed May 31, 2009.
25. Monheit G. Skin rejuvenation procedures. In: Miloro M, Ghali GE, Larsen PE, Waite PD (eds). Peterson's Principles of Oral and Maxillofacial Surgery, ed 2, vol 2. Hamilton, ON: BC Decker, 2004: 1420–1428.
26. Mandy SH, Monheit GD. Dermabrasion and chemical peels. In: Papel I (ed). Facial Plastic and Reconstructive Surgery. New York: Thieme, 2002: 223–239.

INDEX

Page numbers followed by "f" denote figures; those followed by "t" denote tables

C

D

E

F

G

H

I

O

P